Statistical Methods for Hospital Monitoring with R

STATISTICS IN PRACTICE

Series Advisors

Human and Biological Sciences
Stephen Senn
CRP-Santé, Luxembourg

Earth and Environmental Sciences
Marian Scott
University of Glasgow, UK

Industry, Commerce and Finance
Wolfgang Jank
University of Maryland, USA

Founding Editor
Vic Barnett
Nottingham Trent University, UK

Statistics in Practice is an important international series of texts which provide detailed coverage of statistical concepts, methods and worked case studies in specific fields of investigation and study.

With sound motivation and many worked practical examples, the books show in down-to-earth terms how to select and use an appropriate range of statistical techniques in a particular practical field within each title's special topic area.

The books provide statistical support for professionals and research workers across a range of employment fields and research environments. Subject areas covered include medicine and pharmaceutics; industry, finance and commerce; public services; the earth and environmental sciences, and so on.

The books also provide support to students studying statistical courses applied to the above areas. The demand for graduates to be equipped for the work environment has led to such courses becoming increasingly prevalent at universities and colleges.

It is our aim to present judiciously chosen and well-written workbooks to meet everyday practical needs. Feedback of views from readers will be most valuable to monitor the success of this aim.

A complete list of titles in this series appears at the end of the volume.

Statistical Methods for Hospital Monitoring with R

Anthony Morton
Princess Alexandra Hospital
Brisbane, Australia

Kerrie Mengersen
Science and Engineering Faculty
Queensland University of Technology
Brisbane, Australia

Michael Whitby
Greenslopes Clinical School
University of Queensland
Brisbane, Australia

Geoffrey Playford
Princess Alexandra Hospital
Brisbane, Australia

WILEY

This edition first published 2013
© 2013 John Wiley & Sons, Ltd

Registered office
John Wiley & Sons Ltd, The Atrium, Southern Gate, Chichester, West Sussex, PO19 8SQ, United Kingdom

For details of our global editorial offices, for customer services and for information about how to apply for permission to reuse the copyright material in this book please see our website at www.wiley.com.

Library of Congress Cataloging-in-Publication Data

Morton, Anthony Park, 1933– author.
   Statistical methods for hospital monitoring with R / Anthony Morton, Kerrie Mengersen, Geoffrey Playford, Michael Whitby.
      p. ; cm.
   Includes bibliographical references and index.
   ISBN 978-1-118-59630-2 (cloth)
   I. Mengersen, Kerrie L., author.   II. Playford, Geoffrey, author.   III. Whitby, Michael, 1950– author.   IV. Title.
   [DNLM: 1. Hospital Administration.   2. Statistics as Topic.   WX 150.1]
   RA971
   362.11068–dc23

2013008301

A catalogue record for this book is available from the British Library.

ISBN: 978-1-118-59630-2

Set in 10/12pt Times by Aptara Inc., New Delhi, India.
Printed and bound in Malaysia by Vivar Printing Sdn Bhd

1   2013

Contents

R Libraries

arm	gee	PropCIs
bmem	geepack	psy
chron	hglm	qAnalyst
Epi	Kendall	qcc
epibasix	lme4	rmeta
epicalc	MASS	spc
epiR	meta	splines
epitools	mgcv	surveillance
exactci	MKmisc	tseries

R Functions

1. bardenom() – rate data bar chart.
2. barnodenom() – count data bar chart.
3. bbar() – binomial data bar chart.
4. bbaradj() – risk-adjusted binary data bar chart.
5. bewma() – binomial data Shewhart/EWMA chart.
6. bewmacusum() – binary data EWMA/CUSUM chart.
7. bewmaqtr() – binomial data Shewhart/EWMA chart, quarterly data or data with no date column (requires first column e.g. 1:20).
8. bfunnelcusum() – cumulative funnel plot with CUSUM for binary data.
9. bgam() – binomial data generalized additive model (GAM) spline chart.
10. bgamqtr() – binomial data generalized additive model (GAM) spline chart, quarterly data, data with no date column (requires first column e.g. 1:20).
11. bgroupfunnelinstitution() – aggregated binary data funnel plot with institutions on horizontal axis.
12. bgroupfunnelprocedure()– aggregated binary data funnel plot with numbers of procedures on horizontal axis.
13. binarl() – average run length for binomial data.
14. binarladj() – average run length for risk-adjusted binary data.
15. binmonths() – arrange daily binary data by months.
16. binmonthsra() – arrange daily risk-adjusted binary data by months.
17. binqtrs() – arrange daily binary data by quarters.
18. binqtrsra() – arrange daily risk-adjusted binary data by quarters.
19. boecusum() – binary data Cumulative Observed – Expected (O-E) with CUSUM for binary data.
20. boecusumqtr()– binary data Cumulative Observed – Expected (O-E) with CUSUM for binary data (requires first column e.g. 1:100).
21. bshew() – binomial data Shewhart chart.
22. bshewqtr() – binomial data Shewhart chart, quarterly data, data with no date column (requires first column e.g. 1:20).
23. CCMenu() – control chart menu.
24. countewma() – count data Shewhart/EWMA chart.
25. countewmacusum – count data EWMA/CUSUM for uncommon AEs.
26. countewmao() – count data Shewhart/EWMA chart with overdispersion correction.

27. countewmaqtr() – count data Shewhart/EWMA chart, quarterly data, data with no date column (requires first column e.g. 1:20).
28. countewmaqtro() – count data Shewhart/EWMA chart, quarterly data, data with no date column (requires first column e.g. 1:20), with overdispersion correction.
29. countgam() – count data GAM chart.
30. countgamauto() – count data GAM chart with autocorrelation.
31. countgamautoqtr() – count data GAM chart with autocorrelation, quarterly data, data with no date column (requires first column e.g. 1:20).
32. countgamqtr() – count data GAM chart, quarterly data, data with no date column (requires first column e.g. 1:20).
33. countoecusum() – cumulative observed minus expected chart with CUSUM for uncommon count data AEs.
34. countquarters() – arranging count data by quarters.
35. countshew() – count data Shewhart chart.
36. countshewo() – count data Shewhart chart, with overdispersion correction.
37. countshewqtr() – count data Shewhart chart, quarterly data, data with no date column (requires first column e.g. 1:20).
38. countshewqtro() – count data Shewhart chart, quarterly data, data with no date column (requires first column e.g. 1:20), with overdispersion correction.
39. do.acf() – plot of ACF & PACF.
40. ebshrinkageb() – binary data empirical Bayes shrinkage analysis.
41. ewmacountdenom() – count data Shewhart/EWMA chart with separate denominators.
42. ewmacountdenomo() – count data Shewhart/EWMA chart with separate denominators, with overdispersion correction.
43. ewmacountdenomqtr() – count data Shewhart/EWMA chart with separate denominators, quarterly data, data with no date column (requires first column e.g. 1:20).
44. ewmacountdenomqtro() – count data Shewhart/EWMA chart with separate denominators, quarterly data, data with no date column (requires first column e.g. 1:20), with overdispersion correction.
45. g.d() – generic function for importing data into R.
46. getc4() – calculates the Shewhart chart constant c.
47. gammapoisson.odc/count.odc – OpenBUGS script for shrinkage analysis.
48. getnegbinparams() – negative binomial parameters with differing sized denominators (Bissell).
49. iewmachart() – Shewhart/EWMA i chart.
50. iewmachartqtr() – Shewhart/EWMA i chart, quarterly data, data with no date column (requires first column e.g. 1:20).
51. IMenu() – menu for Chapters 1 and 4.
52. ishewchart() – Shewhart i chart.
53. ishewchartqtr() – Shewhart i chart, quarterly data, data with no date column (requires first column e.g. 1:20).
54. manyproportions() – more than two independent proportions.
55. manyrates() – more than two independent rates.
56. mg.d(), ms.d() – generic functions for importing data into R and exporting from R (MAC).
57. monthlyaverage() – monthly averages of daily data.
58. monthlycounts() – arranges count data by months.

59. monthlynumbers() – arranges numerical data by months (aggregates).
60. multiplecounts() – confidence intervals for a series of counts.
61. multipleproportions() – confidence intervals for a series of proportions.
62. numgam() – GAM chart for numerical data without autocorrelation.
63. numgamauto() – GAM chart for numerical data with autocorrelation.
64. numgamautoqtr() – GAM chart for numerical data with autocorrelation, quarterly data, data with no date column (requires first column e.g. 1:20).
65. numgamqtr() – GAM chart for numerical data without autocorrelation, quarterly data, data with no date column (requires first column e.g. 1:20).
66. overdispersed() – to calculate Laney's correction for overdispersion in count and rate control charts.
67. pgroupfunnelinstitution() – funnel plot for aggregated rates sorted by institution.
68. pgroupfunnelprocedure() – funnel plot for aggregated rates sorted by number of procedures.
69. poiarl() – count data ARL.
70. proportion() – analysis involving a single proportion.
71. rate() – single count or rate.
72. rateewma() – rate data Shewhart/EWMA chart.
73. rateewmao() – rate data Shewhart/EWMA chart with overdispersion correction.
74. rateewmaqtr() – rate data Shewhart/EWMA chart, quarterly data, data with no date column (requires first column e.g. 1:20).
75. rateewmaqtro() – rate data Shewhart/EWMA chart, quarterly data, data with no date column (requires first column e.g. 1:20), with overdispersion correction.
76. rategam() – rate data GAM chart.
77. rategamauto() – rate data GAM chart with autocorrelation.
78. rategamautoqtr() – rate data GAM chart with autocorrelation, quarterly data, data with no date column (requires first column e.g. 1:20).
79. rategamqtr() – rate data GAM chart without autocorrelation, quarterly data, data with no date column (requires first column e.g. 1:20).
80. ratenegbin() – negative binomial Shewhart with differing sized denominators (Bissell).
81. ratequarters() – arranges rate data by quarters.
82. rateshew() – rate data Shewhart chart.
83. rateshewo() – rate data Shewhart chart, with overdispersion correction.
84. rateshewqtr() – rate data Shewhart chart, quarterly data, data with no date column (requires first column e.g. 1:20).
85. rateshewqtro() – rate data Shewhart chart, quarterly data, data with no date column (requires first column e.g. 1:20), with overdispersion correction.
86. riditewma() – Shewhart/EWMA RIDIT i chart.
87. riditewmaqtr() – Shewhart/EWMA RIDIT i chart, quarterly data, data with no date column (requires first column e.g. 1:20).
88. riditshew() – Shewhart RIDIT i chart.
89. riditshewqtr() – Shewhart RIDIT i chart, quarterly data, data with no date column (requires first column e.g. 1:20).
90. rocchart() – area under receiver operating characteristic (ROC) chart.
91. runchart() – count data run chart.
92. runchartdenom() – count data run chart with denominators.
93. s.d() – generic function for exporting data from R.

For those who seek to understand the complex dynamic systems that are at the heart of hospital safety. We hope our book will provide them with encouragement.

Counting hospital adverse events is obviously important. However, it is more important to realise that the counted adverse events are not the ones that we have been able to prevent.

Any royalties from this book are to go to a fund to aid students from developing countries in their studies of hospital safety at our universities and hospitals.

Preface

This book had its beginnings when, as director of an intensive care unit, I became interested in analysing acute care hospital outcome data and in trying to understand how such monitoring could prevent care from becoming unsafe. Attempts at data analysis were initially made using a spreadsheet. I retired from clinical practice in 1989 and for several years I worked part-time as a research associate at the then Australian Centre in Strategic Management. In 1994 Professor Michael Whitby invited me to work with him in his department, Infection Management Services at the Princess Alexandra Hospital. I then became acutely aware of the challenges presented by the clustering, high variability and sometimes autocorrelation among adverse event data, particularly but not only that which is due to hospital-acquired infection and colonisation.

Professor Kerrie Mengersen and I first became associated when a combined Queensland University of Technology and Princess Alexandra Hospital Australian Research Council Grant was received over a decade ago to study hospital infection adverse events. Since then we have been fortunate to be able to work on these and similar data. In 2011 Michael Whitby left Princess Alexandra Hospital to become Professor of Medicine at Greenslopes Hospital in Brisbane and Geoffrey Playford became his successor as Director of Infection Management Services at Princess Alexandra Hospital.

This book represents a journey of discovery involving infectious diseases physicians and other infection management staff at the Princess Alexandra Hospital, statisticians particularly at the Queensland University of Technology and the Queensland Health Centre for Health Related Infection Surveillance and Prevention (CHRISP), and others interested in what makes hospitals safer places. This journey continues. The work has been described in a series of journal articles that we acknowledge in the chapters and references. Our principal aim in this book is to demonstrate how the R statistical analysis software can be used to analyse these hospital adverse events (AEs). The data come predominantly from the hospital infection area but also from the wider hospital environment and we gratefully acknowledge the people who have made data available to us.

As we become more involved in attempting to understand what causes hospitals to be safe, we are increasingly reminded that the collection of data and their analysis, vital though it may be, does not alone make for a safe environment. We have to admit our ignorance and learn about safe systems, not just concentrate on outcomes that may be the result of unsafe practices; preventing errors should take precedence over counting them. Evans and her colleagues have recently discussed the role of epidemiologically sound clinically relevant data from clinical-quality registries as opposed to the current practice of monitoring numerous indicators. We have to understand that safety is impossible without discipline. We have to act on evidence and to work to improve that evidence. We must understand that AEs may be the result of the interaction of agents that may not appear individually to be of great concern. It is necessary to ensure that the complex system of interacting people, places and processes that make up a hospital is understood and made as safe as possible. The essential components of evidence-based systems to prevent AEs are being gathered together by organisations such as the Institute of Healthcare Improvement (IHI), for example as bundles in the IHI Improvement Map. In some cases a checklist may be valuable and the use of simulators may be able to detect and remedy unsatisfactory knowledge, skill, behaviour or judgement. Increasingly, engineering advancements that physically prevent specific AEs are becoming available.

There needs to be some practically workable surveillance mechanism to measure compliance with evidence-based systems and there must be some form of disciplinary action available to deal with people who persistently fail to implement them. Counting failures and comparing hospitals using conventional indicators do not do these things.

Analysis of aggregated indicator data usually involves displaying rates for individual hospitals together with prediction or precision limits relative to some average value for the group of hospitals to which they belong. The objective is to identify those hospitals with rates that differ from the average to the extent that predictable, mostly random, variation is an unlikely cause. As Mohammed[B] and colleagues point out, this does not necessarily mean that they are unusually good or bad; it means that they may be atypical to the extent that further investigation, often of a non-statistical nature, is required. If it is found that substandard systems exist or individual performance is unsatisfactory, remedial action can then be taken. This process has nothing to do with comparing hospitals. In addition, it has its limitations. The average for the group of hospitals that may differ markedly in the services they provide increasingly involves some form of risk adjustment and for common count data AEs such as bacteraemias it is in the early stages of development. Within-hospital data typically display much less variability. Ideally, when outcomes are worrying it should be possible to identify this quickly, search for causes and institute remedial action. Sequential within-hospital methods of data analysis complemented by such audits as occur with properly performed mortality and morbidity (M&M) meetings, as described, for example, by Singer, frequently aid in such early detection. Data that are aggregated, for example by years, may hide runs of unsatisfactory outcomes or, if this is not the case, causes may be difficult or impossible to determine when considerable time has elapsed prior to reporting.

It is not uncommon to hear that we must collect data from hospitals so people can compare them and choose the safest. However, to make such comparisons, it would be important to adjust for different patient populations within the institutions and for multiple testing among institutions. Ignoring these adjustments may lead to quite erroneous comparisons and decisions. In addition, simple random variation may influence a hospital's ranking from year to year without any change in its systems. Finally, most people just want their local hospital to treat them courteously as individuals and to perform competently and safely. Implementation of appropriate systems based on evidence does this.

AEs in hospitals result in additional suffering and economic loss for their victims, as well as occasional potentially preventable death, and this burden may extend into the community if there is residual discomfort, delay in regaining function and continuing financial difficulty with reliance on family, community or government for support. Hospital-acquired infections are a major, but by no means the only, cause of hospital AEs. During the past 20 or so years, there has been an explosion in hospital complexity in the face of considerable financial constraint. The last thing any hospital needs in this situation is re-work, having to deal with complications, or to re-do surgery that has not resulted in satisfactory outcomes. When bed occupancy is high and beds are scarce, it is not good practice to have any of them occupied by patients recovering from potentially preventable complications. Yet Eshani and colleagues have reported that over 18% of hospital inpatient budgets can be consumed treating patients with adverse outcomes.

As we begin to understand the science of complexity, it has become apparent that making systems super-efficient may not be a good idea. Although efficiency may be desirable, complex system science has shown that with increasing efficiency there tends to be increasing fragility and instability (Cook and Rasmussen). For resilience, some redundancy is needed. If a ward is full, patients become outliers in other wards and staff must traverse extended networks to care for them. If hand hygiene is substandard and high-touch surfaces are imperfectly cleaned, transmission of hospital-acquired organisms will be enhanced. If the ward in question is the infectious diseases ward, it may become impossible to isolate patients who are carriers of potentially dangerous hospital-acquired organisms, thus resulting in increased transmission to other patients. It is well documented that access block in emergency departments is dangerous and that it impairs the functioning of ambulance services. A super-efficient hospital, the aim of current managerialist management practice, may in fact be involved in enough extra re-work to nullify any gains due to its super-efficiency.

AEs are not confined only to hospital-acquired infections. For example, delay in comprehending the seriousness of a patient's condition may result in the patient's potentially preventable collapse and admission to intensive care. Unconscious patients whose backs and airways are not managed effectively can end up with painful pressure ulcers or an inhalation injury. Stroke or dementia patients who are not managed optimally can fall and sustain injury. Errors with medications can harm patients. Harried staff are more likely to sustain a needlestick injury. These are but a small sample from the list of potentially preventable AEs.

There has, of course, been much work done to improve hospital safety. In particular, there are mandated systems of error reporting. These can be driven from within the hospital, with a view to improving its systems, or they can be externally driven for the purposes of independent monitoring and public reporting. However vital the latter may be for transparency and accountability, there is as yet little evidence that in general rates of potentially preventable AEs are declining, although obviously there are exceptions. The increasing implementation of simple evidence-based groups of interventions that have been placed in bundles, for example for minimising complications associated with the use of intravenous devices, appears to be a major improvement. However, strong leadership and discipline are needed to ensure they become habit, implementation must be sustained until this occurs and, when new evidence becomes available, modification must be possible. The increasing use of checklists and, for some specialties, the employment of simulators are positive steps towards achieving a safer environment. Better understanding of complexity and how agents interact will be a major step forward in the future. The idea of root-cause analysis seems inadequate when an AE may represent the emergent behaviour and self-organisation of an unsatisfactory complex system. The Pareto principle which decrees that most problems have few major causes must also be subjected to scrutiny. Excessive numbers of AEs may occur in complex systems because of the interaction of many agents that, when examined individually, may seem relatively innocuous.

At the level of data analysis, there are problems peculiar to hospitals. The most important methods involve the sequential analysis of AE data. This is often accomplished by adapting quality monitoring and improvement tools from manufacturing industry, where they have a long and successful history (Deming). However, this adaptation is not straightforward: in hospitals these time-series AE data frequently display clustering, high variability, marked skewness, many zero counts and occasionally autocorrelation. The transmission of an infectious agent is not an independent process. Patients vary in their susceptibility to the occurrence of an AE and risk adjustment, although useful, is by no means perfect. Length of stay in hospital contributes to occupied bed-days, a frequently employed denominator and it is also frequently a risk factor. Although these issues also arise in manufacturing processes, they need to be carefully understood and accounted for in this new setting of hospital monitoring. Risk adjustment is available for many binary AEs such as complications of surgical procedures and, although very useful, it is not infallible. With count data AEs, where risk adjustment usually involves the hospital's services rather than individual patient characteristics, it is in the early stages of development. When patients with differing potential to be harmed are in the wards of a hospital, such grouping is often not random, and this can result in AE variation that is sufficiently excessive to invalidate elementary approaches.

Control charts are the most frequently employed quality monitoring tools. These rely on there being some sort of expected value, perhaps a mean value during a known period of stability, and some measure of variability, that is, there are available data that behave predictably and that enable location and spread to be estimated. It is then possible to determine whether or not this month's result is within those predictable limits. If it is not, an audit can be performed to search for causes. A problem with some hospital data is that such expected values may not exist. For example, how can it be possible to determine the expected usage of an antibiotic or the expected prevalence or burden of colonisation with an organism each month? When a quality improvement activity is instituted, the count of AEs may actually increase due to better reporting. Another difficulty arises with some highly skewed data like ICU length of stay that appear, at least approximately, to sometimes follow fractal (power law) distributions and to have no mean value in the usual sense. When this is the case, using familiar control charts can give meaningless misinformation. In addition, we once again mention the limitations of finding obvious causes for apparent signals in the control charts when so many trends and other changes represent emergent behaviour.

This book has been written in light of the above considerations. The aim is to provide statistical tools for monitoring the type of processes that are typically encountered in a hospital context. We devote much attention to addressing the difficulties described above, but we acknowledge that our approaches can certainly be improved. We hope that our book will stimulate interest in improving the methods that are currently available. During the past decade we have published several papers to illustrate how available methods can be adapted to monitor hospital AE data, especially AEs due to hospital-acquired organisms. Spreadsheet software is no longer adequate for analysing hospital AE data and in these notes we endeavour to show how the R statistical analysis system can be employed to undertake these analyses.

Thus we aim to introduce hospital scientists to the statistical software program R for the analysis of their data. Since specialised statistical software can require considerable training and continuity of use, some method has to be found to make software like R useful to hospital scientists who increasingly have postgraduate degrees but often little training in statistics, or continuity of use of statistical software. We have endeavoured to address these difficulties by providing simple to use functions for getting data into and out of R in a standard format and for analysing those data. The earlier parts of Chapters 1 and 4 should be of use to hospital scientists who often have to analyse proportions and rates. Chapters 3 and 6 and parts of Chapter 7 deal with control charts and charts based on generalised additive models. In each case, a menu is provided. Chapters 2 and 5 deal with aggregated data and will be of less interest to hospital scientists. However, we feel that these chapters are necessary for continuity and that they may prove to be of interest to staff whose job it is to present analysed data from groups of hospitals, or units within them that perform similar functions. The Introduction describes how hospital scientists might use R. Chapter 8 is a summary of the very important non-statistical aspects of hospital safety.

In conclusion, it is of interest to speculate on what future developments will occur in this area.

New insights into effective monitoring tools and approaches are being developed by hospital-based researchers such as Mr Ian Smith at St Andrews Hospital and Medical Institute (Smith and colleagues). Of particular importance is their experience regarding implementation and uptake of these approaches. As more AE data collection is mandated by central authorities and punitive action like withholding funding or administering fines may be involved, it is very important that the corresponding statistics are presented fairly. Good performance is dependent on justice, learning and discipline and without justice there cannot be the trust that is vital for high levels of performance. Systems of reward and punishment that are based on random variation in the data, or inappropriate statistical analysis or interpretation, or that involve AEs that occur as a result of high-level decisions or that seek scapegoats, destroy trust and morale and guarantee mediocre performance.

Risk adjustment is another important area that, while relatively well developed, still needs statistical attention. This is particularly true for count data adverse events (AEs) where risk adjustment is still undergoing development. Edward Tong's bacteraemia study was the first we were involved with and the work is being continued by Ms Mohana Rajmokan MSc (Biostats), statistician at the Queensland Health Centre for Health Related Infection Surveillance and Prevention (CHRISP) who has recently applied Tong's methods for risk adjusting hospital antibiotic usage.

As hospital complexity continues to increase in tandem with financial restraint necessitated by increasing population, depletion of resources, environmental degradation and deteriorating climate, change in many areas will become necessary. Understanding hospitals as complex systems within a complex environment will assume ever increasing importance. Our early work on this, employing a Bayesian network, involved Dr Mary Waterhouse (Waterhouse and colleagues) with St Andrews Medical Institute and the Wesley Research Institute in Brisbane and has again been continued and extended by Ms Rajmokan at CHRISP.

Hospitals vary greatly in the specialist services they provide and this can have a large effect on expected rates. For example, one hospital may have a large haematology/oncology or renal dialysis unit and another may have a large maternity unit. Bacteraemias are uncommon in maternity units. A major difficulty for us has been the limited number of hospitals available to us, for example Queensland has one spinal injuries unit so the possible effect of such units on bacteraemia rates or antibiotic use cannot easily be established. In addition, many smaller hospitals have few bacteraemias due, for example, to *Staphylococcus aureus*, so they are of little use in determining which services are associated with these infections. It would seem to be sensible to omit hospitals reporting only a few AEs each year and require them to perform M&M audits when those AEs occur. It would also seem desirable for a standardised evidence-based bundle to be devised for performing an M&M audit, such as that described by Singer. Another area of potential interest is the development of charts for composite measures. For example, track, trigger and report (TTR) systems (Mitchell and colleagues) for the early detection of acute deterioration may benefit from the development of a composite measure that encompasses changes in blood pressure, pulse rate, temperature, respiratory rate, oxygenation and level of consciousness. These are but a few of the areas where future developments could be beneficial.

We wish to acknowledge the valued collaboration of Dr David Cook, Dr David Looke, Dr Margaret Lindsay, Ms Mohana Rajmokan, Professor Tony Pettitt and Dr Anna Barker. We must also acknowledge the selfless work performed by those who developed and sustain R. We are indeed fortunate to be able to take advantage of their work. We also include a list of the libraries we have employed and thank their authors. R can be a wonderful gift to those of us who work with clinical people to make hospitals safer places.

When R starts it indicates that R is free software and comes with no warranty. The R scripts and functions to accompany this book that are available on the internet are similarly free software and come with no warranty (`www.wiley.com/go/hospital_monitoring`). Our primary aim is to show how a complex statistical analysis package can be used by hospital scientists who are not statisticians and who often have to deal with atypical data and we hope that others will build on these notes, scripts and functions. We recommend that before our functions are implemented users seek specialist advice. Hospital adverse event data from other hospital systems may have characteristics that we have not encountered. Inevitably, in spite of our best efforts, errors will be found and we ask that they be brought to our attention so that corrections can be made available via the internet. Further aims are to suggest possible solutions to problems such as the analysis of very low rate adverse events and data that lack predictable measures of location and spread. We hope that others will investigate and build on these proposals.

Anthony Morton, Tarragindi, February 2013

Introduction

0.1 Overview and rationale for this book

0.1.1 Motivation for the book

Quality management (QM) and quality improvement (QI) are fundamental tenets of almost every business, industry, government and institutional enterprise. Established in the 1920s and popularised by Shewhart, Deming and Juran, among others, QM is now recognised as aiming to produce a consistent outcome of interest, whereas QI seeks to improve the consistency and/or quality of the outcome. This often involves changing the physical, technical, environmental or human factors or processes that generate, or impact on, the desired quality and consistency. The importance and pervasiveness of QI are illustrated by the many QI standards that have been established across the world that include ISO guidelines, the Japanese Kaizen program, Six Sigma, Taguchi methods, and others (Wadsworth and colleagues). In the hospital setting, QM and QI mean achieving safety primarily by the disciplined application of systems based on evidence.

One of the more recent applications of QI is in the improvement of hospital acquired infection (HAI) rates and other adverse events that occur in hospitals such as patient falls, pressure ulcers, medication errors, needlestick injuries, complications of treatment and mortality. HAIs are a major contributor to hospital adverse events (AEs): approximately one in every 20 hospitalised patients will contract an HAI (US Centers for Disease Control www.cdc.gov/hai/). They can hinder patient recovery, increase hospital stay, increase costs and can lead to death. The cost of HAIs is considerable: in the United States the annual overall direct cost to hospitals is in the order of 30 billion dollars. In that country in 2002 the estimated number of HAIs was 1.7 million with 99,000 deaths. Graves[A] and colleagues have predicted that in Australia there are approximately 175,000 cases annually resulting in an additional 850,000 bed-days. In another paper, Graves[B] and colleagues express caution concerning the estimation of costs. Nevertheless, reducing HAIs would clearly make available badly needed hospital beds.

Effective infection management (IM) includes understanding the factors involved in the acquisition and spread of the organisms responsible for HAIs, and implementation of systems for managing and reducing infections in hospitals. This requires a strong evidence base, which

Statistical Methods for Hospital Monitoring with R, First Edition. Anthony Morton, Kerrie Mengersen, Michael Whitby and George Playford.
© 2013 John Wiley & Sons, Ltd. Published 2013 by John Wiley & Sons, Ltd.

in turn requires the collection of epidemiologically sound and clinically relevant data (Evans and colleagues), and employment of appropriate statistical methods for their analysis.

These ideas apply equally to other AEs such as patient falls, medication errors and pressure ulcers. An example is the reduction in patient falls resulting in injury following the determined implementation of a suitable evidence-based system (Barker and colleagues).

In the past, spreadsheets have been used regularly for statistical analysis in QI in general, and for IM in hospital departments in particular. This practice can be constraining and possibly misleading due to the limited statistical capabilities of the spreadsheet software, particularly for typical HAI data which can be characterised by small rates, a large number of zeros, and variation within and between hospital units and patient cohorts. This excessive variation occurs because infections are not biologically independent. Frequently, a stable average value is lacking, for example, in antibiotic usage and some prevalence and other data, they may be correlated over time and they are sometimes highly skewed. This means that the well-known statistical approaches, for example simple normal approximation methods for calculating confidence intervals and performing significance tests for proportion and rates may not be appropriate.

A major focus of the book is to provide a suite of methods that we have found to be useful in analysing these types of data. Moreover, we provide the software tools to implement these methods using the freely available statistical package, R. Although the approaches presented in the book are mainly focused on IM, the methods and software tools may be generally applicable across a range of situations for which QI in hospitals is a focus.

0.1.2   Why R?

We choose the software package R (R Core Team (2012). R: A language and environment for statistical computing. R Foundation for Statistical Computing, Vienna, Austria. ISBN 3-900051-07-0, URL http://www.R-project.org/.) because it is freely available and includes very powerful methods such as those based on the beta and gamma distributions. Wherever possible, we employ the functions already available in R and its libraries. We acknowledge that it takes an investment of time to learn R, but we suggest to the reader that this investment is worthwhile. In order to facilitate the learning and implementation of this package, we have developed two menus (IMenu() and CCMenu(), in rprogs.RData) that enable the selection of frequently required methods for the AEs of interest. Each function in these menus is accompanied by a script available in the accompanying code file on the internet that includes the corresponding lines of R code. The functions in the menus can be modified if required for access to other R functions if different analyses are of interest. There is a short Appendix entitled Menus that explains the use of these menus.

0.1.3   Other reading for R

There is excellent R documentation available from the R website http://cran.r-project.org/. For example there are *R for Beginners* by Emmanuel Paradis and Simple R by John Verzani, both available at cran. Other documentation that may be of interest includes *Analysis of Epidemiological Data Using R and Epicalc* by Virasakdi Chongsuvivatwong, *Statistics Using R with Biological Examples* by Kim Seefeld and Ernst Linder, *An Introduction to R: Software for Statistical Modelling and Computing* by Petra Kuhnert and Bill Venables, all available at

cran. There is a useful download by Lawrence Joseph available at www.medicine.mcgill
.ca/epidemiology/joseph/EPIB-621.html together with a downloadable introductory statistics
textbook http://www.medicine.mcgill.ca/epidemiology/Joseph/courses/EPIB-621/rosenberg
.joseph.barkun.pdf).

Excellent introductory books are available such as *Dalgaard's Introductory Statistics with
R* 2nd Edition (2008), *Using R for Introductory Statistics* by Verzani (2004*), Statistics, An
Introduction Using R* by Crawley (2005), *The R Book* also by Crawley (2007), *A Handbook
of Statistical Analysis Using R* 2nd Edition by Everitt and Hothorn (2010), and *Data Analysis
and Graphics Using R* by Maindonald and Braun 3rd Edition (2010). Books at a higher
level include *Statistical Computing* by Crawley (2003), *Modern Applied Statistics with S* by
Venables and Ripley (2002) and *Data Analysis Using Regression and Multilevel/Hierarchical
Models* (Gelman and Hill 2007). Myatt's *Open Source Solutions–R* (2005) explains the use
of R for analysing epidemiological data including advice on the use of logistic regression
for analysing outbreaks and epidemics (www.brixtonhealth.com). The R meta, rmeta, Epi,
epicalc, epibasix, epiR, epitools and other packages mentioned in these notes have functions
that may prove useful to hospital epidemiologists and scientists in IM and QI departments.

Other possibly useful programs are Abramson's WINPEPI (www.brixtonhealth.com/),
CIA (Altman, Machin, Bryant and Gardner 2000), EpiInfo 3.5.4 (Dean, Arner, Sunki,
Friedman, Lantinga, Sangam, Zubieta, Sullivan, Brendel, Gao, Fontaine, Shu, Fuller, Smith,
Nitschke and Fagan. Epi Info™, a database and statistics program for public health profes-
sionals. Centers for Disease Control and Prevention, Atlanta, Georgia, USA, 2007. www.cdc
.gov/epiinfo/) and EpiData (www.epidata.dk/).

Several R libraries are required in addition to those in the basic installation. These include
chron, exactci, PropCIs, mgcv, geepack, arm and others as well as the libraries on which
they depend. For example, for arm lme4 several other libraries are needed and will usually be selected automatically when the arm package is installed. In addition, qAnalyst, spc
and qcc are libraries with statistical process control functions and the library surveillance
provides functions for outbreak and syndromic surveillance. To employ an installed library
use for example library(chron) and to remove a library from the workspace use for example, detach(package:"chron"). This will occasionally be necessary as some libraries disable
functions that may subsequently be required.

0.2   What methods are covered in the book?

The statistical methods that are presented in the book, in particular those that are available
via IMenu() and CCMenu() reflect the monitoring performed at a large tertiary referral
hospital. For example, based on our experience, scientists working in IM and QI departments
are frequently called upon to present summary AE data and AE data on a monthly basis,
for example, in control charts or other time-series graphics such as generalised additive
model (GAM) charts. Similarly, they may be required to model bacteremias; since these are
usually independent events, analysis can generally be assumed to be based on the Poisson
distribution. However, this may not always be the case as patients can differ greatly in their
susceptibility to developing a bacteraemia and, since they may not be distributed randomly
within the hospital, variation can be increased. Moreover, new colonisations and infections
with multiple antibiotic resistant organisms (MROs) are often not independent and can display
excessive variation; we then use the negative binomial distribution or the methods described

by Laney (Mohammed and Laney[A]) or Spiegelhalter[D] for their analysis. Antibiotic usage and MRO prevalence data may display autocorrelation and determination of an average value may be difficult or impossible. Sequential analysis of these data can often be accomplished with a generalised additive model (GAM) chart (Morton[B] and colleagues).

We have found that staff working in IM and QI departments understand proportion and rate methods that employ differences better than the ratio estimators that are more familiar in Epidemiology. An important Evidence Based Medicine (EBM) estimator, the Number Needed to Treat (NNT) (Campbell and Swinscow) and its confidence interval are derived from the difference between proportions. For these reasons, we describe the calculation of proportions and rates and their differences together with corresponding confidence intervals. Frequently used statistical methods such as odds ratios, t-tests, analysis of variance and linear regression are described elsewhere, for example in the book by Kirkwood and Sterne.

Mainstream Biostatistics is still predominantly frequentist. There is now increasing interest in likelihood (van der Tweel) and Bayesian approaches (Woodworth). We believe that these methods have particular appeal in the areas of hospital QI and IM, and we introduce and use the likelihood approach in a natural manner as it emerges during the course of the book.

As an example of the motivation for likelihood analysis in surveillance work in a hospital, there is often no large population from which random samples could have been drawn for an experiment. Instead, there is often an expected value such as a surgical site infection (SSI) rate of say 3%. Surveillance yields data, often the entire sample of relevant patients in a hospital for a particular time period. It is then natural to use the likelihood approach that is based on the support those data provide for the expected value. If they provide little support it can be inferred that a probable difference exists.

We prefer the likelihood approach and we believe that its use will increase. In particular, the likelihood counterpart of the confidence interval, the supported range, has a much simpler and more logical definition than the frequentist confidence interval. However, we mostly continue to use the more familiar term confidence interval. Numerically, they are usually similar. In addition, we report the likelihood ratio (LR) or Bayes factor as described by Goodman. This indicates the relative support that exists for a real difference. For example, a frequentist p-value of 0.05 (1/20) corresponds to an LR of 1/7. This then suggests that there is just seven times as much support for the observed data value as there is for the corresponding expected value.

0.3   Structure of the book

Chapters 1 and 4 deal with basic issues and functions that are most likely to be of use to hospital scientists are available via IMenu(). In Chapters 3, 6 and 7, we provide a series of functions in R that we anticipate will assist scientists in IM and QI departments to use this software package to perform the regular data analyses for which they are responsible; these are available via CCMenu(). In addition, there are chapters in which the analysis of data from multiple institutions is discussed (Chapters 2 and 5). This analysis will usually be performed by staff with a higher level of statistical expertise than most hospital scientists in IM and QI departments. We hope that the discussion in these two chapters will be of interest to them. There is an overview of the chapters in the following box.

1. Chapter 1 is an introduction to binary data (AE data where a complication has or has not occurred). Surgical site infections (SSIs) are frequently used to illustrate the statistical methods that include significance tests and confidence intervals for proportions and their differences, including data that are stratified.

2. Chapter 2 extends the analysis to binary data from multiple institutions such as SSIs for procedures performed in groups of hospitals.

3. Chapter 3 deals with sequential binary data, for example, data in control charts.

4. Chapter 4 is similar to Chapter 1 but for count and rate data such as bacteraemias and multiple antibiotic resistant organism (MRO) infections and colonisations.

5. Chapter 5 is similar to Chapter 2 but for count and rate data.

6. Chapter 6 is similar to Chapter 3 but for count and rate data.

7. Chapter 7 deals with miscellaneous IM and QI issues such as length of stay (LOS), antibiotic usage, MRO prevalence, assessing agreement, making decisions and dealing with outbreaks.

8. Chapter 8 is a brief non-statistical overview of QI.

We recognise that there will always be better ways to achieve our objective: better code or better approaches. We hope that people who are more proficient in the use of R and who have an interest in hospital AEs will respond by producing better, more user-friendly functions. We recognise that those who are unqualified in the analysis of complex data can make serious errors without realising this (a classical example is the continued use of correlation coefficients to assess agreement or causality). Nevertheless, hospital scientists increasingly have postgraduate training, for example, in Microbiology or Public Health, and are well aware of their limitations and the need, on occasion, to seek expert advice. In addition, at regular intervals they are required to produce reports that involve the use of control charts and related methods and they are competent to understand these analyses. For the most part we employ the default settings of existing R functions.

0.4   Using R

In this section, we provide a very introductory overview of the R statistical software package. In Windows, after loading R, click on File Change dir, select the required directory and then choose File Load Workspace and click on rprogs.RData. Alternatively click on rprogs.RData in its folder and R will load and include rprogs.RData at the same time. For other operating systems, consult the documentation at cran.

Although we have written functions to perform routine analyses, there are numerous examples of R code in the book chapters and the code files on the internet. Lines of R code can be run as a group up to a space, a BOX or # for example by copying and pasting the code at the R prompt. Responses from R, comments or inputs from the user are shown in a BOX or preceded by # (R ignores letters on a line after #). In some cases adjacent scripts are separated by # and a space. If modifying code, always beware of using a capital F or other special letter such as T (stands for TRUE) or t (stands for transpose) when naming variables. For example, F will overwrite F for FALSE and cause some functions to malfunction (if necessary use e.g. if(F!=FALSE){rm(F)} to restore). For character data use the correct quotation mark symbol. Your word processor may use an alternative symbol such as " " & R will record an error message unless you change to" ".

When using rprogs.RData some of the functions have unwieldy names. It may be useful to type ls() and RETURN/ENTER at the R prompt, select the required function without the quotes with the mouse and employ Edit and then Copy and Paste to get it to the R prompt.

First, we describe simple, consistent ways for getting data to and from R.

0.4.1   Entering data

Data are usually entered as data frames (data may occasionally need to be entered manually in the scripts shown in the various chapters). A data frame is a two dimensional array with rows for units such as individual patients undergoing a surgical procedure and columns for relevant data such as whether or not a surgical site infection (SSI) occurred. The function g.d() (short for get data) can be used for entering data. A text file can be read using g.d(), for example using a comma or space delimited text file; example files are mostly comma delimited .csv files. The R function file.choose() in g.d() enables the selection of the required folder. The data will be placed in R workspace in the data frame datain. Users are asked if the first column contains dates and if that is the case, the format should be entered; the date format "dd-mmm-yyyy" is then selected by g.d() and it becomes the first column of datain as a date (dates otherwise enter R as factors). This ensures that data going to control chart and similar functions usually have a standard date format that is "dd-mmm-yyyy". It is also possible to copy data in a spreadsheet using the clipboard, for example with EDIT COPY in the spreadsheet, and g.d() will paste the data into the data frame datain in the R workspace. You may then need to type mydata<-datain if you require the data frame to have another name. It is convenient to use head(datain) at the R prompt to view the first six rows of datain and tail(datain) for the last six rows. The command read.table(...) is an alternative to using g.d() that is described in the R reference material. For example, to use the clipboard when the data columns in a spreadsheet file have headings enter at the R prompt: name<-read.table("clipboard",T), or read.table("clipboard",F) if the columns lack headings (do not press ENTER/RETURN in R until you have copied the data in the spreadsheet to the clipboard). Department scientists in hospitals may be most comfortable using g.d() and the clipboard throughout. Mac users require read.table(pipe("pbpaste"),T or F). For the Mac use mg.d()instead of g.d(). If you use an operating system other than Windows, consult the relevant documentation at cran.

Make sure that numerical and date data are correctly specified in the spreadsheet, for example using FORMAT CELLS NUMBER or FORMAT CELLS CUSTOM for dates before copying or they may not copy correctly. For the former, ensure that the correct number of decimal places is specified. A convenient date format is "dd-mmm-yyyy" but .csv file dates are often in the shorter "d-mmm-yy" format. The date format in the spreadsheet need not be changed provided the data are genuine dates (dates transferred to a spreadsheet from another program may need formatting). There must be no spaces in the data to be imported. This may be a problem if headings consist of more than one separate word. For example, change "Observed counts" to something like "ObservedCounts" or "Observed.Counts". The basic version of R does not import files like those produced for example by Microsoft Excel and it is usually simplest to use the clipboard or convert the worksheet data to a text file such as a .csv comma-delimited text file. The use of g.d() is illustrated using the file allorthssi.csv. Beware of missing data in a data file. These should be uncommon with hospital surveillance data. Replace any missing data with for example NA.

```
g.d() # load allorthssi.csv via the clipboard
```

```
Loading data.
Data from clipboard (C) or file (F) c
Do data column(s) have heading(s) (Y/N) y
Is column 1 a date column (Y/N) y
Date format.
 13-Jan-05
Date format.
Enter the required date format dd-mmm-yy
```

```
head(datain) #view first 6 rows
```

```
  ProcedureDate Hospital SSI      RIAdj
1   13-Jan-2005        A   0 0.037132
2   21-Jan-2005        A   0 0.039545
3   24-Jan-2005        A   1 0.041217
4   25-Jan-2005        A   0 0.039545
5   28-Jan-2005        A   0 0.041999
6   01-Feb-2005        A   0 0.037132
```

```
tail(datain) # view last 6 rows
```

```
     ProcedureDate Hospital SSI      RIAdj
5617   28-Dec-2006        Q   0 0.041217
5618   28-Dec-2006        Q   0 0.039545
5619   29-Dec-2006        I   0 0.053374
5620   29-Dec-2006        Q   0 0.039545
5621   29-Dec-2006        Q   0 0.039545
5622   30-Dec-2006        I   0 0.044003
```

```
rm(datain) # removes datain from workspace
g.d() # load allorthssi.csv as .csv text file
```

```
Loading data.
Data from clipboard (C) or file (F) f
Do data column(s) have heading(s) (Y/N) y
Are data columns separated by spaces (S) or commas (C) c
A menu appears from which to select the folder and file required
 (uses built in R function file.choose()).
Is column 1 a date column (Y/N) y
Date format.
 13-Jan-05
Date format.
Enter the required date format dd-mmm-yy
```

```
# to see function g.d(), use fix(g.d)
fix(g.d)
```

```
function(){
library(chron)
q<-readline("Loading data.\nData from clipboard (C) or file (F) ")
if (q=="F"|q=="f"){q<-"F"}else{q<-"C"}
if (q=="C"){q1<-readline("Do data column(s) have heading(s) (Y/N) ")
if (q1=="Y"|q1=="y"){q1<-"H"}else{q1<-"N"}}
if (q=="C"){
if (q=="C"&q1=="H"){datain<<-read.table(file="clipboard",header=T)}
if (q=="C"&q1=="N"){datain<<-read.table(file="clipboard",header=F)}}
if (q=="F"){
q2<-readline("Do data column(s) have heading(s) (Y/N) ")
if (q2=="Y"|q2=="y"){q2<-"Y"}else{q2<-"N"}
q3<-readline("Are data columns separated by spaces (S) or commas (C) ")
if (q3=="c"|q3=="C"){q3<-"C"}else{q3<-"S"}
if (q2=="Y"&q3=="C"){datain<<-read.csv(file.choose(),header=T)}
if (q2=="N"&q3=="C"){datain<<-read.csv(file.choose(),header=F)}
if (q2=="Y"&q3=="S"){datain<<-read.table(file.choose(),header=T)}
if (q2=="N"&q3=="S"){datain<<-read.table(file.choose(),header=F)}
}
q4<-readline("Is column 1 a date column (Y/N) ")
if (q4=="Y"|q4=="y"){
library(chron)
n<-names(datain)
cat("Date format.\n",as.character(datain[1,1]),"\n")
x<-readline("Date format.\nEnter the required date format ")
d<-as.character(datain[,1])
d0<-datain[,-1]
d<-chron(d,format=x,out.format="dd-mmm-yyyy")
g<-data.frame(d,d0)
names(g)<-n
datain<<-g
}
}
```

Code for each function in the book, such as g.d(), is included in the accompanying code file on the internet. We have recently found that when R reads a single column .csv file it adds a second column of NAs so the above code is being modified and tested. We recommend use of the clipboard with those data.

0.4.2 Dates

Since so much of the work in IM and QI departments involves sequential data, dealing with dates is crucial. When there are dates but they are not in the first column, or g.d() is not employed for data entry, they may need to be placed in the required format. When entered into an R data.frame, dates are factors. The function g.d() converts them to dates in the format "dd-mmm-yyyy" when they are in the first column. Otherwise, to convert dates as factors to usable dates they must first be converted to characters. An alternative is to use a marker for the first column of data to be used in a control chart function (e.g. 1 to N for the number of rows of data) and employ a function with its name ending in qtr. However, the data must be properly ordered before employing these functions.

```
rm(datain) # removes datain from workspace

datain<-read.table("clipboard",T)# allorthssi.csv
#NB always copy the above line to the R prompt first but do
#not press ENTER/RETURN. Next, copy the data in the
#spreadsheet to the clipboard. Then press ENTER/RETURN in R.

# formatting dates
class(datain[,1])
#[1] "factor"

x<-1 # in allorthssi.csv column 1 has the dates
d<-datain[,x]
d[1]
#[1] 13-Jan-05
#590 Levels: 1-Apr-05 1-Aug-05 1-Aug-06 1-Dec-05 1-Dec-06 ... 9-Sep-05

library(chron) # in these notes chron is the key to formatting dates
Times<-chron(as.character(d),format="dd-mmm-yy",out.format="dd-mmm-yyyy")
#replace format="dd-mmm-yyyy" with required date format if differ-
ent e.g. may be format="d-mmm-yy", format="m/d/y", format="d/m/y"
datain[,1]<-Times
head(datain)
```

	ProcedureDate	Hospital	SSI	RIAdj
1	13-Jan-2005	A	0	0.037132
2	21-Jan-2005	A	0	0.039545
3	24-Jan-2005	A	1	0.041217
4	25-Jan-2005	A	0	0.039545
5	28-Jan-2005	A	0	0.041999
6	01-Feb-2005	A	0	0.037132

```
class(datain[,1])
# [1] "dates" "times"
```

0.4.2.1   Note on chron

When re-starting an analysis following a break, a date column may revert to being represented as the number of days since 1970-01-01, with negative values for earlier dates and it is necessary to convert it back to the required format. This will usually be corrected by entering library(chron) at the R prompt.

```
# date conversion
#from columns A and B of the file dateconversion.csv
#dates in one of the usual formats entered as factors
datain<-read.table("clipboard",T)

datain[1,]
#       Month Proportion
#1 1-Jul-93       0.091
class(datain[1,1])
#[1] "factor"

library(chron)
n<-names(datain)
```

```
d<-datain[,1] # factor d must be converted to character before date
d<-chron(as.character(d),format="d-mmm-yy",out.format="dd-mmm-yyyy")
datain1<-data.frame(d,datain[,-1])
names(datain1)<-n
datain1[1,]
#          Month Proportion
#1 01-Jul-1993        0.091
class(datain1[1,1])
#[1] "dates" "times"

#from columns E and F of the file dateconversion.csv in numeric format
datain1<-read.table("clipboard",T)

datain1[1,]
#  Month Proportion
#1  8582        0.091
class(datain1[1,1])
#[1] "integer"

library(chron)
n<-names(datain1)
d<-datain1[,1]
d<-chron(d,out.format="dd-mmm-yyyy")
datain1<-data.frame(d,datain1[,-1])
names(datain1)<-n
datain1[1,]
#          Month Proportion
#1 01-Jul-1993        0.091
class(datain1[1,1])
#[1] "dates" "times"
```

0.4.3   Exporting data

To export data, for example to Microsoft Excel, use the function s.d(dataout) (short for save data) where dataout is the name of the data.frame to be exported (Mac users can employ ms.d(dataout) as pipe("pbcopy","w") is required instead of "clipboard" in Windows). These functions may be used to transfer data via a comma-delimited text file (do not add .csv) or, if the data.frame is small, via the clipboard. For other operating systems, consult the relevant documentation at cran.

```
Names<-LETTERS[1:5]
# N.B. for character data use correct quotation mark symbol
#your wordprocessor may use an alternative symbol such as "" &
#R will record an error message unless you change to "".
Results<-c(100,200,150,250,50)
dataout<-data.frame(Names,Results)

s.d(dataout) #transfer to spreadsheet via clipboard
#Use clipboard (c) or a data file (d) c
#use EDIT PASTE in spreadsheet

s.d(dataout) #.csv text file
```

```
Use clipboard (c) or a data file (f)  f
Enter a file name e:/test
```

```
#data in test.csv on E drive
#comma-delimited file with .csv extension automatically appended.
# Note that R uses / rather than \ that is required for formatting.
#to see function s.d(), use fix(s.d)

fix(s.d)
```

```
function(d){
q<-readline("Use clipboard (c) or a data file (f) ")
if (q=="c"|q=="C"){write.table(d,"clipboard",sep="\t",row.names=F)
}else{
q1<-readline("Enter a file name ")
q1<-paste(q1,".csv",sep="")
write.table(d,file=q1,sep=",",row.names=F)
}
}
```

The code in the functions we describe may be viewed by typing fix(function name). It may then be modified if required. The code for each function described in the book is to be found in the corresponding code file on the internet.

0.5   Further notes

It is suggested that the R functions available on the internet that accompany the book be placed in a suitable folder or directory, for example it could be called e:\rprogs in Windows (the R functions dir(), getwd() and setwd() are useful for examining the files in the working directory, obtaining the name of the working directory and changing the working directory; see the R documentation for further details). We like to keep the rprogs.RData functions on a separate USB disk that in our system is the e:\drive in Windows in a directory (folder) called rprogs. Note that R, like Linux, uses / rather than \ for referring to disks and directories as it uses \ for formatting output. Note also that in R case matters; R is not the same as r. When R has been opened, the directory needs to be changed, for example to e:/rprogs in Windows using File and Change dir in the R menu (for other operating systems, see the relevant documentation at cran). Then at the R prompt enter load("rprogs.RData") or select File Load Workspace and click on rprogs.RData. This will ensure that all the required R functions are in memory. An alternative is to select the folder containing rprogs in Windows and click on rprogs.RData; R will then load with rprogs in memory.

When selecting a function in rprogs, there may be difficulty as some of the function names are long and misspelling can easily occur. Use ls() to display the function names, select the required function with the mouse (do not include the quotation marks), and in the R menu select Edit and Paste. The required function name then appears at the R prompt.

0.6   A brief introduction to rprogs charts and figures

There is excellent R documentation available on using charts, for example *R for Beginners* by Emmanuel Paradis (http://cran.r-project.org/) and Dalgaard's *Introductory Statistics with R*.

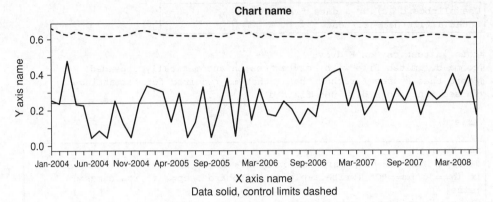

Figure 0.1   General control chart function, illustrates use of locator().

The R Reference Card by Tom Short is also useful (http://cran.r-project.org/). The purpose of this note is to summarise briefly some of the basic anatomy of the charting methods commonly used in rprogs.RData. These are illustrated in figures 0.1 to 0.6.

Many of the charts and figures are control charts. The CONTROLCHARTS worksheet in the chart1.xls file has five columns: rate per 1000 bed-days, mean, months, upper control limit and lower control limit. It is derived from the data in the IVDBACTS worksheet that refers to intravenous device related bacteraemias. The lower control limit is, in this case, zero because the underlying counts are small.

```
library(chron) # for manipulating dates
g.d()# chart1.xls CONTROLCHART sheet
```

```
Loading data.
Data from clipboard (C) or file (F) c
Do data column(s) have heading(s) (Y/N) y
Is column 1 a date column (Y/N) n
```

```
# Figure 0.1
library(chron)
chartout<-datain
d<-chartout[,3] # months column
#reads dates as factors and need changing to dates via characters
d<-chron(as.character(d),format="dd-mmm-yyyy",out.format="dd-mmm-yyyy")
#format may need changing, eg to d/m/y or m/d/y.
up<-max(c(chartout[,1],chartout[,4]))
#to get upper end of vertical axis of chart
lo<-0
#to get lower end of vertical axis of chart
#counts do not go below zero
if (min(chartout[,5]>0)){lo<-min(chartout[,5])}
#to get the minimum when the lower control limit is greater than zero
x<-months(d)
y<-years(d)
xy<-paste(x,y,sep="")
#converts the dates into months and years character strings
#present better on the horizontal axis than the whole dates
```

```
ma<-"Data blue, control limits red"
#explanatory text for the bottom of the chart
par(xaxs="i") # fits horizontal axis to data,
#to leave space at ends use default par(xaxs="r")
#remember to change back to default after charting if necessary
a<-chartout[,1]
#rates per 1000 bed-days per month
plot(a,axes=F,lwd=2,type="l",col="blue",ylim=c(lo,up),
main="Chart Name",ylab="Y Axis Name",xlab=ma)
#type="l" is for lines, default is points, "b" is for both
#axes included later
#lwd line widths increased
#color of data blue
#ylim - limits of vertical axis
#main main heading, xlab, ylab data description & vertical axis headings
box()
axis(side=1,labels=xy,at=1:length(xy))
#horizontal axis labels & their positions
axis(side=c(2,3,4))
#other axes information - especially vertical axis on left
m<-chartout[,2] #center line of chart
abline(h=m) # draws center line
u<-chartout[,4] #upper control limit
l<-chartout[,5] #lower control limit
#attribute data limits calculated using pbeta() and pgamma() in a search
#in most charts there are more than one upper and lower control limit
lines(u,col="red",lwd=2,lty=1)
#upper control limit, lwd=2 makes it thicker
#lty=1 indicates a solid line, 2 if dashed, 3 if dotted
if (lo>0){lines(l,col="red",lwd=2,lty=1)}
#lower control limit drawn if above zero
mtext("X Axis Name",side=1,line=2)
#places "X Axis Name" at line=2 to keep clear of xlab data description

locator() # large third data value selected with left click
#locator can be used to identify points of interest
#it gives their approximate coordinates
#left click on points of interest
#right click to stop.
#$x
#[1] 2.955244
#
#$y
#[1] 0.4800128
a[3]
#[1] 0.4804
```

The next chart illustrates superimposing charts and using the locator() and text() functions to place a message on the chart.

```
library(chron) # for manipulating dates
g.d()# chart1.xls IVDBACTS sheet
```

```
Loading data.
Data from clipboard (C) or file (F) c
Do data column(s) have heading(s) (Y/N) y
Is column 1 a date column (Y/N) y
```

```
Date format.
 01-Jan-2004
Date format.
Enter the required date format dd-mmm-yyyy
```

```
# Figure 0.2
chartout1<-datain
d<-chartout1[,1] # dates
d<-chron(as.character(d),format="dd-mmm-yyyy",out.format="dd-mmm-yyyy")
#format may need changing as described above.
a<-chartout1[,2] #counts of bacteraemias
b<-chartout1[,3] #bed-days denominators
x<-months(d)
y<-years(d)
xy<-paste(x,y,sep="")
#tidying dates for horizontal axis, see above
sspl<-smooth.spline(a,spar=.25) # may use EWMA
ssplk<-smooth.spline(b,spar=.25) # may use EWMA
#see help(smooth.spline)for spar documentation
#smoothing is valuable for showing trends
mb<-"Bed-days Denominators"
par(xaxs="i")
#fits horizontal axis to data, to leave space at ends use par(xaxs="r")
barplot(a,xlab="Data Blue, Median Green, Smooth Red, Denomina-
tors & Smooth Brown.",ylim=c(0,max(a)*1.05),main="Chart
Name",col="blue",ylab="Y Axis Name")
#commands are similar to those for plot() described above
par(new=T)
#to superimpose smoothed outcome data using plotted line
plot(sspl,ylim=c(0,max(a)*1.05),type="l",axes=F,xlab="",ylab="",
 col="red",lwd=3)
abline(h=median(a),lwd=2,lty=1,col="green4")
axis(side=1,tick=T,labels=xy,at=1:length(xy))
par(new=T)
#to superimpose denominator data with smoothing using right vertical axis
plot(b,type="l",axes=F,ylab="",xlab="",ylim=c(0,max(b)),
 col="brown4",lty=1,lwd=3)
lines(ssplk,type="l",lwd=3,col="brown4",lty=4)
```

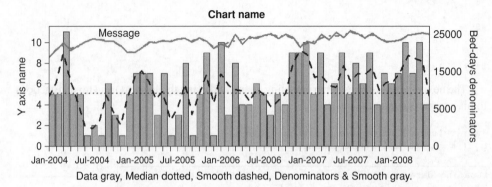

Data gray, Median dotted, Smooth dashed, Denominators & Smooth gray.

Figure 0.2   Bar and run charts, placing a message.

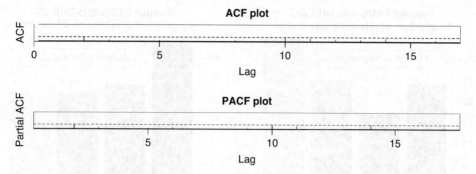

Figure 0.3   Above and below charts, autocorrelation functions.

```
axis(side=4,tick=F)
#selecting right vertical axis
mtext(mb,side=4)
box()
par(new=F) # turn off changes made in par()
text(locator(1),"Message")
#allows a message to be stamped in a suitable place on the chart
```

Placing charts one above another is sometimes desirable although they tend to be narrow. The next chart illustrates the use of layout(matrix()) for this purpose.

```
# Figure 0.3
library(chron) #using above data
a<-chartout1[,2]/chartout1[,3]
#gets rate
layout(matrix(1:2,2,1))
#to put two charts one above the other
par(xaxs="i")
acf(a,axes=F,ylim=c(0,1),main="ACF Plot")
#autocorrelation function
box()
axis(side=c(1,2,3,4))
par(xaxs="r")
pacf(a,axes=F,ylim=c(0,1),main="PACF Plot")
#partial autocorrelation function
box()
axis(side=c(1,2,3,4))
layout(matrix(1:1,1,1))
#to return the layout to normal.
```

Placing charts side by side is often useful for making comparisons. For example, one might wish to compare an observed with a corresponding theoretical distribution. The next chart compares length of stay (LOS) for two hospitals using then (1994–95) ANDRG252 (heart failure and shock) data. LOS is notoriously difficult to analyse because the distribution of these data frequently has a long right tail and, in this case, the percentages of LOS values exceeding the quartiles derived from reference data are plotted. In addition, we illustrate the legend(locator()) function for placing explanatory information on the chart (legend can also use x,y coordinates instead of locator()).

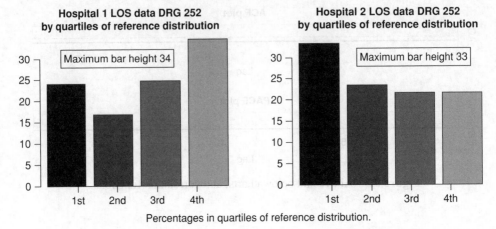

Figure 0.4   Side by side bar charts, messages placed with locator().

```
# Figure 0.4, charts side by side
#when using read.table("clipboard",T or F)
#copy command to the R prompt before copying from the data file
#do not press RETURN/ENTER
#until the data in the spreadsheet are copied to the clipboard
#using chart1.xls DRG252LOS sheet
#reference database (column A)
#using chart1.xls DRG252LOS sheet
#reference database (column A)
drg252ref<-read.table("clipboard",T)

#hospital 1 data (column C)
drg252h1<-read.table("clipboard",T)

#hospital 2 data (column E)
drg252h2<-read.table("clipboard",T)

graphics.off() #cancels existing graphic
d<-drg252ref[,1]
a<-drg252h1[,1]
b<-drg252h2[,1]
#LOS data
f<-fivenum(d)
#gets minimum and maximum, quartiles, median
f[1]<-0
#needs to be below minimum
f[5]<-f[5]+1
#needs to be above maximum
aa<-cut(a,f)
bb<-cut(b,f)
# cut divides the data at median and quartiles
x<-100*as.numeric(table(aa))/length(a)
y<-100*as.numeric(table(bb))/length(b)
# percentages
l<-c("1st","2nd","3rd","4th")
```

```
ll<-1:4
k1<-max(x)
k2<-max(y)
k<-max(c(k1,k2))
m1<-"Hospital 1 LOS data DRG 252\nby quartiles of reference distribution"
m2<-"Hospital 2 LOS data DRG 252\nby quartiles of reference distribution"
mat<-matrix(1:2,1,2)
#sets up for side by side charts
layout(mat)
barplot(x,main=m1,col=c("red","orange","yellow","brown"),ylim=c(0,k))
axis(side=1,labels=l,at=ll)
barplot(y,main=m2,col=c("red","orange","yellow","brown"),ylim=c(0,k))
axis(side=1,labels=l,at=ll)
mat<-matrix(1:1,1,1)
#returns to default
layout(mat)
mtext("Percentages in quartiles of reference distribution.",side=1,line=3)
msg<-"Figures side-by-side"
mtext(msg,side=3,line=3)
mh1<-paste("Maximum bar height ",round(k1,0))
mh2<-paste("Maximum bar height ",round(k2,0))
legend(locator(1),mh1,cex=.75) # cex makes the legend smaller
legend(locator(1),mh2,cex=.75)
#allows text to be placed on charts
```

Next, we illustrate the use of arrows and labels beside data values. These can be very useful for displaying confidence intervals, credible intervals or supported ranges.

```
# Figure 0.5
#continues with data for previous chart data
m<-median(d)
#median of reference data
q1<-length(a[a>m])
#number in A above reference median
n1<-length(a)
#totl in A
q2<-length(b[b>m])
```

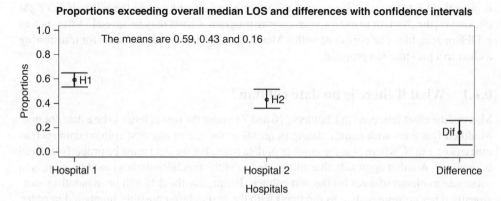

Figure 0.5   Using arrows for confidence intervals, using locator().

```
n2<-length(b)
p1<-prop.test(q1,n1)
#to get A rate & its confidence interval
p1e<-p1$estimate
p1u<-p1$conf.int[1]
p1l<-p1$conf.int[2]
p2<-prop.test(q2,n2)
p2e<-p2$estimate
p2u<-p2$conf.int[1]
p2l<-p2$conf.int[2]
x<-c(q1,q2)
y<-c(n1,n2)
p3<-prop.test(x,y)
#to get difference between A and B and its confidence interval
p3e<-p3$estimate[1]-p3$estimate[2]
p3u<-p3$conf.int[2]
p3l<-p3$conf.int[1]
e<-c(p1e,p2e,p3e)
u<-c(p1u,p2u,p3u)
l<-c(p1l,p2l,p3l)
msg=paste("The means are ",round(e[1],2),", ",round(e[2],2)," and ",
  round(e[3],2),sep="")
#message to show values
plot(e,axes=F,ylim=c(0,1),main="Proportions exceeding overall
  median LOS and differences with confidence intervals",xlab="Hospitals",
  ylab="Proportions",lwd=2,col="blue")
box()
axis(side=1,labels=c("Hospital 1","Hospital 2","Difference"),at=1:3)
axis(side=c(2,3,4))
arrows(1:3,l,1:3,u,angle=90,code=3,lwd=2,col="blue")
par(font=2)
text(e,labels= c("H1","H2","Dif"),pos=4,offset=.3,cex=.8)
par(font=1)
text(locator(1),msg)
```

This brief note can serve only as an introduction to the charting functions commonly used in rprogs.RData. Refer to *The R Reference Card* by Tom Short (http://cran.r-project.org/) and do not hesitate to use the excellent help available in R, for example, help(plot), help(par).

A further issue is getting charts from R into a word processor or presentation program. It is possible in R to save to a file or copy to the clipboard either by using the File menu or right clicking on the chart, or to use a screen capture program. Charts may be saved to a file such as a TIFF or Jpeg file. The clipboard with a Metafile is convenient, for example, for transferring a chart to a presentation program.

0.6.1 What if there is no date column?

Many of the chart functions in Chapters 3, 6 and 7 require the first column to be a date column. Modified functions with names ending in qtr allow the use of any first column data such as quarters or 1 to N, where N is the number of data rows, but the data must be properly ordered beforehand. Another approach, that allows the use of the functions without modification, is to substitute a column of dates for the first column. Frequently the data will be in months (occasionally other groupings such as quarters) with the first column possibly numbered in order. Suppose the data are as follows: (32,43,50,33,24,31,52,48,55,42,34,30,51,48,39,53,51,38)

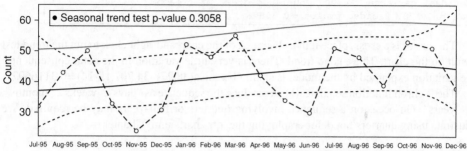

Dates demonstration
GAM chart from Jul 1995 t0 Dec 1996.

Data dashed, Fitted GAM solid, 95% CI dotted, Control limit gray.

Figure 0.6   Dates, GAM chart, Seasonal MannKendall trend test.

and that they represented monthly counts of new MRSA isolates between July 1995 and December 1996. We wish to get them into a suitable format for analysis using the usual functions of Chapter 6.

```
# Figure 0.6
d<-c(32,43,50,33,24,31,52,48,55,42,34,30,51,48,39,53,51,38)
library(chron)
fst<-chron("7/1/95")
lst<-chron("12/31/96")
s<-seq.dates(from=fst,to=lst,by="months")
S<-chron(s,out.format="dd-mmm-yyyy")
datain<-data.frame(S,d)
names(datain)<-c("Months","Counts")
head(datain)
```

```
  Months Counts
1 01-Jul-1995     32
2 01-Aug-1995     43
3 01-Sep-1995     50
4 01-Oct-1995     33
5 01-Nov-1995     24
6 01-Dec-1995     31
```

```
countgam(datain) # chart function from Chapter 6
```

```
Chart heading.
Enter heading for chart Dates demonstration
Change degrees of freedom (Y/N) n
```

An abbreviated summary is as follows:

```
The model is in mmg. Type summary(mmg)/predict(mmg,se=T) to see.
glm(formula = d2 ~ bs(id, df = df1), family = quasipoisson)
                  Estimate Std. Error t value Pr(>|t|)
(Intercept)        3.61638    0.19642  18.412 3.29e-11 ***
```

```
(Dispersion parameter for quasipoisson family taken to be 2.421391)
    Null deviance: 38.278  on 17  degrees of freedom
Residual deviance: 34.707  on 14  degrees of freedom
tau = 0.178, 2-sided pvalue =0.30576
```

The cursor is a cross, place it in a clear area of the chart and right click to put the trend test result on the chart. There is no trend. There is very little variation in the data; consequently the variation explained by the model is small (1-pchisq(38.278-34.707,17-14)=0.3116697).

The R chron function seq.dates() can produce the sequence as "days", "weeks", "months", or "years". On occasion a sequence involving quarters or half-years may be required. We illustrate using quarters but defer employing the .qtr charts until Chapter 6.

```
# data with quarters in first column
# insufficient rows for a control chart
library(chron)
d<-datain[,1]
e<-datain[,2]
a<-rep(1,length(d))
d<-chron(as.character(d),format="dd-mmm-yyyy",out.format="dd-mmm-yyyy")
Year<-years(d)
m<-as.numeric(months(d))
Qtrs<-rep(0,length(m))
Qtrs[m>=1&m<=3]<-1
Qtrs[m>=4&m<=6]<-2
Qtrs[m>=7&m<=9]<-3
Qtrs[m>=10&m<=12]<-4
Table<-as.data.frame(xtabs(e~Qtrs+Year))
aa<-as.data.frame(xtabs(a~Qtrs+Year))
Table<-data.frame(Table,aa[,3])
Table1<-Table[Table[,4]!=0,]
Table1<-Table1[,-4]
Qtr<-paste(Table1[,2],"Q",Table1[,1],sep="")
Table2<-data.frame(Qtr,Table1[,3])
names(Table2)<-c("Quarters","Counts")
Table2
```

```
  Quarters Counts
1     95Q3    125
2     95Q4     88
3     96Q1    155
4     96Q2    106
5     96Q3    138
6     96Q4    142
```

0.7 Appendix menus

0.7.1 IMenu()

This menu enables selection of the univariate methods which department scientists frequently require. Its first sub-menu is for selection of methods for proportions or rates. Each then enables selection of methods for a single proportion or rate, confidence intervals for a series of proportions or rates, two proportions or rates, more than two proportions or rates or weighted averages of proportions or rates. Except for single proportions or rates, data from a data.frame can be entered, for example, IMenu(d) where d is the data.frame containing the data for the relevant function. The data.frame d must be in a suitable format for the function required to do the analysis.

To start, select IMenu() in R. There may optionally be the name of a data.frame, for example, IMenu(d), except for a single proportion or a single count or rate. It is recommended that data be entered as a data.frame if possible; see the documentation in Chapter 1 for multipleproportions(), twoproportions(), manyproportions() and stratifiedproportionsn(), and in Chapter 4 for multiplecounts(), tworates(), manyrates() and stratifiedratesn() for details.

Introductory Menu

1. Proportion data.

2. Count and rate data.

Proportion data menu

1. Single proportion.

2. Confidence intervals for a series of proportions.

3. Two proportions.

4. More than two proportions.

5. Weighted average of proportions.

Count and rate data menu

1. Single count or rate.

2. Confidence intervals for a series of counts or rates.

3. Two counts or rates.

4. More than two counts or rates.

5. Weighted average of rates.

0.7.2   CCMenu()

CCMenu() is a simple guide for hospital surveillance staff to select the chart that they require for displaying sequential adverse event (AE) data when performing routine monthly reporting. Currently those AEs most commonly displayed, for example, in monthly reports at one large tertiary referral hospital, are included but the list can be widened to include other AEs that may require display. The usage is CCMenu(datain). The data.frame datain must be in a suitable format for the function required to do the analysis. Note that at this time the first column of datain must contain valid dates. Modified functions with names ending in qtr allow the use of any first column data such as quarters or 1 to N, where N is the number of data rows, but the data must be properly ordered beforehand. At present CCMenu() does not access these functions.

The rprogs.RData functions must be in the R memory. Next, the required data must be read into R, for example, using the function g.d(). Then enter CCMenu(datain) at the R prompt. The first menu is:

1. Yes/No data e.g. SSI, Mortality.

2. Count data e.g. Bacteraemia (independent), MRO Colonisation (non-independent).

3. Antibiotics/MRO Burden.

Select 1 for binary/binomial data, data where an AE either does or does not occur. These include surgical site infection (SSI) data, mortality or other complication data, length of stay (LOS) data that have been dichotomised, for example, at the mode or median, treatments or documentation that are either correct or not correct. These data are often risk-adjusted. Usually they will consist of a column of dates (e.g. procedure dates) and a column of zeros and ones to indicate the non-occurrence or occurrence of the complication (plus a third column of predicted outcome probabilities if there is risk-adjustment). When the data are numerous (e.g. mortality data from an ICU that has a hundred or so admissions each month), they may be aggregated by months. The first column will then have a date (e.g. the first of each month), the second column a count of the AEs, the third column a count of the patients or procedures and, if there is risk-adjustment there will be a fourth column of expected outcome counts in that month.

When 1 is selected a further sub-menu will appear:

1. O-E/CUSUM.

2. Shewhart Control Chart.

3. Shewhart/EWMA Control Chart.

4. GAM Chart.

Select 1 for data that consist of a column of dates (e.g. procedure dates) and a column of zeros or ones to indicate the non-occurrence or occurrence of the complication (plus a third column of predicted outcome probabilities if there is risk-adjustment). If the data are aggregated by months, select 2 for a Shewhart Chart, 3 for a Shewhart/EWMA Chart or 4 for a GAM Chart. It would be uncommon for aggregated binary data to display autocorrelation so this option is not provided with the GAM chart.

To return to the first menu, select 2 for count data. These data include bacteraemias, needlestick injuries, patient falls, pressure ulcers, multiple antibiotic-resistant (MRO) new in-hospital colonisations and infections; any count data AE where the denominator is a space such as the hospital or a hospital ward. Denominator data such as occupied bed-days (OBDs) per month may be available. These data may be independent (one patient's bacteraemia usually does not result in another patient's bacteraemia) or they may not be independent (colonisation with an MRO requires a source such as another carrier from whom transmission occurs). This is a complex issue and is dealt with in more detail in Chapters 5 and 6. When 2 is selected from the first menu the following sub-menu appears:

1. Rare events.

2. Counts.

3. Rates.

Select 1 for rare events. Bacteraemias due to methicillin-resistant *Staphylococcus aureus* (MRSA) or intravenous device-related bacteraemias due to *Staphylococcus aureus* occur in some hospitals at a rate that is equal to or less than one per month. This rate is too low for aggregating the data by months. The data will be in a single column of dates that indicate the times when these AEs occurred. Care must be taken to ensure that the correct starting and ending dates of the time series are entered as described in Chapter 6. Select 2 for monthly count AE data when denominator data are unavailable or 3 when denominator data are available. The data will have a column of dates (e.g. the first of each month), a column of AE counts and, if denominators are available, a column of denominators such as OBDs.

When 2 or 3 is selected, a further sub-menu appears as follows:

1. Shewhart Chart.

2. Shewhart/EWMA Chart.

3. GAM chart with autocorrelation.

4. GAM chart no autocorrelation.

Select the required function from this sub-menu. When 2 has been selected in the previous menu count data functions appear and rate data functions appear when 3 is selected.

To return to the first menu, select 3 for antibiotic data or MRO Burden (prevalence) data. The former must be in two columns, the first being the date, for example, for the first of the month and the second for the antibiotic in defined daily doses (DDDs). If the data are not so arranged, this needs to be done before the data are entered into CCMenu(). See Chapter 7 for more details. A linear regression with a cubic regression spline is used to produce the chart. MRO Burden data are frequently available as daily counts of all known patients colonised with that MRO in the hospital on that day. The data to enter into CCMenu() must be monthly averages of these daily counts in two columns, the first for the date (e.g. first of month) and the second for the average for that month. As these are averages, a linear regression with a cubic regression spline is used to produce the chart. A sub-menu appears as follows:

1. Autocorrelation present.

2. Autocorrelation absent.

When data are aggregated by months, autocorrelation is not a common problem. Nevertheless, when analysing new count or numerical data, it may be wise to check. The autocorrelation present option can be selected and if significant autocorrelation is not found the analysis can then proceed without this option.

Throughout these notes we emphasise the value of tabulations and we show examples. Since it may be difficult to anticipate the tabulation requirements of particular IM and QI departments, we have not included this option in CCMenu() at this time. We anticipate that most potential users will have begun by employing the cross-tabulation facilities of a spreadsheet. If they wish at a later date to perform tabulations in R, the code we have shown in the chapters may prove helpful.

1

Introduction to analysis of binary and proportion data

Binary data occur frequently in infection management (IM) and quality improvement (QI) work. Two examples are surgical site infections (SSIs) and patient mortality: an SSI occurs or doesn't occur, and similarly a patient does or does not survive. The number of such outcomes in a sample of patients, or over a period of time, is often described using a binomial distribution. The dominant assumptions underlying this distribution are that each outcome is independent and has the same probability of occurrence. Note that these assumptions may not always hold. For example, we describe data in Chapter 7 that appear to be binomial but tend to display too much or too little variability due to measurement error, repeated measurements on the same individual, clustering and so on. This has an impact on conclusions about the true level of infection rates and whether these have changed unexpectedly during a monitoring period or between groups. However, the binomial distribution is applicable, at least approximately, to many hospital IM and QI outcomes. In this chapter, we focus on the following problems that are commonly encountered in the analysis of grouped binary data.

```
1. Estimation and testing of a single proportion,
2. Estimation for a series of proportions,
3. Comparison of two proportions,
4. Evaluation of more than two proportions.
5. The analysis of stratified data.
```

1.1 Single proportion, samples and population

Consider the scenario in which 14 SSIs were observed in 74 consecutive major lower limb vascular operations. Based on these data, what can we say about the true population proportion

Statistical Methods for Hospital Monitoring with R, First Edition. Anthony Morton, Kerrie Mengersen,
Michael Whitby and George Playford.
© 2013 John Wiley & Sons, Ltd. Published 2013 by John Wiley & Sons, Ltd.

of infection (p) in the population of patients undergoing such operations, commonly called the infection rate? We consider three common approaches to estimating this value.

The first is a moment-based approach, in which the population infection rate is estimated by the sample proportion. The sample proportion, usually labeled $\hat{p}$, is calculated as the number of complications (X) divided by the number of operations (N), so that $\hat{p} = X/N$. In the above scenario, $\hat{p} = 14/74 = 0.19$, so the sample percentage is 19%. (Note that in many texts, N is used to denote the population size and n is used to denote the sample size. Here we use N to indicate the sample size. Note also that later in these notes we may drop the notation where the context is obvious, or use other symbols where it is relevant, e.g. R=X/N.)

The second is a maximum likelihood approach. The likelihood is the chance of obtaining the observed data (e.g., 14 SSIs in 74 operations) given a certain value of p. The estimate of p is then taken to be the value that maximises this likelihood. For example, suppose that only two population rates were under consideration in the above example: p=0 or p=0.20. It is much more likely to observe 14 outcomes in 74 operations if the underlying population infection rate is 0.20 compared to the chance of observing these outcomes if the rate is 0, so the value of 0.20 would be chosen as the maximum likelihood estimate (MLE).

The third is a Bayesian approach, which estimates a (posterior) distribution for p based on the data (via the likelihood) and a prior distribution for p. This prior can be noninformative if nothing is known about p apart from the information provided in the data, or it can be based on information available about the population rate obtained from sources other than the data.

Regardless of the approach, the estimated value of p is just that: an estimate of the population rate based on a sample. The value of $\hat{p}$ is obviously dependent on the sample taken from the population. In particular, when samples are small, as they often are in QI and IM studies, there is a great deal of variation in the observed rates and corresponding uncertainty about the true population rate: for example, if p=0.5 then in a sample of four patients it would be equally probable to observe 1 out of 4 outcomes (moment-based estimated proportion $\hat{p}=0.25$) and 3 out of 4 outcomes ($\hat{p}=0.75$). Moreover, there is a question of representativeness in small samples: for example, if there were four patients and two had complications, it would be difficult to believe that these four patients with their observed 50% complication rate were representative of all such patients. If the next two patients studied did not have complications, the observed rate would fall from 50% to 30%.

The most common method of describing uncertainty is through some form of confidence interval (CI). A wider CI indicates greater uncertainty in the estimation of p. Under a moment-based approach, the CI is usually based on the variance of the binomial distribution, given by $\hat{p}(1-\hat{p})/N$. The width of the CI is thus determined by the magnitude of $\hat{p}$ and the sample size (N). Under a likelihood-based approach, the CI (usually called a supported range) tells us the range of possible values for p that are supported by the data ($\hat{p}$). Under a Bayesian approach, a range of values (a 95% credible interval) is found from the posterior distribution of p. These approaches are described in more detail in the following section. Under the frequentist idea of repeated sampling from a population, a 95% CI implies that on average, for every 100 samples drawn randomly from a population, 95 of the corresponding CIs computed from these samples will contain the true value of p (i.e. the true underlying complication rate). Under the Bayesian approach, a 95% credible interval is interpreted more directly, as a range of values that encompass the true value of p with 95% probability, given the observed data.

Another common objective is to use the observed data to test an hypothesis. For example, as we have described, we may know what SSI rate to expect based on published literature or from local data obtained when the vascular surgery SSI rate was considered satisfactory.

We wish then to determine whether the observed infection rate from a sample of patients is consistent with this value of p. If the data support a higher rate, we may need to examine our system of wound care in vascular surgery. The hypothesis test is usually evaluated using a form of P-value under a frequentist approach, likelihood ratio (LR) under a likelihood approach, or Bayes Factor (BF) under a Bayesian approach. As Goodman describes, these measures are inter-related. For example, a likelihood ratio of 1/7 coincides approximately with a 95% supported range that is numerically similar to a 95% CI. Although P-values that we discuss below and LRs are not strictly comparable, Goodman points out that, when testing certain hypotheses, a P-value of 0.05 (1/20) that corresponds to a 95% CI matches an LR of 1/7. The LR suggests that there is seven times as much support for the observed value $\hat{p}$ as there is for the population value p. If we are testing the hypothesis that the population rate is equal to a certain value (e.g., p=0) compared with an alternative (e.g., p=0.20), and we find that the P-value is small, the LR is large or the range of values supported by the data does not include p, it is reasonable to reject the hypothesis in favour of the alternative.

An important point to note at this stage is that although we use a 95% level of confidence in the above discussions, other confidence levels should also be considered, such as 68%, 95.5% or 99.7% (approximately equivalent to 1, 2 and 3 standard deviations (SDs) for normally distributed data). These may sometimes be more useful in surveillance and monitoring for detecting poor outcomes which can then be followed up through other means such as Morbidity and Mortality (M&M) meetings, as discussed in Chapter 8.

It is also important to understand the difference between CIs (often called precision limits) and control limits in control charts (often called prediction limits). The former surround an observed value such as $\hat{p}$ whereas the latter surround a mean value such as p and are thus analogous to significance tests that we describe for example in section 1.2 of this chapter. Often, if $\hat{p}$ does not differ greatly from p, precision and prediction limits do not differ greatly and are used interchangeably either because of availability or ease of calculation. Thus confidence limits are occasionally used to obtain approximate control chart limits. In addition, as Altman and Bland describe, confidence limits may, with symmetrical data, be employed to obtain approximate P-values (see below) and vice versa. Control charts are described in Chapters 3, 6 and 7.

1.1.1   Calculating the confidence interval

How do we calculate a CI for the unknown population rate p, based on binomial data? Under a frequentist approach, the most common approach is to assume that $\hat{p}$ is normally distributed and to calculate a CI as $\hat{p} \pm Z \times \sqrt{(\hat{p} \times (1-\hat{p})/N)}$, where N is the sample size and Z is the standard normal value corresponding to the confidence level (e.g. Z=1.96 for a 95% CI). For the example of 14 SSIs in 74 operations, the 95% CI obtained by this approach is 0.1 to 0.28). This approximation is suitable for large values of N and moderate values of p (i.e. not very small or very large). In many situations in IM and QI work, both p and N are small, so this common approximation is not sufficiently accurate.

An alternative method that is applicable to a much wider range of p and N values, and that avoids the normality approximation, is to describe p by a beta distribution; a common choice is p~Beta(X+1,N-X+1), where ~ means 'is distributed as'. We can then take the middle 95% of this probability distribution as the range for a 95% CI. This is consistent with both likelihood and Bayesian approaches. Moreover, the ready availability of beta distribution functions in computer software makes the use of the normal approximation unnecessary even when samples are large. This calculation is easily performed in R. The required commands for a 95% CI are qbeta(0.025,X,N-X+1) and qbeta(0.975,X+1,N-X). Employing these formulas for the above scenario, qbeta(0.025,14,61)=0.107 or 10.7% and qbeta(0.975,15,60)=0.297 or 29.7%.

Another approach is to calculate so-called exact intervals. For the running example, results identical to those obtained above are found with binom.exact() in the R exactci library. However, these can be conservative for proportion and count data due to the discrete nature of the binomial distribution. (This also applies to hypergeometric and Poisson distributions.) Wilson score or exact mid-P intervals have been advocated to deal with this difficulty (Armitage and colleagues, Campbell and Swinscow, Altman and colleagues, Kirkwood and Sterne, Clayton and Hills). The Wilson formula is $(N/(N+Z^2))\times(X/N+Z^2/(2\times N)\pm Z\times((X\times(N-X)/N^3)+Z^2/(4\times N^2))^{.5})$, where for a 95% CI Z=1.96. It is available as scoreci() in the R PropCIs library. The mid-P method is slightly more complicated and is available as midPci() in the R PropCIs library.

```
# comparison of CI methods
# using the beta distribution
qbeta(0.025,14,61)   # [1] 0.107
qbeta(0.975,15,60)   # [1] 0.297
# exact intervals
library(exactci)
binom.exact(14,74)$conf.int
# [1] 0.107, 0.297
library(PropCIs)
# Wilson score intervals
scoreci(14,74,conflev=.95)
#   lowlim  uplim
#   0.116, 0.293
# mid-P exact intervals
midPci(14,74,alpha=.05)
#   lowlim  uplim
#   0.112, 0.290
```

For these data the limits based on the beta distribution are similar to the exact limits while the Wilson score and mid-P limits are similar and narrower than the exact and beta distribution limits. Following the recommendation of Armitage and colleagues, we have generally quoted both mid-P and exact intervals but give more emphasis to the former, particularly in functions that employ Newcombe's CI method. For example mid-P intervals are employed in section 1.4.1 of this chapter that deals with the CI for the difference between independent proportions.

1.1.2   Comparison with an expected rate

As discussed above, a frequent requirement is to compare an observed rate ($\hat{p}$) with a reference rate (p). For example, one hospital's SSI rate for a certain procedure may be compared with a rate obtained for a group of hospitals that is regarded as the achievable background rate for that procedure. Clearly a difference between $\hat{p}$ and p may be due to predictable (mostly random) variation in the single hospital's rate due to the particular sample taken and its size. We thus wish to determine whether the difference between $\hat{p}$ and p is so large that predictable variation is unlikely to be able to explain it. Note that the population rate, described above, may not necessarily be a reference rate. For example, the same approach may be used to evaluate whether there has been a change in the previously stable process rate (p) within the hospital (e.g. in a control chart as described in Chapter 3). In all these cases, we can again use the beta distribution to assess the expected rate p.

To illustrate the method, suppose a rate of 10% was expected for the SSIs. We wish to determine whether the observed 19% rate (X=14, N=74) is so large that predictable variation is unlikely to have produced it. This is easily calculated by using pbeta(), the beta distribution function in R. If the observed rate exceeds the expected rate, as it does with the SSI data (19% observed, 10% expected), pbeta(p,X,N-X+1) is employed in R, where p is the expected 10% rate and pbeta(0.10,14,61) equals 0.014. This is analogous to a one tailed P-value (so it needs to be multiplied by 2 to be equivalent to the widely used conventional two-sided P-value of 0.028). When the observed proportion is less than expected, 1-pbeta(p,X+1,N-X) is used and the result must also be multiplied by 2 for a two tailed result (the differing positions of 1 in these formulas occur because of the discrete nature of the binomial distribution). The binom.exact() function mentioned above gives identical results. Approximate mid-P P-values can be calculated by getting the P-value for the next more extreme case, for example, X=15 in this case, and obtaining the average of that and the exact P-value for the observed X=14 (Vollset). These calculations are in the R function proportion() in rprogs that may also be accessed through IMenu().

```
# Proportion CI and P-value
library(exactci)
library(PropCIs)
#Enter numerator
x<-14
# Enter denominator
n<-74
p<-0 #if no reference proportion
# Enter reference proportion if available
p<-0.1
if (p!=0){jj<-"y"}else{jj<-"n"}
lo<-binom.exact(x,n)$conf.int[1]
up<-binom.exact(x,n)$conf.int[2]
midplo<-midPci(x,n,alpha=0.05)[1]
midpup<-midPci(x,n,alpha=0.05)[2]
cat("Proportion = ",round(x/n,3),", lower 95% limit =
",round(lo,3),", upper limit = ",round(up,3),"\nMid-p lower
95% limit = ",round(midplo,3),", upper limit =
",round(midpup,3),".\n",sep="")
#Proportion = 0.189, lower 95% limit = 0.107, upper limit = 0.297
#Mid-p lower 95% limit = 0.112, upper limit = 0.29.
if (jj=="y")
{
q<-binom.exact(x,n,p)$p.value
z<-qnorm(q/2)
lr0<-paste("1/",as.character(round(1/exp(-z^2/2),0)),sep="")
q1<-0
if (x!=0){
if (x/n>p){q1<-binom.exact(x+1,n,p)$p.value}else{q1<-
binom.exact(x-1,n,p)$p.value}
q1<-(q+q1)/2
z1<-qnorm(q1/2)
lr1<-paste("1/",as.character(round(1/exp(-z1^2/2),0)),sep="")
```

```
}
if (p!=x/n){
cat("P = ",round(q,3),", LR = ",lr0,sep="")
cat(".\n",sep="")
if (x!=0){
cat("Mid-P P = ",round(q1,3),", LR = ",lr1,sep="")
cat(".\n",sep="")
}
}
}
#P = 0.028, LR = 1/11.
#Mid-P P = 0.02, LR = 1/15.

#proportion function (also via IMenu(), select 1 and 1)
proportion()
```

```
Enter numerator 14
Enter denominator 74
Is a reference proportion available? y
Enter reference proportion .1
Proportion = 0.189, lower 95% limit = 0.107, upper limit = 0.297
Mid-P lower 95% limit = 0.112, upper limit = 0.29.
P = 0.028, LR = 1/11.
Mid-P P = 0.02, LR = 1/15.
```

1.2   Likelihood ratio (Bayes factor) & supported range

We have referred in the Introduction to the usefulness of the likelihood ratio (LR) concept. Goodman describes how an approximate LR can be obtained by converting the P-value (P) to a standard normal deviate. This can be accomplished in R by using Z<-abs(qnorm(P/2)) and then employing cat(paste("1/",as.character(round(1/exp(-Z^2/2),0)),sep=""),"\n"). For a two-sided P-value of 0.028, the LR is 1/11. (Although they are not strictly comparable, Goodman notes the difference implied by a P-value=0.028 or about 1/36 and a LR of 1/11.) This LR suggests that there is 11 times the support for the observed rate of 19% as there is for the expected rate of 10%, making predictable variation an unlikely explanation for the observed 19% rate. In addition, the supported range (CI) for R=14/74=19% suggests that the possible values of p supported by the data at the 95% level range from 10.7% (mid-P 11.2%) that are above the expected value of 10%. However, although predictable variation would be an unlikely cause for the observed difference, thus indicating for example, that an M&M audit should be performed, we cannot be absolutely certain since the LR indicates that there is some support for a 10% rate.

It is important to note that the above tests indicate whether a difference is unlikely to have arisen by chance; it does not tell whether the difference is of practical importance. In small samples, it may be difficult to be sure that large differences that may be of practical importance have not occurred by chance and in very large samples, differences of no practical importance may be conventionally statistically significant. It is useful to employ a combination of practical experience and the CI, P-value and LR to make informed decisions. In addition, the consequences of making a wrong decision are important: are they trivial or potentially serious? A practically important difference in a small sample that fails to reach conventional statistical significance requires further attention.

The Camp-Poulson approximation (Gebhardt), an accurate method for approximating the F-distribution that is related to the beta distribution, is a useful alternative for performing the significance test. If X/N>p, set X=X-1. Then $F=(N-X)\times p/((X+1)\times(1-p))$. $A=F^{(1/3)}\times(9-1/(N-X))+1/(X+1)-9$. $B=3\times(F^{(2/3)}\times(1/(N-X))+1/(X+1))^{-5}$, and Z=-A/B. It is also useful, with some adjustment, for a significance test for overdispersed count data analysed using the negative binomial distribution (section 4.10 of Chapter 4).

```
# Camp-Poulson approximation
X<-14;N<-74
X<-X-1
p<-.1
FF<-(N-X)*p/((X+1)*(1-p))
A<-FF^(1/3)*(9-1/(N-X))+1/(X+1)-9
B<-3*(FF^(2/3)*(1/(N-X))+1/(X+1))^.5
Z<--A/B
Z
#[1] 2.188263
#P-value
P<-2*(1-pnorm(Z))
P
#[1] 0.02865046
#
#mid-P
X<-15;N<-74
X<-X-1
p<-.1
FF<-(N-X)*p/((X+1)*(1-p))
A<-FF^(1/3)*(9-1/(N-X))+1/(X+1)-9
B<-3*(FF^(2/3)*(1/(N-X))+1/(X+1))^.5
Z1<--A/B
Z1
#[1] 2.50614
#P-value
P1<-2*(1-pnorm(Z1))
P1
#[1] 0.01220573
#
(P+P1)/2 #mid-p value
#[1]0.02042809
```

1.3   Confidence intervals for a series of proportions

Calculating confidence intervals for a series of proportions for a report is often a job for hospital scientists, for example, SSI rates for different procedures with differing expected rates. This can be time-consuming and prone to error. The file hosprops.csv has columns for procedure codes, procedure dates, risk-indexes and SSI codes for a group of hospitals. Our interest is in the in-hospital (Infection Type 1) SSI rates for each of the procedures.

```
# getting the hosprops.csv data with function g.d()
g.d()
```

```
Loading data.
Data from clipboard (C) or file (F) c
Do data column(s) have heading(s) (Y/N) y
Is column 1 a date column (Y/N) n
```

Tabulations are performed using tapply() and confidence interval calculations using binom.exact(). The tabulations can also be performed using the xtabs() function. Calculation of the overall rate and its confidence interval need to be performed separately.

The confidence interval calculations can be performed using the function multipleproportions(). The function multipleproportions() may also be accessed via IMenu().

```
# tabulate by procedure code using tapply()
Proc<-datain[,1]
SSI<-rep(0,length(datain[,1]))
SSI[datain[,4]==1]<-1
SSIs<-tapply(SSI,Proc,sum)
Procedures<-tapply(SSI,Proc,length)
ProcCode<-names(SSIs)
Table<-data.frame(ProcCode,SSIs,Procedures)
row.names(Table)<-1:length(SSIs)
Table
```

	ProcCode	SSIs	Procedures
1	1	20	508
2	3	78	4897
3	4	19	521
4	5	69	6269
5	6	8	348
6	7	44	702
7	8	65	12724
8	9	153	16654
9	10	90	8129
10	11	159	9479
11	12	6	568
12	13	8	673
13	14	3	589
14	15	52	3474

```
#calculate 95% & 99.7% confidence intervals
#mid-P values not calculated
library(exactci)
a<-Table[,2]
b<-Table[,3]
x<-length(a)
s<-0;l<-0;u<-0
ll<-0;uu<-0
for (i in 1:x){s[i]<-binom.exact(a[i],b[i])$estimate
l[i]<-binom.exact(a[i],b[i])$conf.int[1]
u[i]<-binom.exact(a[i],b[i])$conf.int[2]
ll[i]<-binom.exact(a[i],b[i],conf.level=.997)$conf.int[1]
uu[i]<-binom.exact(a[i],b[i],conf.level=.997)$conf.int[2]
}
```

```
Proc<-Table[,1]
ss<-data.frame(Proc,s,l,ll,u,uu)
# adding average rate and CIs
a0<-sum(Table[,2])
b0<-sum(Table[,3])
Mean<-a0/b0
l0<-binom.exact(a0,b0)$conf.int[1]
u0<-binom.exact(a0,b0)$conf.int[2]
ll0<-binom.exact(a0,b0,conf.level=.997)$conf.int[1]
uu0<-binom.exact(a0,b0,conf.level=.997)$conf.int[2]
ssall<-data.frame("All",Mean,l0,ll0,u0,uu0)
names(ssall)<-c("Proc","s","l","ll","u","uu")
ss<-rbind(ss,ssall)
#print(ss), see multipleproportions() below

#using the multipleproportions() function
multipleproportions(Table)
```

	Proc	s	l	ll	u	uu
1	1	0.039370	0.024211	0.0184405	0.060151	0.07203
2	3	0.015928	0.012610	0.0111286	0.019840	0.02199
3	4	0.036468	0.022096	0.0166802	0.056366	0.06778
4	5	0.011007	0.008574	0.0074982	0.013909	0.01551
5	6	0.022989	0.009976	0.0060866	0.044792	0.05792
6	7	0.062678	0.045908	0.0387491	0.083232	0.09457
7	8	0.005108	0.003945	0.0034334	0.006507	0.00728
8	9	0.009187	0.007794	0.0071453	0.010755	0.01160
9	10	0.011071	0.008912	0.0079378	0.013591	0.01497
10	11	0.016774	0.014285	0.0131226	0.019566	0.02107
11	12	0.010563	0.003886	0.0021197	0.022849	0.03045
12	13	0.011887	0.005146	0.0031365	0.023287	0.03021
13	14	0.005093	0.001052	0.0003735	0.014812	0.02113
14	15	0.014968	0.011199	0.0095739	0.019583	0.02215
15	All	0.011810	0.010997	0.0105966	0.012667	0.01312

```
[1]    "The results are is ss"
```

```
#l & u are equivalent to a 95% & ll & uu a 99.7% interval
#approximately equivalent to two and three standard
#deviations respectively
#producing a more attractive output
ss<-cbind(ss[,1],round(ss[,c(2:6)],4))
names(ss)<-c("Proc","SSI","L95","L99.7","U95","U99.7")
ss
```

	Proc	SSI	L95	L99.7	U95	U99.7
1	1	0.0394	0.0242	0.0184	0.0602	0.0720
2	3	0.0159	0.0126	0.0111	0.0198	0.0220
3	4	0.0365	0.0221	0.0167	0.0564	0.0678
4	5	0.0110	0.0086	0.0075	0.0139	0.0155
5	6	0.0230	0.0100	0.0061	0.0448	0.0579
6	7	0.0627	0.0459	0.0387	0.0832	0.0946
7	8	0.0051	0.0039	0.0034	0.0065	0.0073
8	9	0.0092	0.0078	0.0071	0.0108	0.0116
9	10	0.0111	0.0089	0.0079	0.0136	0.0150

```
10  11 0.0168 0.0143 0.0131 0.0196 0.0211
11  12 0.0106 0.0039 0.0021 0.0228 0.0304
12  13 0.0119 0.0051 0.0031 0.0233 0.0302
13  14 0.0051 0.0011 0.0004 0.0148 0.0211
14  15 0.0150 0.0112 0.0096 0.0196 0.0221
15 All 0.0118 0.0110 0.0106 0.0127 0.0131
```

```
s.d(ss) # if required, export to office program using the clipboard
```

```
# also use IMenu()
IMenu(Table)
```

```
Introductory Menu

1. Proportion data,
2. Count and rate data.
1
1. Single proportion,
2. Confidence intervals for a series of proportions,
3. Two proportions,
4. More than two proportions,
5. Weighted average of proportions.
2
```

These data refer to different procedures with differing expected SSI rates so the need for comparisons does not arise. The use of multiple confidence intervals for the same procedure within differing institutions, their comparison with a reference value and corrections for multiple testing are discussed when we deal with aggregated data obtained from several institutions in Chapter 2.

1.4   Difference between two proportions

In IM and QI studies one occasionally compares two independent proportions. The odds ratio, as described by Kirkwood and Sterne, is often used for this purpose. However, NNT, the number needed to treat to prevent one complication, also described by Kirkwood and Sterne, is useful in IM and QI work; this is the reciprocal of the risk difference. Thus, if a complication rate is 20% and a new process is able to reduce it to 10%, the difference would be 10%. By using the new method for the next 10 patients, one complication could potentially be averted; NNT is therefore 10 (i.e. the reciprocal of the risk difference is $1/0.1 = 10$). Calculation of the CI for NNT involves the reciprocals of the confidence limits for the difference between proportions so the risk difference is often a better estimator for IM and QI work than the odds ratio. However, the odds ratio is mathematically a more natural estimator and we employ it, for example, via logistic regression. We also describe calculations for the ratio of two independent proportions (risk ratio).

1.4.1   Confidence intervals

Newcombe's method for the CI for the difference between two independent proportions is recommended by Altman and colleagues. First, one must obtain the confidence limits for each proportion as described above. Let P_1 and P_2 be the two sample proportions, L_1 and L_2 their lower and U_1 and U_2 their upper confidence limits. Let D be the difference between the two proportions and U and L the required upper and lower difference confidence limits. Then the formulas are $U=D+\sqrt{[(P_2-L_2)^2+(U_1-P_1)^2]}$ and $L=D-\sqrt{[(P_1-L_1)^2+(U_2-P_2)^2]}$.

Nam describes an accurate score method for the calculation of the confidence interval for the risk ratio. It involves the solution of a complicated cubic equation. A difficulty occurs if there is a zero numerator; when this happens 0.5 can be added to each of the numerators and 1 to each of the denominators. The function riskscoreci() in the PropCIs library implements this method.

```
# Ratio (Nam)
z<-1.96
x1<-14
n1<-74
x2<-8
n2<-114
if (x2/n2>x1/n1){v<-x1;x1<-x2;x2<-v;v<-n1;n1<-n2;n2<-v}
if (x1/n1!=x2/n2)
{
if (x1==0 | x2==0){x1<-x1+0.5;x2<-x2+0.5;n1<-n1+1;n2<-n2+1}
xd<-x2+x1
nd<-n2+n1
a1<-n2*(n2*nd*x1+n1*(n2+x1)*z^2)
a2<--n2*(n2*n1*xd+2*nd*x2*x1+n1*(n2+x2+2*x1)*z^2)
a3<-2*n2*n1*x2*xd+nd*x2^2*x1+n2*n1*xd*z^2
a4<--n1*x2^2*xd
b1<-a2/a1
b2<-a3/a1
b3<-a4/a1
c1<-b2-b1^2/3
c2<-b3-b1*b2/3+2*b1^3/27
th<-acos(27^0.5*c2/(2*c1*(-c1)^0.5))
P<-pi
ca<-cos(P/3-th/3)
t1<--2*(-c1/3)^0.5*ca
cb<-cos(P/3+th/3)
t2<--2*(-c1/3)^0.5*cb
cc<-cos(th/3)
t3<-2*(-c1/3)^0.5*cc
t1<-t1-b1/3
t2<-t2-b1/3
t3<-t3-b1/3
ta<-t1;tb<-t2
if (t1>t2 & t1>t3){ta<-t2;tb<-t3}
if (t2>t1 & t2>t3){ta<-t1;tb<-t3}
upr<-(1-(n1-x1)*(1-ta)/(x2+n1-nd*ta))/ta
lor<-(1-(n1-x1)*(1-tb)/(x2+n1-nd*tb))/tb
if (lor>upr){y<-upr;upr<-lor;lor<-y}
if (x2>0){cat("Ratio ",round(x1*n2/(n1*x2),2),".\n",sep="")}
cat("Ratio 95% confidence limits are ",round(lor,2)," and
",round(upr,2),".\n",sep="")
}
#Ratio 2.7.
#Ratio 95% confidence limits are 1.22 and 6.
```

For the risk difference, Newcombe recommends that using Wilson score intervals for the two proportions gives better results than exact intervals as the latter for proportion and count data can be conservative due to the discrete nature of the binomial, hypergeometric and Poisson distributions. Wilson score or exact mid-P intervals have been advocated to deal with this difficulty (Armitage and colleagues, Campbell and Swinscow, Altman and colleagues). We have employed mid-P intervals using the R function midPci() in the PropCIs library.

Consider the vascular surgical unit SSIs. In 74 consecutive Class 1 operations there were 14 SSIs, a rate of 19%. Since this rate was considered unacceptably high, the processes of wound care were carefully revised and in the following 114 operations there were eight SSIs, giving a rate of 7%.

1.4.2   Hypothesis test

If there is indeed no real difference between the population rates in the two groups, what is the probability of observing the sample data? Although frequently used with case-control data, the Fisher Exact test may be employed to answer this question. The data are arranged in a 2×2 table. The test involves computing the exact probability of the observed data assuming no difference between the two groups and adding to this the probability of all possible less likely data arrangements, conditional on the row and column totals of the table remaining fixed. To illustrate the calculation for the observed data, let the four cell counts of the 2×2 table be a=14, b=8, c=74-14=60 and d=114-8=106. N=74+114=188 is the total and the marginal totals of the 2×2 table are m1=a+c=14+60=74, m2=b+d=8+106=114, m3=a+b=14+8=22 and m4=c+d=60+106=166.

The probability of the observed result if there is no difference between the groups is then P=(N!×a!×b!×c!×d!)/(m1!×m2!×m3!×m4!)=0.0094, where ! stands for factorial (because factorials rapidly become large numbers, logs are used and added and for large counts Stirling's approximation log(N!)≈log(N)*N-N+log($\sqrt{(2 \times \pi \times N)}$) is employed). The exact two-sided P-value is obtained by adding to this the values for all less probable cell counts conditional upon the marginal totals m1, m2, m3, m4 of the resulting 2×2 table remaining fixed. It is considered to be conservative so may fail to indicate significance at the 5% level when the lower 95% confidence limit for the difference is greater than zero. The mid-P method has been advocated by Armitage and colleagues and Campbell and Swinscow to overcome this problem. To obtain the mid-P value, half the probability of the observed result is taken from the fisher.test P-value.

```
# calculating difference between and ratio of two proportions
library(PropCIs)
z<-1.96
x1<-8
n1<-114
x2<-14
n2<-74
y<-0
if (x2/n2>x1/n1){y<-x1;x1<-x2;x2<-y;y<-n1;n1<-n2;n2<-y}
q1<-n1-x1
q2<-n2-x2
diff<-x1/n1-x2/n2
lo1<-midPci(x1,n1,.05)[1]
up1<- midPci(x1,n1,.05)[2]
```

```
lo2<-midPci(x2,n2,.05)[1]
up2<- midPci(x2,n2,.05)[2]
l<-diff-((x1/n1-lo1)^2+(up2-x2/n2)^2)^.5
u<-diff+((x2/n2-lo2)^2+(up1-x1/n1)^2)^.5
diff
#[1] 0.1190138
l;u
#[1] 0.02228644
#[1] 0.2263485
#confidence limits for the risk difference of .119 are .022 & .226.
#
#Risk ratio
#using riskscoreci()
rr<-x1*n2/(x2*n1)
rr
#[1] 2.695946
library(PropCIs)
riskscoreci(x1,n1,x2,n2,.95)
#[1] 1.217218 5.995263
#confidence limits for the risk ratio of 2.7 are 1.2 & 6.

# Fisher Exact test
x1<-14
n1<-74
x2<-8
n2<-114
q1<-n1-x1
q2<-n2-x2
u1 <- c(x1, x2)
u2 <- c(q1, q2)
u3 <- data.frame(u1, u2)
ft <- fisher.test(u3)
ft1 <- ft$p.value
ft1 # Fisher test P-value
#[1] 0.01908641
sw <- T
if (x1 == 0 | x2 == 0) {
sw <- F
}
if (sw == T) {
a <- x1
a[2] <- q1
a[3] <- x2
a[4] <- q2
a[5] <- a[1] + a[2]
a[6] <- a[3] + a[4]
a[7] <- a[1] + a[3]
a[8] <- a[2] + a[4]
a[9] <- a[7] + a[8]
f <- 0
for (i in 1:9) {
if (a[i] > 100) {
f[i] <- a[i] * log(a[i]) - a[i] + log((2 * pi * a[i])^0.5)
}
else {
f[i] <- log(factorial(a[i]))
```

```
}
}
s1 <- sum(f[5:8])
s2 <- sum(c(f[1:4], f[9]))
d0 <- exp(s1 - s2)
fishermidp <- ft1 - d0/2
fishermidp # mid-P value
}
#[1] 0.01437578
```

1.4.3   The twoproportions function

The function twoproportions() incorporates the above calculations in a convenient format. Data may be entered at the keyboard or as twoproportions(data.frame(x_1,n_1,x_2,n_2)) for example, twoproportions(data.frame(14,74,8,114)).

```
#the twoproportions function (also via IMenu())
twoproportions()
```

```
Enter first numerator 14
Enter first denominator 74
Enter second numerator 8
Enter second denominator 114
First proportion 0.189, Second proportion 0.07
Difference between proportions 0.119.
Lower 95% limit 0.022, upper limit 0.226
Fisher Exact P-value = 0.019, LR = 1/16
Fisher Mid-P-value = 0.014, LR = 1/20
Ratio 2.7.
Ratio 95% confidence limits are 1.22 and 6.
```

```
d<-data.frame(14,74,8,114)
IMenu(d)
```

```
Introductory Menu

1. Proportion data,
2. Count and rate data.
1
1. Single proportion,
2. Confidence intervals for a series of proportions,
3. Two proportions,
4. More than two proportions,
5. Weighted average of proportions.
3
First proportion 0.189, Second proportion 0.07
Difference between proportions 0.119.
Lower 95% limit 0.022, upper limit 0.226
Fisher Exact P-value = 0.019, LR = 1/16
Fisher Mid-P-value = 0.014, LR = 1/20
Ratio 2.7.
Ratio 95% confidence limits are 1.22 and 6.
```

Occasionally the confidence intervals and the Mid-P P-value will be discordant, for example, the difference CI may not include zero or the ratio interval may not include one when the P-value is above 0.05. Alternatively, one or the other may not be reported, for example, in a published paper. Approximate CIs can be obtained from the P-value or the approximate P-value from the CIs using the methods described by Altman and Bland. Clearly, in the first instance (when there is discordance), one should adopt a consistent approach. A suitable one could be to use the riskscoreci() interval, that on a log scale is likely to be symmetrical, to obtain a concordant P-value. In the second instance (absence of one or other estimate in a published report), either one may be required, so we illustrate both. Since the interval for the logarithm of the risk ratio (RR) is usually closer to symmetrical than the risk difference (RD), we illustrate the Altman and Bland methods with the former. For the confidence interval $Z \approx 0.862 + (0.743 - 2.404 \times \log(\text{P-value}))^{.5}$, $SE \approx \text{abs}(\log(RR)/Z)$ and $CI \approx \exp(\log(RR) \pm 1.96^* SE)$. For the latter, $SE \approx (\log(U95) - \log(L95))/(2 \times 1.96)$, $Z \approx \log(RR)/SE$ and $P.value \approx \exp(-0.717 \times Z - 0.416 \times Z^2)$, where CI is the confidence interval and U95 and L95 are the upper and lower 95% confidence limits.

```
#adjusting the difference CI using the P-value (Bland and Altman)
P<-0.014
D<-0.119
Z<--0.862+(0.743-2.404*log(P))^.5
Z
#[1] 2.455371
SE<-abs(D/Z)
SE
#[1] 0.04846518
U<-D+1.96*SE
U
#[1] 0.2139918
L<-D-1.96*SE
L
#[1] 0.02400824

#adjusting the ratio CI using the P-value
P<-0.014
R<-2.7
Z<--0.862+(0.743-2.404*log(P))^.5
Z
#[1] 2.455371
SE<-abs(log(R)/Z)
SE
#[1] 0.4045221
U<-exp(log(R)+1.96*SE)
U
#[1] 5.966229
L<-exp(log(R)-1.96*SE)
L
#[1] 1.221877
#the Mid-P P-value and the ratio CIs are in good agreement for these data

#using the CI to recalculate the P-value
#calculating approximate P-value using difference (Altman and Bland)
#difference CIs must be approximately symmetric about the difference
SE<-(0.2263485-0.02228644)/(1.96*2)
```

```
Z<-0.1190138/SE
P.value<-exp(-0.717*Z-0.416*Z^2)
Z;P.value
#[1]  2.286236
#[1]  0.02206832
#this does not agree well with the Fisher Mid-P result
# difference between estimate and CIs
0.1190138-0.02228644
#[1]  0.09672731
0.2263485-0.1190138
#[1]  0.1073348
#there is some asymmetry about the difference

#calculating approximate P-value using ratio (Altman and Bland)
#logs used to obtain approximate symmetry about the risk ratio
SE<-(log(5.995263)-log(1.217218))/(2*1.96)
Z<-log(2.695946)/SE
P.value=exp(-0.717*Z-0.416*Z^2)
Z;P.value
#[1]  2.438317
#[1]  0.0146758
#good agreement with Fisher Mid-P result
```

1.5   Introducing a Bayesian approach

Although Bayesian methods are not the focus of these notes, they are increasingly being used for quality improvement in general and hospital surveillance in particular. There is a growing literature on useful approaches. These need not be complex; for example, as we have seen, a simple Beta distribution can be used to describe a population rate. Interested readers are referred, for example, to the texts by Woodworth and Spiegelhalter[F] and colleagues.

1.6   When the data are not just one or two independent samples

There are several issues when there are a number of samples. For example, is a comparison required or an average? The two common stratifying agents in QI and IM work are hospitals and years. The former are often exchangeable in the sense that their order is unimportant and they may be thought of as random selections from a group of hospitals unless there is prior reason to believe otherwise, for example, that hospital size and AE rates are related. However, with years it is frequently of interest to obtain a weighted average with stronger weighting for more recent years, or some QI activity may have been undertaken and a downwards trend or change point may have been anticipated. Years can therefore usually be thought of as being fixed agents, although it is possible that there may be times when years are exchangeable (although time series data are often not independent, when stratified by years, counts of AEs can usually be analysed as if independent). In the presence of inhomogeneity among the samples, due to excessive variation or interaction or a combination of both, analyses may differ. When this occurs and the stratifying agent is fixed, attention should be directed to the individual within stratum data but when it is random, a random effects analysis may be possible. The issues of exchangeability and fixed and random effects are important, for example, when AEs from several hospitals are analysed in funnel plots in the presence of excessive variability (Spiegelhalter[B,C,D]), or when employing shrinkage analysis, and we return to it in later chapters.

1.6.1   More than two independent proportions

In some cases, there may be more than two proportions to study and compare and sometimes it may make sense to expect that a trend might exist among the proportions. These data may be analysed in a fixed analysis with the R function prop.test() that employs the chi-squared (χ^2) distribution. If a trend test is required, the R prop.trend.test() function is employed and departure from trend can be assessed by subtraction (Armitage and colleagues), that is, the prop.test χ^2 has degrees-of-freedom (DF) equal to the number of proportions minus one and the prop.trend.test χ^2 has one DF. Subtracting the latter χ^2 from the former gives a departure from trend χ^2 with DF equal to the number of proportions minus two. If the departure from trend χ^2 is large relative to its DF, we should examine the proportions individually to see which might be different; these are displayed by prop.test. Usually we will be alerted by the prop.test result whether or not a trend test is employed but occasionally there will be both a trend and a departure from the trend. Breslow and Day describe these χ^2 tests. Also, prop.test is unsuitable when samples are small.

For prop.test, let x_i be the numerator and n_i the denominator of the ith of the I proportions, $p_i = x_i/n_i$, $p = \sum x_i / \sum n_i$ and $q = 1-p$. Then $\chi^2 = \sum((n_i \times (p_i-p)^2)/(p \times q))$ with DF=I-1. For prop.trend.test, also let $X = \sum x_i$, $i = 1..I$ and $N = \sum n_i$. Then $a = N \times (N \times \sum(x_i \times i) - X \times \sum(n_i \times i))^2$, $b = X \times (N-X) \times (N \times \sum(n_i \times i^2) - (\sum(n_i \times i))^2)$ and the trend $\chi^2 = a/b$ with 1 DF.

It is useful to investigate those proportions that appear to differ. In cases where there is a reference rate or, as with the present data, risk adjustment values, these can be used for this purpose. For the present, we assume that the average rate for the data can be used to see which, if any, of the proportions differ, for example, by calculating Z-scores. We deal with risk adjusted data in Chapter 2.

1.6.2   Example 1, yearly data

The file ssi0106.csv has SSI data for a group of related surgical procedures from 2001 to 2006. SSI data from hospital G are selected to see if there were yearly variations in SSI rates and, if so, whether a trend existed.

```
#getting ssi0106.csv data via clipboard
g.d()
```

```
Loading data.
Data from clipboard (C) or file (F) c
Do data column(s) have heading(s) (Y/N) y
Is column 1 a date column (Y/N) n
```

```
options(digits=4) # reduce number of decimal places printed
# remember to change back to default (digits=7) if required
# prop.test()
G<-datain[datain$Hospital=="G",c(3,5)]
```

```
Y<-G$ProcedureDate
Y<-chron(as.character(Y),format="d-mmm-yy",out.format="dd-mmm-yyyy")
Yrs<-years(Y)
SSIs<-tapply(G$SSI,Yrs,sum)
Proc<-tapply(G$SSI,Yrs,length)
GYrs<-data.frame(SSIs,Proc)
#prop.test
pt<-prop.test(SSIs,Proc) # prop.test requires SSIs & Totals
pt
```

```
6-sample test for equality of proportions without continuity correction
data:  SSIs out of Proc
X-squared = 25.9, df = 5, p-value = 9.324e-05
alternative hypothesis: two.sided
sample estimates:
 prop 1  prop 2  prop 3  prop 4  prop 5  prop 6
 0.03966 0.05476 0.04711 0.09456 0.03770 0.02778
```

The test suggests that the proportions are likely to differ and that 2004 may be an outlier.

```
# using prop.trend.test
ptt<-prop.trend.test(SSIs,Proc)
ptt
```

```
          Chi-squared Test for Trend in Proportions
data:  SSIs out of Proc ,
 using scores: 1 2 3 4 5 6
X-squared = 1.1741, df = 1, p-value = 0.2786
```

There is no evidence of a trend. The departure from trend is highly significant and we wish to find which proportions differ.

```
# departure from trend
Departure<-pt$statistic-ptt$statistic #departure from trend
DF<-pt$parameter-ptt$parameter # degrees of freedom
P.value<-as.numeric(1-pchisq(Departure,DF))
Departure;DF;P.value
#
#X-squared
#   24.7275
#df
# 4
# P-value
#[1] 5.707159e-05
```

```
# finding which proportions differ
# Z-scores obtained from the fixed analysis expected counts
# assumes average rate from the data
SSI<-GYrs[,1]
Totals<-GYrs[,2]
s1<-sum(SSI)
s2<-sum(Totals)
```

```
mn<-s1/s2
expected<-Totals*mn
Expecteds<-round(expected,2)
GYrs1<-data.frame(GYrs,Expecteds)
library(exactci)
rate<-GYrs1[,1]/GYrs1[,2]
d<-GYrs1[,3]/GYrs1[,2]
Z<-0;p<-0
for (i in 1:length(GYrs1[,1])){p[i]<-
binom.exact(GYrs1[i,1],GYrs1[i,2],d[i])$p.value;if(rate[i]>d[i])
{Z[i]<--qnorm(p[i]/2)}else{Z[i]<-qnorm(p[i]/2)}}
Z<-round(Z,2)
GYrs2<-data.frame(GYrs1,Z)
GYrs2
```

	SSIs	Proc	Expecteds	Z
2001	14	353	17.39	−0.69
2002	19	347	17.10	0.38
2003	22	467	23.01	−0.08
2004	40	423	20.84	3.78
2005	19	504	24.83	−1.11
2006	14	504	24.83	−2.26

Although not always strictly correct since the proportions may not be independent (e.g. as here by calculating the expected counts from the overall SSI rate), multiple confidence intervals or Z-scores are often used with these data to identify outliers. Here, we illustrate the use of Z-scores for this purpose. There are Z-scores greater |2| in 2004 and 2006. In the absence of risk adjustment or a reference rate, this analysis could be used to identify areas requiring further study, for example, using an M&M audit.

Although these data do not display a trend, inspection of GYrs3 suggests a trend during the latter three years and repeating prop.trend.test with GYrs[4:6,] confirms this. Had there been a QI response to the relatively high SSI rate in 2004, for example, an M&M audit with implementation of an evidence-based bundle, this could have been evidence of a subsequent downward trend.

```
prop.trend.test(SSIs[4:6],Proc[4:6])$p.value
#
#[1] 6.509e-06
```

The function manyproportions() can be used to perform the calculations using prop.test. It includes the option to calculate P-values by Monte Carlo simulation and Z-scores modified for multiple significance testing using the Benjamini-Hochberg procedure. Data may be entered manually using manyproportions() or from a data.frame.

```
SSI<-c(14,19,22,40,19,14)
Proc<-c(353,347,467,423,504,504)
manyproportions(data.frame(SSI,Proc))
```

```
6-sample test for equality of proportions without continuity correction.
Chisq = 25.9, DF = 5, P-value = 0.
P-value by Monte Carlo simulation = 0.
Is a trend expected (Y/N) y
```

```
Chi-squared Test for Trend in Proportions.
Chisq = 1.174, DF = 1, P-value = 0.279.
Departure from trend chisq = 24.73, DF = 4, P-value = 0.
```

	Successes	Totals	Proportions	Expecteds	Z	ZAdj
1	14	353	0.04	17.39	−0.69	−0.34
2	19	347	0.05	17.10	0.38	0.20
3	22	467	0.05	23.01	−0.08	−0.08
4	40	423	0.09	20.84	3.78	3.31
5	19	504	0.04	24.83	−1.11	−0.62
6	14	504	0.03	24.83	−2.26	−1.81

```
# via IMenu()
d<-data.frame(SSI,Proc)
IMenu(d)
```

```
Introductory Menu

1. Proportion data,
2. Count and rate data.
1
1. Single proportion,
2. Confidence intervals for a series of proportions,
3. Two proportions,
4. More than two proportions,
5. Weighted average of proportions.
4

6-sample test for equality of proportions without continuity correction.
Chisq = 25.9, DF = 5, P-value = 0.
P-value by Monte Carlo simulation = 0.
Is a trend expected (Y/N) y
Chi-squared Test for Trend in Proportions.
Chisq = 1.174, DF = 1, P-value = 0.279.
Departure from trend chisq = 24.73, DF = 4, P-value = 0.
```

	Successes	Totals	Proportions	Expecteds	Z	ZAdj
1	14	353	0.04	17.39	−0.69	−0.34
2	19	347	0.05	17.10	0.38	0.20
3	22	467	0.05	23.01	−0.08	−0.08
4	40	423	0.09	20.84	3.78	3.31
5	19	504	0.04	24.83	−1.11	−0.62
6	14	504	0.03	24.83	−2.26	−1.81

1.6.3   Example 2, hospital data

Orthopaedic SSI data from a group of hospitals are in the file orthcomp0106.csv. These data were collected between 2001 and 2006. We will examine the data for the earlier period of data collection 2001 to 2004 and the later period of 2005 and 2006. For the present we ignore risk stratification and restrict the analysis to hospitals reporting 10 or more SSIs in the later period. We assume that the hospitals are exchangeable.

```
g.d # orthcomp0106.csv
```

```
Loading data.
Data from clipboard (C) or file (F) c
Do data column(s) have heading(s) (Y/N) y
Is column 1 a date column (Y/N) n
```

```
head(datain)
```

```
    Hospital    ProcedureDate    SSI
1       A            1-Feb-01      0
2       A            5-Feb-01      0
3       A            7-Feb-01      0
4       A            8-Feb-01      0
5       A           12-Feb-01      0
6       A           14-Feb-01      0
```

```
# ordering by hospital
o<-order(datain[,1])
datain<-datain[o,]
# getting before and after end of 2004
d<-datain[,2]
library(chron)
d<-chron(as.character(d),format="d-mmm-yy",out.format="dd-mmm-yyyy")
Before<-datain[d<"01-Jan-2005",]
After<-datain[d>"31-Dec-2004",]
ssib<-tapply(Before[,3],Before[,1],sum)
procb<-tapply(Before[,3],Before[,1],length)
nameb<-names(ssib)
OrthSSIb<-data.frame(nameb,ssib,procb)
lb<-1:length(OrthSSIb[,1])
row.names(OrthSSIb)<-lb
ssia<-tapply(After[,3],After[,1],sum)
proca<-tapply(After[,3],After[,1],length)
namea<-names(ssia)
OrthSSIa<-data.frame(namea,ssia,proca)
la<-1:length(OrthSSIa[,1])
row.names(OrthSSIa)<-la
Group2<-OrthSSIa[OrthSSIa[,2]>10,]
Group1<-
OrthSSIb[OrthSSIb[,1]=="A"|OrthSSIb[,1]=="B"|OrthSSIb[,1]=="E"|
OrthSSIb[,1]=="F"|OrthSSIb[,1]=="G"|OrthSSIb[,1]=="I"|
OrthSSIb[,1]=="J"|OrthSSIb[,1]=="K"|OrthSSIb[,1]=="N"|OrthSSIb[,1]=="Q",]
options(digits=4)
prop.test(Group2$ssia,Group2$proca)
```

```
X-squared = 29.13, df = 9, p-value = 0.0006173
sample estimates:
 prop 1  prop 2  prop 3  prop 4  prop 5  prop 6  prop 7  prop 8  prop 9
0.08264 0.03325 0.05288 0.06180 0.03274 0.06849 0.04950 0.04898 0.06007
prop 10
0.02634
```

INTRODUCTION TO ANALYSIS OF BINARY AND PROPORTION DATA

```
prop.test(Group1$ssib,Group1$procb)
```

```
X-squared = 58.35, df = 9, p-value = 2.783e-09
sample estimates:
 prop 1  prop 2  prop 3  prop 4  prop 5  prop 6  prop 7  prop 8
0.09631 0.03687 0.02926 0.05108 0.05975 0.06303 0.03650 0.07759
 prop 9 prop 10
0.06863 0.02609
```

These data are not homogeneous. This is not surprising as post-discharge SSI data collection was optional. We concentrate on the more recent data. In Chapter 2 we use expected numbers of outcomes derived from the NNIS risk index to determine which institutions differ from expected but here we obtain expected numbers from the unadjusted data.

```
# finding which proportions differ in Group2, 2005-2006 data
# assumes average rate from the data
SSI<-Group2$ssia
Totals<-Group2$proca
s1<-sum(SSI)
s2<-sum(Totals)
mn<-s1/s2
expected<-Totals*mn
Expecteds<-round(expected,2)
Group2a<-data.frame(Group2,Expecteds)
library(exactci)
rate<-Group2a[,2]/Group2a[,3]
d<-Group2a[,4]/Group2a[,3]
Z<-0;p<-0
for (i in 1:length(Group2a[,1])){p[i]<-binom.exact(Group2a
[i,2],Group2a[i,3],d[i])$p.value;if(rate[i]
>d[i]){Z[i]<--qnorm(p[i]/2)}else{Z[i]<-qnorm(p[i]/2)}}
Z<-round(Z,2)
Group2b<-data.frame(Group2a,Z)
Group2b
```

	namea	ssia	proca	Expecteds	Z
1	A	20	242	10.66	2.54
2	B	13	391	17.23	−0.91
5	E	22	416	18.33	0.77
6	F	11	178	7.84	0.98
7	G	33	1008	44.42	−1.72
9	I	25	365	16.08	2.04
10	J	15	303	13.35	0.36
11	K	12	245	10.80	0.26
14	N	17	283	12.47	1.16
17	Q	25	949	41.82	−2.75

```
# random effects analysis
# data as individual observations
Bbefore<-
Before[Before[,1]=="A"|Before[,1]=="B"|Before[,1]=="E"|Before[,1]=="F"|
Before[,1]=="G"|Before[,1]=="I"|Before[,1]=="J"|Before[,1]=="K"|
Before[,1]=="N"|Before[,1]=="Q",]
```

```
s.d(Bbefore)
#
#Use clipboard (c) or a data file (f) f
#Enter a file name d:/Before
#

Bafter<-
After[After[,1]=="A"|After[,1]=="B"|After[,1]=="E"|After[,1]==
"F"|After[,1]=="G"|After[,1]=="I"|After[,1]=="J"|After[,1]=="K"
|After[,1]=="N"|After[,1]=="Q",]

s.d(Bafter)
#
#Use clipboard (c) or a data file (f) f
#Enter a file name d:/After
#

g.d() # After.csv

library(hglm)
h<-
hglm(fixed=datain$SSI~1,random=~1|datain$Hospital,fix.disp=1,
family=binomial(link=logit))
Diffs<-data.frame(Group2b,round(h$ranef/h$SeRe,2))
names(Diffs)<-c("Name","SSI","Proc","Exp","Zfixed","Zrandom")
row.names(Diffs)<-1:length(Diffs[,1])
Diffs
```

	Name	SSI	Proc	Exp	Zfixed	Zrandom
1	A	20	242	10.66	2.54	1.72
2	B	13	391	17.23	−0.91	−1.05
3	E	22	416	18.33	0.77	0.33
4	F	11	178	7.84	0.98	0.56
5	G	33	1008	44.42	−1.72	−1.73
6	I	25	365	16.08	2.04	1.30
7	J	15	303	13.35	0.36	0.07
8	K	12	245	10.80	0.26	0.04
9	N	17	283	12.47	1.16	0.67
10	Q	25	949	41.82	−2.75	−2.44

We see, from this seemingly simple data set, how difficult such aggregated hospital AE data can be to analyse. When hospitals that are members of a group of hospitals and are exchangeable are compared, this difficulty may be compounded. It seems much better if institutions implement evidence-based bundles and monitor their own data sequentially (Chapters 3 and 6). Sometimes average rates for several years appear in reports. For the After data the average rate was $100 \times \sum SSIs/\sum Proc=4.41\%$. This differs from the rates for most of the hospitals (8.26, 3.32, 5.29, 6.18, 3.27, 6.85, 4.95, 4.90, 6.01 and 2.63 per cent respectively). It is difficult to see how, in this case, such an average could be interpretable. Also, we should bear in mind the advice of Mohammed and colleagues: look first for data or analysis error, then for problems with risk adjustment if used, then for system errors, and finally for problems involving staff. For example, was data collection different among the hospitals? We know that collection of post-discharge SSI data was optional at the time these data were collected and those who chose to collect these data would have higher rates. In addition, we should consider variations related to regression to the mean; an institution's AE rate may vary randomly within predictable limits from year to year without any system change and this may be of particular concern with smaller institutions.

1.6.4   Prop test and small samples

When there are small expected values, the prop.test χ^2 can become artificially large, it provides a warning message and its result can be ignored. This will often be the case with SSI and similar adverse event (AE) data. When samples are small, prop.test() can be replaced with fisher.test(). We illustrate with similar data from a smaller hospital Q. Although it will usually be unnecessary, it is possible to obtain a 2 DF χ^2 value corresponding to the fisher.test() P-value ($\chi^2{}_2$=-2×log(P-value)). The prop.trend.test() is less affected by small sample numbers than prop.test() and its $\chi^2{}_1$ value could be compared with the $\chi^2{}_2$ value from the fisher.test() to obtain an approximate departure from trend analysis. The Z-scores should remain useful. Although there is no suggestion of a significant difference or a trend among the yearly data from hospital Q, we use them to illustrate the calculations employing the Fisher exact test.

```
#getting ssi0106.csv data via clipboard
g.d()

#data from hospital Q
Q<-datain[datain$Hospital=="Q",c(3,5)]
Y<-Q$ProcedureDate
Y<-chron(as.character(Y),format="d-mmm-yy",out.format="dd-mmm-yyyy")
Yrs<-years(Y)
SSIs<-tapply(Q$SSI,Yrs,sum)
Proc<-tapply(Q$SSI,Yrs,length)
QYrs<-data.frame(SSIs,Proc)
QYrs<-QYrs[-1,] #remove single 2001 procedure
#
#Fisher test
ft<-fisher.test(data.frame(QYrs$SSIs,QYrs$Proc-QYrs$SSIs))
ft$p.value
#
#[1] 0.1596462
#
FT<--2*log(ft$p.value)
FT #fisher.test χ², DF=2
#
#[1] 3.66959
#
TT<-prop.trend.test(QYrs$SSIs,QYrs$Proc)
TT$statistic #prop.trend.test X2, DF=1
#X-squared
#0.08975511
as.numeric(1-pchisq(TT$statistic,1)) # trend test P-value
#0.7644887
DT<-FT-TT$statistic
DT #departure from trend X2, DF=1
#X-squared
#3.579835
as.numeric(1-pchisq(DT,1)) # departure from trend P-value
#0.05848496
```

Since the departure from trend χ^2 result of 0.06 is close to conventional statistical significance, further scrutiny of these data might be warranted. Comparing the first (2002) and second (2003) yearly data gives the following result.

```
twoproportions(data.frame(7,165,5,393))
```

```
First proportion 0.042, Second proportion 0.013
Difference between proportions 0.03.
Lower 95% limit 0.002, upper limit 0.07
Fisher Exact P-value = 0.048, LR = 1/7
Fisher Mid-P-value = 0.035, LR = 1/9
Ratio 3.33.
Ratio 95% confidence limits are 1.13 and 9.81.
```

A logistic regression analysis can be performed. The year 2003 appears to differ from the 2002 reference year but the overall test for the model gives a P-value of 0.17, similar to that of the Fisher exact test. The test involving just the 2002 and 2003 data is suggested by the data and fails to provide information about the overall group of years. Post-hoc analyses of this kind can mislead. It would only be of interest if, at the end of 2002, the test had been performed because of prior interest in these two years, for example, there may have been a change in the management of surgical wounds in 2003. Also, there were more procedures performed that year and this apparent increase in workload could have produced an interest in its influence on SSI rates at that time.

```
# logistic regression
YEARS<-c(rep(1,165),rep(2,393),rep(3,476),rep(4,477),rep(5,472))
SSIS<-c(rep(1,7),rep(0,165-7),rep(1,5),rep(0,393-5),rep(1,15),rep(0,476-
15),rep(1,10),rep(0,477-10),rep(1,15),rep(0,472-15))
g<-glm(SSIS~as.factor(YEARS),family=binomial)
summary(g)
```

```
Coefficients:
                    Estimate Std.   Error   z value  Pr(>|z|)
(Intercept)          -3.1167  0.3862  -8.069  7.08e-16  ***
as.factor(YEARS)2    -1.2349  0.5931  -2.082  0.0373    *
as.factor(YEARS)3    -0.3087  0.4669  -0.661  0.5086
as.factor(YEARS)4    -0.7271  0.5013  -1.450  0.1470
as.factor(YEARS)5    -0.2999  0.4669  -0.642  0.5206
     Null deviance: 481.30 on 1982 degrees of freedom
Residual deviance: 474.84 on 1978 degrees of freedom
1-pchisq(481.3-474.84,4) #deviance χ² test
[1] 0.1673282
```

1.7   Summarising stratified proportion data

Frequently, rather than seeking differences in annual AE rates, there is an interest in obtaining an overall average value. However, in doing so it often makes sense to give more weight to the most recent data, for example last year's data could receive half the weight of this year's data with each preceding year receiving half the weight of its successor. The result is a directly standardised rate. We illustrate the necessary calculations using Newcombe's square-and-add procedure.

The function stratifiedproportionsn() employs Newcombe's procedure as follows: X_i and N_i are the numerators and denominators for stratum i and W_i are the weights. The upper and lower limits u_i and l_i for each stratum are calculated, for example using midPci() in the PropCIs library as previously described. $p_i=X_i/N_i$ and $W_i=W_i/\sum W_i$ (so the weights sum to one). Then the weighted average is $A_W=\sum W_i p_i$. The lower (L) limit is $L=A_W-\sqrt{l}$ and the upper limit (U) is $U=A_W+\sqrt{u}$, where $l=\sum(((p_i-l_i)\times W_i)^2)$ and $u=\sum(((u_i-p_i)\times W_i)^2)$.

We now illustrate with data from the smaller hospital. Data may be entered into the R editor from the keyboard or as a data.frame. Once again, we should check that the proportions are reasonably homogeneous.

```
# check of homogeneity
x1<-c(7,5,15,10,15)
n1<-c(165,393,476,477,472)
fisher.test(data.frame(x1,n1-x1))$p.value
#
#[1] 0.1596 (suggests proportions are reasonably homogeneous
#stratified proportion data calculations
library(PropCIs)
I<-length(n1)
w<-1
for (i in 2:I){w[i]<-w[i-1]*2}
i1<-1:I
N<-rep(0,I)
up<-rep(0,I)
lo<-rep(0,I)
up1<-rep(0,I)
lo1<-rep(0,I)
s<-data.frame(i1,x1,n1,w)
#default weights geometrically decreasing, may be changed
s<-edit(s) # to R data editor for checking & editing data

#click on right top cross to return to the analysis
w<-s$w/sum(s$w)
u11<-0;l11<-0
for (i in 1:I){
l11[i]<-midPci(s$x1[i],s$n1[i],.05)[1]
u11[i]<-midPci(s$x1[i],s$n1[i],.05)[2]
}
p1<-s$x1/s$n1
a1<-sum(p1*w)
a0<-a1/sum(w)
a22<-sum((((p1-l11)*w)^2)
a33<-sum((((p1-u11)*w)^2)
l011<-a0-a22^.5;u011<-a0+a33^.5
cat("Weighted average = ",round(a0,3),".\nLower 95% limit =
",round(l011,3),", upper limit = ",round(u011,3),".\n",sep="")
#Weighted average = 0.028.
#Lower 95% limit = 0.021, upper limit = 0.039.

# using stratifiedproportionsn()
#to enter data from the keyboard, use stratifiedproportionsn()
#the R data editor will appear for manual data entry
#illustrating entry as a data.frame
x1<-c(7,5,15,10,15)
```

```
n1<-c(165,393,476,477,472)
w<-c(1,2,4,8,16)
s<-data.frame(x1,n1,w)
stratifiedproportionsn(s) #entry from data.frame

#check data in editor revise weights if required then click on close.
```

```
Weighted average = 0.028.
Lower 95% limit = 0.021, upper limit = 0.039.
```

The function stratifiedproportionsn() may also be accessed via IMenu().

```
x1<-c(7,5,15,10,15)
n1<-c(165,393,476,477,472)
w<-c(1,2,4,8,16)
s<-data.frame(x1,n1,w)
IMenu(s)
```

```
Introductory Menu

1. Proportion data,
2. Count and rate data.
1
1. Single proportion,
2. Confidence intervals for a series of proportions,
3. Two proportions,
4. More than two proportions,
5. Weighted average of proportions.
5
Weighted average = 0.028.
Lower 95% limit = 0.021, upper limit = 0.039.
```

1.8 Stratified proportion data, differences between rates

It may occasionally be necessary to assess the difference between two sets of stratified rates, for example, rates of SSIs for two units doing the same procedures. Once again we may need to distinguish between data that are stratified by fixed and random agents. Here we employ some hypothetical small-sample data to illustrate the former using Newcombe's method. When the rates and CIs for each of the sets of stratified rates have been determined, as in the previous section, Newcombe's method for the difference between them can be applied as described in the section describing the difference between two independent proportions. Data may be entered into the R editor from the keyboard or as a data.frame.

```
# differences between rates, hypothetical data
GroupA<-c(1,32,4,43,2,21);GroupB<-c(0,97,3,142,2,49)
ssi2<-data.frame(GroupA,GroupB)
row.names(ssi2)<-
c("Stratum1Failures","Stratum1Procedurers","Stratum2Failures",
"Stratum2Procedurers","Stratum3Failures","Stratum3Procedurers")
ssi2
```

	GroupA	GroupB
Stratum1Failures	1	0
Stratum1Procedurers	32	97
Stratum2Failures	4	3
Stratum2Procedurers	43	142
Stratum3Failures	2	2
Stratum3Procedurers	21	49

```
Group<-c(rep(1,3),rep(0,3))
Stratum<-gl(3,1,6)
AE<-c(1,4,2,0,3,2)
Total<-c(32,43,21,97,142,49)
Hypothdat<-data.frame(Group,Stratum,AE,Total)
x1<-Hypothdat[1:3,3]
n1<-Hypothdat[1:3,4]
x2<-Hypothdat[4:6,3]
n2<-Hypothdat[4:6,4]
I<-(length(Hypothdat[,1]))/2
w<-rep(1,I) #equal weights
i1<-1:I
s<-data.frame(i1,x1,n1,x2,n2,w)
s<-edit(s) #to R data editor for checking & editing data

# click on right top cross to return to the analysis
#stratified risk difference using Newcombe's method
library(PropCIs)
x1<-s$x1;x2<-s$x2;n1<-s$n1;n2<-s$n2;w<-s$w
s$y1<-s$n1+s$n2
w<-w/sum(w)
u11<-0;l11<-0
for (i in 1:I){
l11[i]<-midPci(x1[i],n1[i],.05)[1]
u11[i]<-midPci(x1[i],n1[i],.05)[2]
}
u22<-0;l22<-0
for (i in 1:I){
l22[i]<-midPci(x2[i],n2[i],.05)[1]
u22[i]<-midPci(x2[i],n2[i],.05)[2]}
p1<-x1/n1
a1<-sum(p1*w)
a0<-a1/sum(w)
a22<-sum(((p1-l11)*w)^2)
a33<-sum(((p1-u11)*w)^2)
l011<-a0-a22^.5;u011<-a0+a33^.5
p2<-x2/n2
b1<-sum(p2*w)
b0<-b1/sum(w)
b22<-sum(((p2-l22)*w)^2)
b33<-sum(((p2-u22)*w)^2)
l022<-b0-b22^.5;u022<-b0+b33^.5
d<-a0-b0
lomh1<-d-((a0-l011)^2+(u022-b0)^2)^.5
upmh1<-d+((b0-l022)^2+(u011-a0)^2)^.5
N1<-paste("\nNewcombe's method using mid-P binomial 95% confidence
limits.\n")
```

```
N2<-paste("Weighted average in first group ",round(a0,3),".",sep="")
N3<-paste("\nFirst group confidence limits ",round(l011,3),"
to ",round(u011,3),".",sep="")
N4<-paste("\nWeighted average in second group ",round(b0,3),".",sep="")
N5<-paste("\nSecond group confidence limits ",round(l022,3),"
to ",round(u022,3),".",sep="")
N6<-paste("\nWeighted difference ",round(d,3),".",sep="")
N7<-paste("\nDifference confidence limits ",round(lomh1,3),"
to ",round(upmh1,3),".",sep="")
cat(N1,N2,N3,N4,N5,N6,N7,"\n",sep="")
```

```
Newcombe's method using mid-P binomial 95% confidence limits.
Weighted average in first group 0.073.
First group confidence limits 0.038 to 0.155.
Weighted average in second group 0.021.
Second group confidence limits 0.008 to 0.054.
Weighted difference 0.053.
Difference confidence limits 0.005 to 0.135.
```

```
#stratified risk ratio using Newcombe's method
P1<-a0
P2<-b0
U1<-u011
L1<-l011
U2<-u022
L2<-l022
U=exp(log(P1)-log(P2)+((log(U1)-log(P1))^2+(log(P2)-log(L2))^2)^.5)
L=exp(log(P1)-log(P2)-((log(P1)-log(L1))^2+(log(U2)-log(P2))^2)^.5)
R1<-paste("\nRatio ",round(P1/P2,3),".",sep="")
R2<-paste("\nApproximate 95% ratio confidence limits
",round(L,3)," to ",round(U,3),".",sep="")
cat(R1,R2,"\n",sep="")
```

```
Ratio 3.544.
Approximate 95% ratio confidence limits 1.119 to 11.575.
```

1.8.1 Yearly data

The function stratified2proportionsn() performs the calculations described in section 1.8. Data may be entered via the R editor from the keyboard (leave the space between () blank and use the R data editor for data entry), or enter the data as a data.frame. The former method is tedious and can be prone to error so the latter is recommended. The analysis using stratified2proportionsn() is illustrated with yearly SSI data from two hospitals. Note that when the larger rates are in the second group, the groups are interchanged.

```
#using function stratified2proportionsn()
Year<-2002:2006
SSI1<-c(7,5,15,10,15)
Proc1<-c(165,393,476,477,472)
SSI2<-c(19,22,40,19,14)
Proc2<-c(347,467,423,504,504)
I<-length(Year)
```

```
w<-1:I # weights can be changed in the R Editor
TYrs<-data.frame(Year,SSI1,Proc1,SSI2,Proc2,w)
TYrs
```

```
  Year SSI1 Proc1 SSI2 Proc2 w
1 2002    7   165   19   347 1
2 2003    5   393   22   467 2
3 2004   15   476   40   423 3
4 2005   10   477   19   504 4
5 2006   15   472   14   504 5
```

```
stratified2proportionsn(TYrs[,-1]) #weights 1 to 5
#Enter required confidence level .95
```

```
The two groups have been interchanged so the larger is first.
Newcombe's method using mid-P binomial 95% confidence limits.
Weighted average in first group 0.04815626.
First group confidence limits 0.0403548 to 0.05852714.
Weighted average in second group 0.02701087.
Second group confidence limits 0.02098259 to 0.03603815.
Weighted difference 0.02114539.
Difference confidence limits 0.009214145 to 0.03314103.
Ratio 1.782847.
Ratio confidence limits 1.271269 to 2.452981.
```

An approximate P-value can be calculated using the method of Bland and Altman. As shown in section 1.9 that deals with heterogeneity, the CI may be too narrow and the P-value may be too small.

```
#calculating approximate P-value (Altman and Bland)
SE<-(log(2.452981)-log(1.271269))/(2*1.96)
Z<-log(1.782847)/SE
P.value=exp(-0.717*Z-0.416*Z^2)
Z;P.value
#[1] 3.448394
#[1] 0.0005995516
```

```
#calculating 3 SD equivalent limits using stratified2proportionsn()
stratified2proportionsn(TYrs[,-1])
#Enter required confidence level .997
```

```
The two groups have been interchanged so the larger is first.
Newcombe's method using mid-P binomial 99.7% #confidence limits.
Weighted average in first group 0.04815626.
First group confidence limits 0.03714774 to 0.06479125.
Weighted average in second group 0.02701087.
Second group confidence limits 0.01867971 to 0.0417506.
Weighted difference 0.02114539.
Difference confidence limits 0.002748458 to 0.03974999.
Ratio 1.782847.
Ratio confidence limits 1.073857 to 2.862108.
```

1.8.2   Hospital data

The previous section dealt with stratified yearly data where the stratifying agent, years, is fixed so that in the presence of heterogeneity among the strata, it will usually be best to study the within stratum rate differences and ratios individually. When the stratifying agent is hospitals, a random effects approach may be feasible and this is illustrated by Spiegelhalter[B,C,D] with funnel plots displaying data from groups of hospitals (Chapter 2). In this case, we are unlikely in advance to consider the hospitals as having special characteristics that would make them fixed agents. In the following section we discuss the role of Mantel-Haenszel, Homogeneity, Trend Tests and the derSimonian-Laird random effects method in the analysis of data stratified by years and by hospitals.

1.9   Mantel-Haenszel, homogeneity and trend tests

We are primarily interested in risk differences, and to a lesser extent risk ratios, because they seem to us to be the most useful for analysing routine surveillance data. The natural estimator for binomial data is the odds ratio (OR), and this is especially employed for case-control studies as well as being reported generally in analyses based on models such as logistic regression. While such studies are frequently performed in IM and QI departments for research, they are performed less frequently when analysing routine surveillance data (a relatively uncommon exception is the investigation of an outbreak, for example, of food poisoning, as described in Chapter 7). These notes are primarily for staff in IM and QI departments in hospitals as an aid to their analysis of routine surveillance data. Consequently, we have given less emphasis to the OR. However, it is employed in the following section.

We include an exact Mantel-Haenszel (MH) analysis (Rosner), an alternative to the Newcombe method for combining and comparing two sets of data in different strata that is based on the OR. The MH test is a generalisation of the Fisher exact test to data in several strata using weights derived from the data. The weights for the MH test for stratum i are $N_{1i} \times N_{2i}/(N_{1i}+N_{2i})$ where N_{1i} and N_{2i} are the denominators for that stratum (Armitage and colleagues). These weights have the desirable property of being inversely proportional to the stratum i variance. The MH method is more conservative than the Newcombe method described above as the latter is based on mid-P binomial intervals and the OR is based on the hypergeometric distribution. In addition, the ability to weight the data in the strata to obtain a directly standardised rate as described above no longer applies.

The stratification methods that employ the OR such as the MH method may be especially useful in routine IM and QI work when there may be heterogeneity (unusual variation) among the strata with the results in the individual strata differing. Tests for heterogeneity are often called homogeneity tests and they may include a test for a trend. In addition, there are random-effects modifications for dealing with heterogeneity such as the derSimonian-Laird method. The latter comes from meta-analysis where a number of related studies are analysed as a group and it is reasonable to regard them as random selections of such studies (i.e. they are in a sense exchangeable).We should ensure that it is reasonable to regard our stratifying agent as a random agent before using the derSimonian-Laird method; for example, this would not be the case if the stratifying agent were sex or, usually, years as more recent years should in general receive greater weight. Since the stratifying agent will often be hospitals among a group of hospitals or units within a hospital performing similar work, it will often be the case that it is reasonable to regard the stratifying agent as being random. Although the Newcombe and MH methods differ, if there is evidence of heterogeneity of the ORs among the strata, the

Newcombe analysis may be invalid and it may be preferable to concentrate on the differences within the individual strata if they are fixed. (The Newcombe analysis with weighting would not be suitable if the stratum agent were random.)

The homogeneity test seeks evidence of unusual variability among the strata; for example, the effect of the group variable may differ among them. In most cases the strata will not be ordered; for example, they could represent hospitals or the wards of a hospital that could be regarded as exchangeable and therefore as random agents. Some stratifying agents such as sex or years, where more recent ones should in general receive greater weight, would not be exchangeable and should therefore be treated as being fixed. Occasionally, they may be ordered, for example, patients' ages that have been placed in ordered groups, and a homogeneity trend test may then be required. Ordered strata would be fixed as they would not be exchangeable. When there is unusual variability among the strata and they may be regarded as being random, a random effects analysis may be appropriate. This is illustrated by Spiegelhalter[B,C,D] when analysing highly variable AE data among groups of hospitals using funnel plots. We illustrate these methods in Chapters 2 and 5. When there is heterogeneity among the strata and the stratifying agent is fixed, analysis of the data within the separate strata will usually be needed.

The MH CI method requires finding the fitted values in the first group cases or AEs given the MH OR; this is described by Breslow and Day. The homogeneity test requires large samples and typically has low power. An alternative although less powerful approach, on which the derSimonian and Laird method of moments random-effects analysis is often based, employs the Woolf log(OR). We illustrate the use of the log(OR) with the yearly data from the two hospitals. The analysis is further illustrated in the Outbreak Investigation in Chapter 7.

The Woolf and derSimonian-Laird procedures are described by Kirkwood and Sterne and Rosner. To illustrate the calculation of the former for the yearly SSI data from hospitals G and Q, the group 1 AEs in the first stratum (2002) were $x1=7$ (hospital Q) and in the second group there were $x2=19$ AEs (hospital G). The corresponding totals were $N1=165$ and $N2=347$. Therefore the four cell counts in the resulting stratum one 2×2 table are $a=7$, $b=19$, $c=165-7=158$ and $d=347-19=328$.

The marginal totals of the 2×2 table are $m1=N1$, $m2=N2$, $m3=a+b=7+19=26$ and $m4=c+d=158+328=486$. The data in the remaining strata are arranged in a similar manner. The odds ratio for stratum i ($i=1..I$) is $OR_i=(a_i \times d_i)/(b_i \times c_i)$. The approximate variance of $\log(OR_i)$ is $V_i=1/a_i+1/b_i+1/c_i+1/d_i$. To avoid division by zero when there are zero AEs, 0.5 is usually added to a_i, b_i, c_i and d_i. A weight $w_i=1/V_i$ is defined and the stratified $\log(OR)$ is then $\sum(w_i \times \log(OR_i))/\sum w_i$ with variance $V=1/\sum w_i$. The homogeneity of the stratum $\log(ORs)$ is assessed by $\chi^2=\sum(w_i \times (\log(OR_i)-\log(OR))^2)$ with $DF=I-1$. For a 1 DF trend test define $x=1..I$ and $lor_i=\log(OR_i)$. Then $\chi^2_1=Lxy^2/Lxx$ where $Lxy=a-b \times d/e$ with $a=\sum(w_i \times x_i \times lor_i)$, $b=\sum(w_i \times lor_i)$, $d=\sum(x_i \times w_i)$ and $e=\sum w_i$; and $Lxx=f-d/e$, where $f=\sum(w_i \times x_i^2)$. The homogeneity test described by Breslow and Day mentioned above is more powerful but the Woolf log(OR) procedure is in common use. The former is available in the function epi.2by2() in the epiR library that we employ in Chapter 4.

If the homogeneity test suggests heterogeneity among the strata, the approximate additive method of moments random effects analysis described by derSimonian and Laird can then be employed provided it is reasonable to regard the levels of the stratifying agent as being exchangeable and therefore the stratum agent as being random. The within stratum variance V_i is widened to include the between stratum variance $tau=max(0,(Q-I+1)/W)$ where Q is the homogeneity χ^2 and $W=\sum w_i-\sum w_i^2/\sum w_i$. Then $V^*_i=V_i+tau$, $\log(OR_{Adj})=\sum(w^*_i \times \log(OR_i))/\sum w^*_i$, and $V^*=1/\sum w^*_i$ where $w^*_i=1/V^*_i$.

1.9.1 Yearly data

The hospital G and hospital Q data for 2002 to 2006 are shown analysed by stratum (year), converted to individual observations and placed in a .csv file using s.d() (twosamplestratified.csv) and tabulated. We illustrate converting to individual observations here as they are used later in this chapter.

```
# converting data to individual observations
Group<-c(rep(1,5),rep(0,5))
Stratum<-gl(5,1,10)
AE<-c(19,22,40,19,14,7,5,15,10,15)
Total<-c(347,467,423,504,504,165,393,476,477,472)
NoAE<-Total-AE
dta<-data.frame(Group,Stratum,AE,NoAE)
I<-(length(dta[,1]))/2
dta1<-data.frame(Group,Stratum,AE,Total)
dta2<-cbind(dta1[1:I,],dta1[(I+1):(2*I),])
group<-c(rep(1,sum(dta2[,4])),rep(0,sum(dta2[,8])))
stratum<-0
for (i in 1:length(dta2[,1])){stratum<-c(stratum,rep(dta2[i,2],dta2[i,4]))}
stratum<-stratum[-1]
for (i in 1:length(dta2[,1])){stratum<-c(stratum,rep(dta2[i,6],dta2[i,8]))}
outcome<-0
for (i in 1:length(dta2[,1])){outcome<-c(outcome,rep(1,dta2[i,3]),
rep(0,dta2[i,4]-dta2[i,3]))}
outcome<-outcome[-1]
for (i in 1:length(dta2[,1])){outcome<-c(outcome,rep(1,dta2[i,7]),
rep(0,dta2[i,8]-dta2[i,7]))}
dta4<-data.frame(group,outcome,stratum)
```

Next, the Mantel-Haenszel analysis is illustrated. A logistic regression analysis shows that stratification by years is necessary. The stratified analysis is repeated using the Woolf method. Homogeneity and trend tests are illustrated and it can be seen that there is some evidence of heterogeneity among the strata but no evidence of a trend. Since years are here regarded as fixed, no random effects analysis is performed.

```
# logistic regression, is stratification necessary?
g1<-glm(outcome~group,family=binomial)
g<-glm(outcome~group+as.factor(stratum),family=binomial)
a<-anova(g1,g)
p<-1-pchisq(a$Deviance[2],a$Df[2])
a;cat("P-value=",round(p,4),"\n",sep="")
#the P-value is highly significant, stratification is required
```

```
Analysis of Deviance Table
Model 1: outcome ~ group
Model 2: outcome ~ group + as.factor(stratum)
  Resid. Df Resid. Dev Df Deviance
1     4226     1382.9
2     4222     1364.1  4   18.776
P-value=9e-04
```

```
#Mantel-Haenszel analysis
mant2<-mantelhaen.test(table(group,outcome,stratum),exact=T,alternative="t")
mant2$p.value
```

```
#
#[1] 2.731074e-05

# Woolf stratified analysis
dta3<-data.frame(dta[1:I,2:4],dta[(I+1):(2*I),3:4])
names(dta3)<-c("Stratum","Group1AE","Group1NoAE","Group2AE","Group2NoAE")
lor<-0;vlor<-0
for (i in 1:I){
x<-c(dta3$Group1AE[i],dta3$Group1NoAE[i])
y<-c(dta3$Group2AE[i],dta3$Group2NoAE[i])
ta<-data.frame(x,y)
ta1<-ta+.5
or1<-ta1[1,1]*ta1[2,2]/(ta1[1,2]*ta1[2,1])
lor[i]<-log(or1)
vlor[i]<-sum(1/ta1)
}
alor<-sum(lor/vlor)/sum(1/vlor)
valor<-1/sum(1/vlor)
OR<-exp(alor)
L95<-exp(alor-1.96*valor^.5)
U95<-exp(alor+1.96*valor^.5)
Z.score<-alor/valor^.5
P.value<-2*(1-pnorm(Z.score))
cat("OR=",round(OR,2),"\nL95=",round(L95,2),"\nU95=",round(U95,2),
"\nZ-score=",round(Z.score,2),"\nP-value=",round(P.value,5),"\n",sep="")
```

```
OR=1.89
L95=1.35
U95=2.65
Z-score=3.73
P-value=2e-04
```

```
# homogeneity and trend tests
ch<-sum((1/vlor)*(lor-alor)^2)
p<-1-pchisq(ch,(I-1))
H<-paste("\nHomogneity test chi-squared = ",round(ch,2))
P<-paste("\nP-value = ",round(p,3))
if (I>2){
xx<-1:I
w<-1/vlor
aa<-sum(w*xx*lor);bb<-sum(w*lor);dd<-sum(xx*w);ee<-sum(w);ff<-sum(w*xx^2)
Lxy<-aa-bb*dd/ee
Lxx<-ff-dd^2/ee
ch.sq<-Lxy^2/Lxx
pp<-1-pchisq(ch.sq,1)
TR<-paste("\nTrend test chi-squared = ",round(ch.sq,2))
PT<-paste("\nP-value = ",round(pp,3))
}
cat("\n")
cat(H,P,"\n")
if (I>2){cat(TR,PT,"\n")}
```

```
Homogneity test chi-squared =  9.73
P-value =  0.045
Trend test chi-squared =  1.73
P-value =  0.189
```

It may be of interest to compare logistic regression including group by stratum interaction in a fixed effects analysis. There is evidence of group by stratum interaction. For the standard logistic regression the OR is exp(0.7043)=2.02 and the P-value is 0.00004, similar to the MH values of OR=2.02 and P-value=0.00003 (the group effect is difficult to assess when an interaction term is included). Thus the most appropriate approach may be to analyse these data within the strata separately.

```
# logistic regression and interaction
G<-glm(outcome~group+as.factor(stratum),family=binomial)
#adding interaction term
G1<-glm(outcome~group*as.factor(stratum),family=binomial)
A<-anova(G,G1)
P<-1-pchisq(A$Deviance[2],A$Df[2])
A; cat("P-value=",round(P,4),"\n",sep="")
```

```
Analysis of Deviance Table
Model 1: outcome ~ group + as.factor(stratum)
Model 2: outcome ~ group * as.factor(stratum)
  Resid. Df Resid. Dev Df Deviance
1      4222     1364.1
2      4218     1354.1  4   10.033
P = 0.0399
```

```
# examining the individual strata
Group<-c(rep(1,5),rep(0,5))
Stratum<-gl(5,1,10)
AE<-c(19,22,40,19,14,7,5,15,10,15)
Total<-c(347,467,423,504,504,165,393,476,477,472)
NoAE<-Total-AE
dta<-data.frame(Group,Stratum,AE,NoAE)
I<-(length(dta[,1]))/2
dta1<-data.frame(Group,Stratum,AE,Total)
dta2<-cbind(dta1[1:I,],dta1[(I+1):(2*I),])
#individual strata using twoproportions
for (i in 1:I){cat("\n",i,"\n",sep="");twoproportions(dta2[i,c(3,4,7,8)])}
```

```
1. First proportion 0.055, Second proportion 0.042
Difference 0.012, L95 -0.032, U95 0.049
Fisher Exact P-value = 0.669, LR = 1/1
Fisher Mid-P-value = 0.595, LR = 1/1
Ratio 1.29, L95 0.57, U95 2.95
```

```
2. First proportion 0.047, Second proportion 0.013
Difference 0.034, L95 0.012, U95 0.058
Fisher Exact P-value = 0.005, LR = 1/51
Fisher Mid-P-value = 0.004, LR = 1/63
Ratio 3.7, L95 1.47, U95 9.39.
```

```
3. First proportion 0.095, Second proportion 0.032
Difference 0.063, L95 0.032, U95 0.096
Fisher Exact P-value = 0, LR = 1/2404
Fisher Mid-P-value = 0, LR = 1/3270
Ratio 3, L95 1.7, U95 5.32.
```

```
4. First proportion 0.038, Second proportion 0.021
Difference 0.017, L95 -0.004, U95 0.038
Fisher Exact P-value = 0.135, LR = 1/3
Fisher Mid-P-value = 0.111, LR = 1/4
Ratio 1.8, L95 0.86, U955 3.77.
```

```
5.First proportion 0.028, Second proportion 0.032
Difference -0.004, L95 -0.026, U95 0.017
Fisher Exact P-value = 0.851, LR = 1/1
Fisher Mid-P-value = 0.781, LR = 1/1
Ratio 0.87, L95 0.43, U95 1.77.
```

Lastly, we could employ a bootstrap analysis of the standardised risk difference and risk ratio. This also appears to give intervals that are too narrow and this is not corrected using bias and acceleration (BCa) adjustments. The outlier SSI rate for hospital G in 2004 has resulted in significant heterogeneity. The practice of making comparisons of these and similar data should be approached with great caution. We have repeatedly urged caution when comparisons are made between hospitals (see section 1.4). This is another example of the potential difficulties entailed in such comparisons.

1.9.2   Data stratified by hospital

We now return to the earlier data in the files Before.csv and After.csv. These may be stratified by hospital and compared to see if there was overall improvement in the later period. In this analysis we employ the random effects method.

```
g.d() # Before.csv

Before<-datain
Group<-rep(1,length(Before[,1]))
Before<-data.frame(Before,Group)

g.d() # After.csv

After<-datain
Group<-rep(2,length(After[,1]))
After<-data.frame(After,Group)

# amalgamating
All<-rbind(Before,After)
stratum<-All[,1]
group<-All[,4]
outcome<-All[,3]

# logistic regression, is stratification necessary?
# is interaction present?
g1<-glm(outcome~group,family=binomial)
g<-glm(outcome~group*as.factor(stratum),family=binomial)
g2<-glm(outcome~group+as.factor(stratum),family=binomial)
a<-anova(g1,g2) # stratification
p<-1-pchisq(a$Deviance[2],a$Df[2])
b<-anova(g2,g) # interaction
```

```
p1<-1-pchisq(b$Deviance[2],b$Df[2])
a;cat("P-value=",round(p,4),"\n",sep="")
#the P-value is highly significant, stratification is required
```

```
Model 1: outcome ~ group
Model 2: outcome ~ group + as.factor(stratum)
  Resid. Df Resid. Dev Df Deviance
1    10920    4266.9
2    10911    4196.7  9   70.262
P-value=0
```

```
b;cat("P-value=",round(p1,4),"\n",sep="")
# interaction P-value is of borderline significance
```

```
Model 1: outcome ~ group + as.factor(stratum)
Model 2: outcome ~ group * as.factor(stratum)
  Resid. Df Resid. Dev Df Deviance
1    10911    4196.7
2    10902    4181.2  9   15.463
P-value=0.079
```

```
#Mantel-Haenszel analysis
mant2<-
mantelhaen.test(table(group,outcome,stratum),exact=T,alternative="t")
mant2$estimate
#
#common odds ratio
#       0.8874502
# reciprocal
1/mant2$estimate
#
#common odds ratio
#       1.126824
mant2$p.value
#
#[1] 0.2133

# Woolf stratified analysis
AE1<-tapply(Before$SSI,Before$Hospital,sum)
AE2<-tapply(After$SSI,After$Hospital,sum)
To1<-tapply(Before$SSI,Before$Hospital,length)
To2<-tapply(After$SSI,After$Hospital,length)
No1<-To1-AE1
No2<-To2-AE2
I<-length(AE1)
AEA<-c(AE1,AE2)
AEA<-as.numeric(AEA)
TotalA<-c(To1,To2)
TotalA<-as.numeric(TotalA)
NoAEA<-TotalA-AEA
GroupA<-c(rep(1,I),rep(0,I))
StratumA<-gl(I,1,2*I)
dta<-data.frame(GroupA,StratumA,AEA,NoAEA)
dta3<-data.frame(dta[1:I,2:4],dta[(I+1):(2*I),3:4])
```

```
names(dta3)<-c("Stratum","Group1AE","Group1NoAE","Group2AE","Group2NoAE")
lor<-0;vlor<-0
for (i in 1:I){
x<-c(dta3$Group1AE[i],dta3$Group1NoAE[i])
y<-c(dta3$Group2AE[i],dta3$Group2NoAE[i])
ta<-data.frame(x,y)
ta1<-ta+.5
or1<-ta1[1,1]*ta1[2,2]/(ta1[1,2]*ta1[2,1])
lor[i]<-log(or1)
vlor[i]<-sum(1/ta1)
}
w<-1/vlor
alor<-sum(lor*w)/sum(w)
valor<-1/sum(w)
OR<-exp(alor)
L95<-exp(alor-1.96*valor^.5)
U95<-exp(alor+1.96*valor^.5)
Z.score<-alor/valor^.5
P.value<-2*(1-pnorm(Z.score))
cat("OR=",round(OR,2),"\nL95=",round(L95,2),"\nU95=",round(U95,2),"
\nZ-score=",round(Z.score,2),"\nP-value=",round(P.value,5),"\n",sep="")
```

```
OR=1.1
L95=0.92
U95=1.32
Z-score=1.03
P-value=0.3026
```

```
# homogeneity test
# trend test not indicated for exchangeable strata
ch<-sum(w*(lor-alor)^2)
p<-1-pchisq(ch,(I-1))
H<-paste("\nHomogeneity test chi-squared = ",round(ch,2))
P<-paste("\nP-value = ",round(p,3))
cat("\n")
cat(H,P,"\n")
```

```
Homogeneity test chi-squared =   14.98
P-value =   0.091
```

```
# derSimonian-Laird random Effects
W<-sum(w)-(sum(w^2)/sum(w))
Q<-max(0,ch-I+1)
Q/W # random effects variance
#[1] 0.05954
qw<-Q/W
rvlor<-vlor+qw
w1<-1/rvlor
rlor<-sum(w1*lor)/sum(w1)
vrvlor<-1/sum(w1)
L<-exp(rlor-1.96*vrvlor^.5)
U<-exp(rlor+1.96*vrvlor^.5)
Z<-rlor/vrvlor^.5
P<-2*(1-pnorm(rlor/vrvlor^.5))
```

Manatel-Haenszel analysis

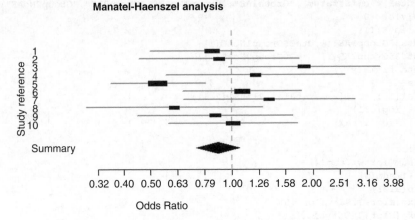

Figure 1.1   Stratified data, Mantel-Haenszel analysis.

```
cat("Adjusted OR=",round(exp(rlor),2),"\nL95=",round(L,2),"\nU95=",
round(U,2),"\nZ-score=",round(Z,2),"\nP-value=",round(P,5),"\n",sep="")
```

```
Adjusted OR=1.06
L95=0.83
U95=1.35
Z-score=0.46
P-value=0.6466
```

A derSimonian and Laird random-effects analysis was performed. This should be suitable as the hospitals could be considered as random agents. It may be convenient to use metaDSL() in the rmeta library to perform this analysis. This has the advantage of providing a plot of the confidence intervals, called a forest plot (Figure 1.1 and Figure 1.2). There is no evidence that, overall, the Before and After proportions differ.

derSimonian-Laird analysis

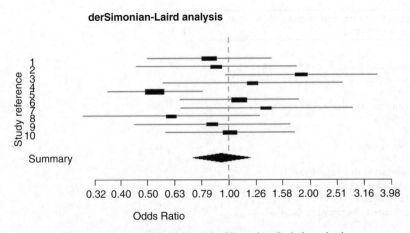

Figure 1.2   Stratified data, derSimonian-Laird analysis.

```
#using the rmeta library
library(rmeta)
SSI1<-AE1 #Before
Proc1<-To1
SSI2<-AE2 #After
Proc2<-To2
ORD<-meta.DSL(Proc2,Proc1,SSI2,SSI1,names=1:10)
ORM<-meta.MH(Proc2,Proc1,SSI2,SSI1,names=1:10)
summary(ORM)
```

```
Fixed effects ( Mantel-Haenszel ) meta-analysis
Call: meta.MH(ntrt = Proc2, nctrl = Proc1, ptrt = SSI2, pctrl = SSI1,
     names = 1:10)
-----------------------------------
      OR (lower 95% upper)
1   0.85    0.50     1.44
2   0.90    0.45     1.78
3   1.85    0.97     3.53
4   1.22    0.57     2.63
5   0.53    0.36     0.80
6   1.09    0.66     1.81
7   1.38    0.66     2.86
8   0.61    0.29     1.30
9   0.87    0.45     1.68
10  1.01    0.58     1.75
-----------------------------------
Mantel-Haenszel OR =0.89 95% CI ( 0.74,1.07 )
Test for heterogeneity: X^2( 9 ) = 15 ( p-value 0.0908 )
```

```
ORD
```

```
Random effects ( DerSimonian-Laird ) meta-analysis
SummaryOR= 0.94   95% CI ( 0.73,1.2 )
Test for heterogeneity: X^2( 9 ) = 14.98 ( p-value 0.0914 )
Estimated random effects variance: 0.06
```

```
plot(ORM,main="Mantel-Haenszel Analysis")
```

```
plot(ORD,main="derSimonian-Laird Analysis")
```

1.10   Stratified rates and overdispersion

One of the methods described by Spiegelhalter[B,C,D] for displaying overdispersed hospital AE data in funnel plots involves modifying prediction limits using the derSimonian-Laird random effects variance and the null variance of the AE rate. Since there is no difference between the Before and After data but considerable differences among the hospitals, we illustrate the methods of Spiegelhalter[B,C,D] and Laney (Mohammed and Laney[A]) using the combined data in the data.frame All. This issue is discussed further in Chapters 2 and 5.

First we obtain the rates for the hospitals, the overall mean rate and the null and non-null variances for the hospital rates. Z-scores and the derSinomian-Laird random-effects variance are then obtained.

$Z_i=(H_i-M)/V0_i^{.5}$, where H_i is the rate for hospital i, M is the mean rate and $V0_i$ is the null variance for that hospital ($V0_i=M\times(1-M)/N_i$, where N_i is the hospital i denominator). The random effects variance is $(Q-(L-1))/W$, where $Q=\sum(Z_i^2)$, L is the number of hospitals and $W=\sum w_i-\sum w_i^2/\sum w_i$, where w_i is the reciprocal of the non-null variance for hospital i ($V_i=H_i\times(1-H_i)/N_i$). The revised Z-score for hospital i is then $Z_i=(H_i-M)/(V0_i+Q)^{.5}$.

```
M<-mean(All$SSI)
S<-tapply(All$SSI,All$Hospital,sum) # observed counts
N<-tapply(All$SSI,All$Hospital,length)
E<-round(M*N,2) # expected counts
L<-length(N)
H<-S/N # observed rates
VH<-H*(1-H)/N
V0<-M*(1-M)/N
ZH<-(H-M)/VH^.5
Z0<-(H-M)/V0^.5
IZ<-sum(Z0^2)
w<-1/VH
W<-sum(w)-sum(w^2)/sum(w)
Q<-(IZ-(L-1))/W
ZHDSL<-(H-M)/(V0+Q)^.5
data.frame(S,N,E,H,Z0,ZHDSL)
```

	S	N	E	H	Z0	ZHDSL
A	80	865	42	0.092	5.928	2.309
B	38	1069	52	0.036	-2.035	-0.724
E	39	997	49	0.039	-1.443	-0.529
F	30	550	27	0.055	0.604	0.283
G	128	2598	127	0.049	0.067	0.016
I	70	1079	53	0.065	2.419	0.857
J	30	714	35	0.042	-0.863	-0.364
K	30	477	23	0.063	1.407	0.697
N	38	589	29	0.065	1.747	0.797
Q	52	1984	97	0.026	-4.700	-1.264

As well as the additive correction (Z0 is the unadjusted Z-score and ZHDSL is the Z-score with the additive adjustment described above), Spiegelhalter describes a multiplicative adjustment that employs the square root of the mean of the squared Z-scores (the Z0s) and Laney advocates using the standard deviation (sd) of the Z-scores for the adjustment (ZS and ZL in the box). For funnel plot control limits using, for example, Laney's correction $U,L=M\pm Z\times sd(Z0)\times\sqrt{V0_i}$, U and L are upper and lower control limits, and Z is for example, 3 for a 3 sd control limit.

```
(mean(Z0^2))^.5 # Spiegelhalter's multiplicative correction

#[1] 2.7

sd(Z0) # Laney's correction

#[1] 2.9

ZS<-Z0/(mean(Z0^2))^.5 # Z-score with Spiegelhalter's
# multiplicative correction
```

```
ZL<-Z0/sd(Z0) # Z-score with Laney's correction
data.frame(Z0,ZHDSL,ZS,ZL)
```

	Z0	ZHDSL	ZS	ZL
A	5.928	2.309	2.158	2.061
B	−2.035	−0.724	−0.741	−0.708
E	−1.443	−0.529	−0.525	−0.502
F	0.604	0.283	0.220	0.210
G	0.067	0.016	0.024	0.023
I	2.419	0.857	0.880	0.841
J	−0.863	−0.364	−0.314	−0.300
K	1.407	0.697	0.512	0.489
N	1.747	0.797	0.636	0.607
Q	−4.700	−1.264	−1.711	−1.634

These corrections can be excessive and Spiegelhalter recommends winsorising, for example, 10% of the outlier Z-scores. Clearly, this adjustment requires considerable expertise and will be beyond the scope of most hospital scientists. There are 10 hospitals in the example and to illustrate we winsorise the largest and smallest Z-scores (20% winsorising).

```
# Z-scores modified using 20% winsorising
Z1<-Z0
Z1[1]<-Z0[6]
Z1[10]<-Z0[2]
(mean(Z1^2))^.5 # Spiegelhalter's multiplicative correction

#[1] 1.7

sd(Z1) # Laney's correction

#[1] 1.8

ZHS1<-Z0/(mean(Z1^2))^.5
ZHL1<-Z0/sd(Z1)
data.frame(Z0,ZHS1,ZHL1)
```

	Z0	ZHS1	ZHL1
A	5.928	3.53	3.380
B	−2.035	−1.21	−1.160
E	−1.443	−0.86	−0.823
F	0.604	0.36	0.345
G	0.067	0.04	0.038
I	2.419	1.44	1.379
J	−0.863	−0.51	−0.492
K	1.407	0.84	0.802
N	1.747	1.04	0.996
Q	−4.700	−2.80	−2.679

These corrections are now more like those from a random effects logistic regression.

```
library(hglm)
h<-hglm(fixed=SSI~1,random=~1|Hospital,family=binomial(link=logit),
fix.disp=1,data=All)
```

```
ZH<-h$ranef/h$SeRe
H<-data.frame(Z0,ZHL1,ZH)
H # Z0 (Basic Z-scores), ZHL1 (Laney's correction with
winsorising), ZH (empirical Bayes random effects)
```

	Z0	ZHL1	ZH
A	5.92783301	3.37951606	3.6637585
B	−2.03541984	−1.16041292	−1.6827657
E	−1.44339214	−0.82289209	−1.2287119
F	0.60432864	0.34453372	0.3373963
G	0.06729646	0.03836637	−0.1533509
I	2.41850576	1.37881399	1.4696057
J	−0.86251894	−0.49173056	−0.7909855
K	1.40749594	0.80242731	0.9370932
N	1.74653449	0.99571654	1.1579940
Q	−4.69992412	−2.67947309	−3.5371427

Spiegelhalter[B,C] notes that with winsorising variances are underestimated but a correction factor does not appear to be used.

2

The analysis of aggregated binary data

Chapter 1 has dealt with grouped binary data. In this chapter we describe aggregated binary data. By this we mean data that come from a number of institutions (hospitals or units within them doing similar work) that we wish to summarise (Morton[E,F,I] and colleagues). The methods include the following:

```
A. Risk-adjustment,
B. Tabulations,
C. Confidence intervals and Z-scores,
D. Corrections for multiple testing,
E. Corrections for excessive variability(Overdispersion),
F. Funnel plots,
G. Random-effects (shrinkage) analysis,
      The lmer() and hglm() libraries in R
      The gamma-Poisson random-effects analysis in OpenBUGS.
```

Aggregated binary outcome data from several institutions or units within them are being analysed with increasing frequency and the results made public. Although it is arguably unlikely that evidence-based systems are much improved by this approach (Fung and colleagues, Ryan and colleagues), it is nevertheless desirable for accountability and transparency. In addition, as Evans and colleagues show, these data can have a useful research role for extending evidence provided epidemiologically sound and clinically relevant data are collected. This requires a rigorous method of collecting, managing and updating that evidence, for example, by using a Bayesian network (Waterhouse and colleagues).

Statistical Methods for Hospital Monitoring with R, First Edition. Anthony Morton, Kerrie Mengersen, Michael Whitby and George Playford.
© 2013 John Wiley & Sons, Ltd. Published 2013 by John Wiley & Sons, Ltd.

The presentation of aggregated data should follow a suitable pattern. Available methods include tabulations, multiple confidence intervals, Z-scores, funnel plots and random-effects (shrinkage) analysis. These data are increasingly risk-adjusted.

2.1   Risk-adjustment

Risk scores may be available, for example, as EuroSCORES for cardiac surgery or APACHE scores for ICU data, or risk-adjustment may need to be performed with available data. In the latter case, a common approach is to use a regression equation, for example, a logistic regression or, if there are few explanatory variables, risk scores may be obtained using stratification.

Available risk scores sometimes predict numbers of AEs that differ substantially from those of the group of hospitals or units of interest. In this case, it will often be desirable to re-calibrate the risk score for local use using logistic regression. We illustrate the derivation of risk scores for a series of orthopaedic SSIs and their re-calibration for a subset of the data used to derive the scores.

2.1.1   Using stratification

The data used to obtain the risk scores comprise 14,126 orthopaedic procedures performed between 2001 and 2006 (Morton[1] and colleagues). There were five procedures (PHR = partial hip replacement, THR = total hip replacement, RTHR = revision of total hip replacement, TKR = total knee replacement and RTKR = revision of total knee replacement). In addition, the CDC NNIS risk index (Horan and colleagues) has been used to stratify SSIs for each procedure into one of three risk categories (the NNIS risk index allocates 1 point if the operation is classified as either contaminated or dirty, 1 point if the patient has an American Society of Anesthesiologists (ASA) score above 2 indicating the presence of severe systemic disease and 1 point if the duration of the operation exceeds the 75th percentile for that procedure). There are thus potentially 15 risk categories. However, surveillance included few risk index two patients. The data are in orth0106.csv. The risk scores, obtained by stratification are shown in Table 2.1. Overall, there were 654 SSIs in 14,216 procedures, a crude rate of 4.6%. Due to small numbers and similar rates in several risk categories some amalgamation was required as shown in the last column of the table. The tabulations may be performed in R and the data can then be returned to a spreadsheet if required.

```
#data from orth0106.csv, the first column is not a date column
g.d()
```

```
Loading data.
Data from clipboard (C) or file (F) c
Do data column(s) have heading(s) (Y/N) y
Is column 1 a date column (Y/N) n
```

```
a<-rep(1,length(datain[,1]))
d<-data.frame(datain,a)
a<-as.data.frame(xtabs(d[,5]~d[,4]+d[,2]))
b<-as.data.frame(xtabs(d[,6]~d[,4]+d[,2]))
ab<-data.frame(a,b[,3])
```

```
e<-ab[,3]/ab[,4]
ssi<-data.frame(ab,e)
names(ssi)<-c("RIs","Procedure","SSI","Procedures","Proportion")
ssi
```

	RIs	Procedure	SSI	Procedures	Proportion
1	0	PHR	12	226	0.05309735
2	1	PHR	20	270	0.07407407
3	2	PHR	5	69	0.07246377
4	0	RTHR	25	364	0.06868132
5	1	RTHR	14	196	0.07142857
6	2	RTHR	3	39	0.07692308
7	0	RTKR	16	235	0.06808511
8	1	RTKR	15	135	0.11111111
9	2	RTKR	2	23	0.08695652
10	0	THR	127	3619	0.03509257
11	1	THR	79	1641	0.04814138
12	2	THR	21	201	0.10447761
13	0	TKR	199	4766	0.04175409
14	1	TKR	97	2102	0.04614653
15	2	TKR	19	240	0.07916667

```
#amalgamation of similar risk categories
Expected<-ssi[,5]
Expected[2:3]<-sum(ssi[2:3,3])/sum(ssi[2:3,4])
Expected[5:6]<-sum(ssi[5:6,3])/sum(ssi[5:6,4])
Expected[8:9]<-sum(ssi[8:9,3])/sum(ssi[8:9,4])
ssi<-data.frame(ssi[,-5],Expected)
ssi
```

	RIs	Procedure	SSI	Procedures	Expected
1	0	PHR	12	226	0.05309735
2	1	PHR	20	270	0.07374631
3	2	PHR	5	69	0.07374631
4	0	RTHR	25	364	0.06868132
5	1	RTHR	14	196	0.07234043
6	2	RTHR	3	39	0.07234043
7	0	RTKR	16	235	0.06808511
8	1	RTKR	15	135	0.10759494
9	2	RTKR	2	23	0.10759494
10	0	THR	127	3619	0.03509257
11	1	THR	79	1641	0.04814138
12	2	THR	21	201	0.10447761
13	0	TKR	199	4766	0.04175409
14	1	TKR	97	2102	0.04614653
15	2	TKR	19	240	0.07916667

```
#tabulation, rates (Table 1)
Rate<-ssi[,3]/ssi[,4]
Table1<-data.frame(ssi[,2],ssi[,1],ssi[,3:4],Rate,ssi[,5])
names(Table1)<-c("Procedure","RiskIndex","SSIs","Procedures","ObservedRate",
"StratumRate")
Table1
```

	Procedure	RiskIndex	SSIs	Procedurs	ObservedRate	StratumRate
				Table 2.1		
1	PHR	0	12	226	0.05309735	0.05309735
2	PHR	1	20	270	0.07407407	0.07374631
3	PHR	2	5	69	0.07246377	0.07374631
4	RTHR	0	25	364	0.06868132	0.06868132
5	RTHR	1	14	196	0.07142857	0.07234043
6	RTHR	2	3	39	0.07692308	0.07234043
7	RTKR	0	16	235	0.06808511	0.06808511
8	RTKR	1	15	135	0.11111111	0.10759494
9	RTKR	2	2	23	0.08695652	0.10759494
10	THR	0	127	3619	0.03509257	0.03509257
11	THR	1	79	1641	0.04814138	0.04814138
12	THR	2	21	201	0.10447761	0.10447761
13	TKR	0	199	4766	0.04175409	0.04175409
14	TKR	1	97	2102	0.04614653	0.04614653
15	TKR	2	19	240	0.07916667	0.07916667

```
# adding expected values to individual subject data
e<-ssi[,5]
RI<-rep(0,length(datain[,1]))
for (i in 1:length(datain[,1])){
if (datain[i,2]=="PHR"&datain[i,4]==0){RI[i]<-e[1]}
if (datain[i,2]=="PHR"&(datain[i,4]==1|datain[i,4]==2)){RI[i]<-e[2]}
if (datain[i,2]=="RTHR"&datain[i,4]==0){RI[i]<-e[4]}
if (datain[i,2]=="RTHR"&(datain[i,4]==1|datain[i,4]==2)){RI[i]<-e[5]}
if (datain[i,2]=="RTKR"&datain[i,4]==0){RI[i]<-e[7]}
if (datain[i,2]=="RTKR"&(datain[i,4]==1|datain[i,4]==2)){RI[i]<-e[8]}
if (datain[i,2]=="THR"&datain[i,4]==0){RI[i]<-e[10]}
if (datain[i,2]=="THR"&datain[i,4]==1){RI[i]<-e[11]}
if (datain[i,2]=="THR"&datain[i,4]==2){RI[i]<-e[12]}
if (datain[i,2]=="TKR"&datain[i,4]==0){RI[i]<-e[13]}
if (datain[i,2]=="TKR"&datain[i,4]==1){RI[i]<-e[14]}
if (datain[i,2]=="TKR"&datain[i,4]==2){RI[i]<-e[15]}
}
ssi0106<-data.frame(datain,RI)
head(ssi0106)
```

	Hospital	Procedure	ProcedureDate	RiskIndex	SSI	RI
1	A	TKR	01-Feb-2001	0	0	0.04175409
2	A	PHR	05-Feb-2001	1	0	0.07374631
3	A	TKR	07-Feb-2001	1	0	0.04614653
4	A	TKR	08-Feb-2001	1	0	0.04614653
5	A	THR	12-Feb-2001	0	0	0.03509257
6	A	TKR	14-Feb-2001	1	0	0.04614653

2.1.2   Using logistic regression

Logistic regression is commonly used to perform risk adjustment. A logistic regression analysis of the orth0106 data produces results that are similar to the stratification described above.

```
#logistic regression
#make large THR group reference group
```

```
datain$Procedure<-relevel(datain$Procedure,ref="THR")
g<-
glm(SSI~Procedure+as.factor(RiskIndex),family=binomial,data=datain)
#fitted values are in g$fitted
summary(g)

#Repeating the analysis with various amalgamations of Procedure,
for example amalgamating THR & TKR makes little difference
to the AIC value so the above analysis has been accepted.
```

	Estimate	Std. Error	z value	Pr(>|z|)	
(Intercept)	−3.24501	0.07533	−43.075	< 2e-16	***
ProcedurePHR	0.36613	0.18522	1.977	0.048076	*
ProcedureRTHR	0.52193	0.17421	2.996	0.002735	**
ProcedureRTKR	0.72045	0.19454	3.703	0.000213	***
ProcedureTKR	0.07100	0.08906	0.797	0.425327	
as.factor(RiskIndex)1	0.22053	0.08675	2.542	0.011022	*
as.factor(RiskIndex)2	0.74396	0.15884	4.684	2.82e-06	***

```
    Null deviance: 5296.3 on 14125 degrees of freedom
Residual deviance: 5249.6 on 14119 degrees of freedom
AIC: 5263.6
```

2.2   Discrimination and calibration

The utility of the risk adjustment is measured by its discrimination and calibration. The former refers to its ability to differentiate between those who have and those who do not have the AE and the latter to its ability to classify outcomes correctly. For example, if the risk adjustment predicts that 10% of patients with certain characteristics will have the AE, approximately 10% of patients with those characteristics should in fact be demonstrated to have the AE.

Figure 2.1 shows the discriminatory ability of the risk adjustment using logistic regression, measured by the area (AUC) under the receiver operating characteristic (ROC) curve. Its discriminatory ability (AUC = 0.57) with these data is little better than chance (0.5) (Clements and colleagues). This is not unexpected as NNIS risk adjustment for some SSIs is known to be

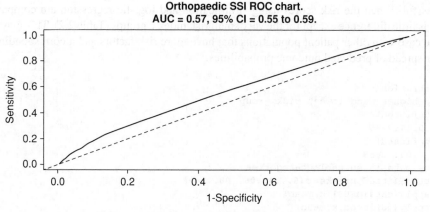

Figure 2.1   AUC chart.

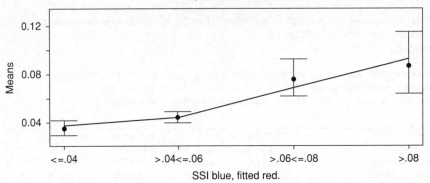

Figure 2.2   Calibration of SSI data.

only moderately successful, the procedures are related and the spread of predicted SSI values is very limited. Superior methods of risk adjustment for specific procedures are becoming available (Farsky and colleagues). However, we illustrate the analysis using these data and the NNIS risk index. The function rocchart() employs the method described by Altman[A] and colleagues.

```
# using function rocchart() to obtain AUC

rocchart(data.frame(datain$SSI,g$fitted)) # Figure 2.1

#Enter a name for the ROC chart Orthopaedic SSI
```

Calibration is usually performed by dividing the data in up to 10 ordered categories using the risk scores, and a goodness-of-fit test of the observed and expected numbers within the groups is frequently employed (Spiegelhalter[A]). Because, with the current data, the observed average outcome rate was about 5% and no risk group differed markedly from this, the calibration can only be illustrated using fewer categories. (Calibration and discrimination are further illustrated in section 3.9 of Chapter 3.) Figure 2.2 shows that calibration is moderately successful. When the risk scores using stratification and logistic regression are compared, there is little difference except for the very small risk index 2 groups (Table 2.2). This may not be the case with other patient populations that have more risk factors and a correspondingly larger spread of predicted outcome probabilities.

```
#Calibration
#find highest and lowest risk groups
max(g$fitted)
#[1] 0.1442285
min(g$fitted)
#[1] 0.03750659
#place data in suitable categories
k<-cut(g$fitted,breaks=c(0,.04,.06,.08,.16))
m<-tapply(datain$SSI,k,mean)
n<-tapply(g$fitted,k,mean)
lo<-tapply(datain$SSI,k,length)
```

```
ss<-tapply(datain$SSI,k,sum)
d<-data.frame(round(m,3),round(n,3),ss,round(n*10,0),10)
names(d)<-c("Observed","Expected","SSIs","Predicted","Procedures")
# Figure 2.2
#calculates precision limits for a column of proportions
a<-ss
b<-10
x<-length(a)
s<-0;l<-0;u<-0
ll<-0;uu<-0
for (i in 1:x){s[i]<-binom.test(a[i],b[i])$estimate
l[i]<-binom.test(a[i],b[i])$conf.int[1]
u[i]<-binom.test(a[i],b[i])$conf.int[2]
ll[i]<-binom.test(a[i],b[i],conf.level=.997)$conf.int[1]
uu[i]<-binom.test(a[i],b[i],conf.level=.997)$conf.int[2]
}
s1<-data.frame(s,l,ll,u,uu)
plot(m,axes=F,ylim=c(.025,.13),col="blue",lwd=2,pch=19,main="Orthopaedic
SSI Calibration.",xlab="SSI blue, Fitted red.",ylab="Means.")
box()
axis(side=1,labels=c("<=.04",">.04<=.06",">.06<=.08",">.08"),at=1:4)
axis(side=c(2,3,4))
lines(n,lwd=2,col="red")
arrows(1:4,l,1:4,u,angle=90,code=3,lwd=2,col="blue")

#goodness-of-fit using Figure 2.2 data (Spiegelhalter[A])
library(exactci)
Pval<-0
for (i in 1:x){Pval[i]<-binom.exact(a[i],b[i],n[i])$p.value}
z<--0.862+(0.743-2.404*log(Pval))^.5 # Bland and Altman
k<-sum(z^2)
p<-1-pchisq(k,3)
cat("Chi-squared=",round(k,3),", P-value=",round(p,3),".\n",sep="")
# Chi-squared=1.503,P-value=0.682.
```

Since there are potentially few ordered categories with these data, they have also been grouped by all 15 possible combinations (three risk indices, five procedures). Some amalgamation is needed because some categories have similar expected outcome probabilities or because numbers in the categories are small. In the logistic regression risk adjustment, RTHR risk index (RI) 1 and THR RI 2 have almost identical predicted values and are amalgamated. In addition PHR RI 2, RTHR RI 2 and RTKR RI 2 have very small numbers and are amalgamated with RTKR RI 1. Figure 2.3 shows the result. It is of note that the stratification and logistic regression predictions for the small RI 2 groups differed. When we concentrate on the 2005 and 2006 data (section 2.3 below), we observe that data in these risk categories were no longer being collected.

```
#goodness of fit using the categories from logistic regression
G<-round(g$fitted,4) #reduce lengths of fitted values
datain1<-data.frame(datain,G)
dd<-as.data.frame(xtabs(datain1[,6]~datain1[,2]+datain1[,4]))
y<-as.data.frame(xtabs(datain1[,5]~datain1[,2]+datain1[,4]))
yy<-rep(1,length(datain1[,1]))
y0<-as.data.frame(xtabs(yy~datain1[,2]+datain1[,4]))
ya<-dd[,3]/y0[,3]
```

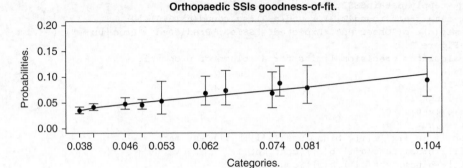

Figure 2.3   Goodness-of-fit SSI data.

```
dd<-data.frame(y,dd[,3],y0[,3],ya)
o<-order(ya)
dd<-dd[o,]
names(dd)<-c("Procedure","RI","Observed","Expected","Procedures",
"Probability")
row.names(dd)<-1:15
dd
```

	Procedure	RI	Observed	Expected	Procedures	Probability
1	THR	0	127	35.7125	3619	0.0375
2	TKR	0	199	91.5932	4766	0.0402
3	THR	1	79	75.9783	1641	0.0463
4	TKR	1	97	04.2592	2102	0.0496
5	PHR	0	12	12.0232	226	0.0532
6	RTHR	0	25	22.4224	364	0.0616
7	PHR	1	20	17.6850	270	0.0655
8	RTKR	0	16	17.4370	235	0.0742
9	RTHR	1	14	14.8372	196	0.0757
10	THR	2	21	15.2358	201	0.0758
11	TKR	2	19	19.4160	240	0.0809
12	RTKR	1	15	12.2580	135	0.0908
13	PHR	2	5	7.2933	69	0.1057
14	RTHR	2	3	4.7346	39	0.1214
15	RTKR	2	2	3.3166	23	0.1442

```
# amalgamating groups
Expected<-tapply(datain1[,6],datain1[,6],sum)
Observed<-tapply(datain1[,5],datain1[,6],sum)
Procedures<-tapply(datain1[,5],datain1[,6],length)
d<-data.frame(Observed,Procedures,Expected)
Probability<-as.numeric(row.names(d))
d<-data.frame(Probability,d)
row.names(d)<-1:15
#in d amalgamate rows 9 & 10 and 12 to 15
O<-c(Observed[1:8],sum(Observed[9:10]),Observed[11],sum(Observed[12:15]))
E<-c(Expected[1:8],sum(Expected[9:10]),Expected[11],sum(Expected[12:15]))
P<-c(Procedures[1:8],sum(Procedures[9:10]),Procedures[11],sum(Procedures
[12:15]))
```

```
# calculating goodness-of-fit
library(exactci)
Pval<-0
l<-length(O)
for (i in 1:l){Pval[i]<-binom.exact(O[i],P[i],E[i]/P[i])$p.value}
z<--0.862+(0.743-2.404*log(Pval))^.5
N0<-as.numeric(E)/as.numeric(P)
gof<-data.frame(N0,as.numeric(z))
names(gof)<-c("Rate","Z")
#goodness-of-fit test
k<-sum(z^2)
k # goodness-of-fit chi-squared
#[1] 2.845058
Pval<-1-pchisq(k,l-1)
Pval # goodness-of-fit P-value
# [1] 0.9848387

# Hosmer-Lemeshow test
library(MKmisc)
HLgof.test(datain1[,6],datain1[,5])$C
```

```
            Hosmer-Lemeshow C statistic
 X-squared = 0.9396, df = 3, p-value = 0.8159
```

```
# confidence limits for observed values, goodness of fit chart
a<-O
b<-P
x<-length(a)
s<-0;l<-0;u<-0
ll<-0;uu<-0
for (i in 1:x){s[i]<-binom.test(a[i],b[i])$estimate
l[i]<-binom.test(a[i],b[i])$conf.int[1]
u[i]<-binom.test(a[i],b[i])$conf.int[2]
ll[i]<-binom.test(a[i],b[i],conf.level=.997)$conf.int[1]
uu[i]<-binom.test(a[i],b[i],conf.level=.997)$conf.int[2]
}
sl<-data.frame(s,l,ll,u,uu)
Op<-O/P
Ep<-E/P
plot(Op~N0,ylim=c(0,.2),col="blue",pch=19,lwd=2,axes=F,main="Orthopaedic
SSIs goodness-of-fit.",xlab="Observed blue, Expected Red.",
ylab="Probabilities.")
box()
axis(side=1,labels=as.character(round(N0,3)),at=N0)
axis(side=c(2,3,4))
arrows(N0,l,N0,u,angle=90,code=3,length=.1,lwd=2,col="blue")
lines(Ep~N0,col="red",lwd=2)
mtext(side=1,line=2,"Categories.") # Figure 2.3
```

The standard libraries of R do not provide a Hosmer-Lemeshow goodness-of-fit test but it is available in the library MKmisc. A test described by Spiegelhalter[A] has also been employed; it does not suggest a poor fit.

The combination of poor discrimination and reasonable calibration appears to have occurred because, with an observed average outcome rate of about 5%, there are few risk groups and no risk group differed markedly from 5%. It would make little difference to the analysis of these data if risk-adjustment were not employed (Clements and colleagues). However, this will not always be the case, especially when complex SSI data are analysed as Anderson and colleagues have shown. In addition, including risk adjustment, even when it is only marginally successful (e.g. AUC greater than 0.6), can increase variation and widen the control limits in sequential cumulative observed minus expected (O-E) charts (Chapter 3) thereby reducing the risk of false signals. Risk adjustment is discussed further in Chapter 3. We employ it in the following analysis to illustrate the methods available.

2.3   Using 2005–06 data

We now examine the 2005–2006 data comprising 5,622 procedures with 227 SSIs (4%). These can be obtained from ssi0106. The stratification risk scores predicted 244.5 SSIs and the logistic regression predicted 244.8. Since the numbers of predicted and observed SSIs differed, these data can be used to illustrate recalibration. The R commands to achieve recalibration are now employed. The re-calibrated risk scores that now add up to 227 are in the data.frame ssi0506adj. If desired, they can be saved to a comma delimited csv file as there are too many rows for the R clipboard. The file can then be opened in a spreadsheet.

```
# SSI data for 2005-2006
LogistRI<-g$fitted # g$fitted from section 2.2 above
ssi0106a<-data.frame(ssi0106,LogistRI)
#dates are imported as factors, converts to dates & select 2005-6 data.
library(chron)
d<-ssi0106a[,3]
d[1] # see date format
#[1] 1-Feb-01
d<-chron(as.character(d),format="d-mmm-yy",out.format="dd-mmm-yyyy")
ssi0506<-ssi0106a[d>="01-Jan-2005",]
names(ssi0506)<-c("Hospital","Procedure","ProcedureDate","RiskIndex","SSI",
"StratRI","LogistRI")
#
length(ssi0506[,1])
#[1] 5622
sum(ssi0506[,5])
#[1] 227 #observed number of SSIs
227/5622
#[1] 0.04037709 #observed rate
sum(ssi0506[,6]) # expected from stratification risk scores
#[1] 244.4994
sum(ssi0506[,7]) # expected from logistic regression risk scores
#[1] 244.7513

#recalibration of stratification risk scores
g<-glm(ssi0506[,5]~ssi0506[,6],family=binomial)
StratRiskAdj<-g$fitted
# recalibration of logistic regression risk scores
g<-glm(ssi0506[,5]~ssi0506[,7],family=binomial)
LogistRiskAdj<-g$fitted
ssi0506adj<-data.frame(ssi0506[,-c(6,7)],StratRiskAdj,LogistRiskAdj)
row.names(ssi0506adj)<-1:length(ssi0506adj[,1])
```

2.3.1   Displaying and analysing data from multiple institutions

Simple tabulations are found to be very useful by many clinicians and are often under-utilised. Multiple confidence intervals (CIs) are often used, for example in league tables, but are best avoided, if possible (Adap and colleagues) unless appropriate adjustment is made for multiple comparisons. CIs provide precision estimates and usually employ only the data for the hospital or unit of interest whereas it is important to view it as a member of a group of institutions. In addition, there is the related issue of false discovery described in section 2.3.3.3 of this chapter. If there is a mean or reference value, approximately one in 20 intervals may on average exclude that value by chance when a 95% interval is employed.

Funnel plots are arguably more useful than CIs as they employ all the data to obtain more stable estimates of mean values and prediction intervals. This may be accomplished by employing risk-adjusted rates (RARs) obtained by indirect standardisation. However, these may overestimate rates when samples are small, and excessive variability (overdispersion) due to patient and institution differences may be a problem that can only partially be overcome with risk-adjustment. In addition, when there are many institutions, there may also be apparent outliers that are due to chance leading to false discovery discussed in section 2.3.3.3 of this chapter. Funnel plots are easy to use, they do not require specialised software and they are well received by clinical staff. They are ideal for initial data screening of aggregated binary data. Provided results that appear abnormal are used to pinpoint potential problem areas for systems analysis using for example, M&M audits and are subjected to the analysis advocated by Lilford and colleagues and Mohammed[B] and colleagues, false discovery should not be a serious problem. They recommend that we should first look for data or analysis error, then problems with risk adjustment, followed by system (structure and process) errors, and finally problems involving staff. If a judgemental approach cannot be avoided, it is probably wise to concentrate on three standard deviation equivalent limits but with small samples this may miss differences that warrant further scrutiny, for example, by using an M&M audit.

The use of RARs with risk-adjusted count data can be biased as we describe for bacteraemia (count) data analysis in Chapter 5. It is possible that this problem may also occur with binary data if the denominators and the risk scores differ markedly among the institutions (Morton[E] and colleagues). When this occurs, it will be preferable to employ Observed/Expected ratios (Standardized Morbidity Ratios or SMRs). Since one is the usual reference value for an SMR, the advantage of using the RARs, their weighted mean and intervals based on it is then lost. However the expected values that form the SMR denominators and that are derived from the risk adjustment scores enable it to have a useful interpretation. If the risk adjustment scores are suitably recalibrated for the group of institutions of interest, an average SMR of one will be expected. When RARs are used the horizontal axis of the funnel plot can be the number of procedures or the institutions sorted by the number of procedures. For the SMR, the horizontal axis must be the expected number of AEs or the institutions sorted by the expected number of AEs. We describe both approaches for binary data in this chapter.

Random-effects (shrinkage) analysis assumes that the institutions of interest can be considered as a collection of institutions having their own distribution. By borrowing strength from the overall distribution, the predicted rate for small institutions is improved. This analysis may usefully be performed if the funnel plot suggests the presence of one or more outliers. However, should the shrinkage analysis also indicate a definite outlier, it is reasonable to assume that it might not be part of the collection and its accompanying distribution. It might therefore not be exchangeable (section 1.6 of Chapter 1). Consideration could be given to removing the outlier and repeating the analysis. The outlier's data should then be audited, bearing in mind the advice of Mohammed[B] and colleagues first to check the data, then the analysis, then the system and lastly the practitioners. The book by Winkel and Zhang discusses the use of hierarchical (random effects) models in QI.

An issue of importance is the influence of variability in the risk-adjustment probabilities. Expected values are often considered as being free of error. This may be the case with large independently derived risk-scores such as EuroSCORE or APACHE score, provided they do not require re-calibration, but it is unlikely to be so when smaller local databases are employed. A further difficulty arises when the institution of interest is also a contributor to the risk-score as there will then be covariation that may be important when that institution provides a large proportion of the data used to calculate the risk scores. There is a further note on this subject in section 2.4 of this chapter. Until further work is done in this area, it is probably wise to regard SMR confidence (precision) and control (prediction) limits as probably being too narrow. However, as Nelson has described, control charts are meant to be practically useful process-improvement tools, not exact statistical tests. If, with our aggregated data, we concentrate on 2.5 or 3 standard deviation equivalent limits (approximately 99% or 99.7%) and use the analysis to learn how to practice more safely, the slightly narrow control limits should not be a serious problem.

2.3.2   Tabulations

Tabulations are valuable for preliminary data analysis. When there are several institutions, it is useful to tabulate the data by institution and by year. Depending on the volume of data, tabulations by half-years, quarters, months or weeks may also be useful, although weekly data are often unstable, as well as sparse, and there are often delays when ordering tests and receiving results. Tabulations by institution and time-period are often too large for displaying in reports but can be valuable for scrolling through to detect institutional data requiring further scrutiny. It is also often useful to incorporate test statistics such as Z-scores. For example, if it is of interest to distinguish time periods in which to search for runs, the Z-scores corresponding to this test could be included; time periods with Z-scores greater than two can be further investigated using a CUSUM. (Note that if there are for example, 12 institutions and 12 outcomes of interest, performing 144 CUSUM charts, most of which would show no abnormality but several might result in false discovery, is to be avoided.) One should look for contiguous time-periods when the observed outcomes exceed their expected values as this may suggest the need for a cumulative observed minus expected chart that incorporates a CUSUM (Chapter 3). Tabulations are also valuable for presenting data to central authorities and the staff of institutions. Beware of persistently low values; they may indicate under-reporting.

Tabulations can be performed using a spreadsheet, for example in an Excel Pivot Table or in a OpenOffice Calc DataPilot. Here we concentrate on using R. Table 2.2 shows the data by hospital or unit, Table 2.3 by quarters and Table 2.4 shows the data for selected hospitals by quarters for the most recent year. There are several apparent outliers in Table 2.2. Post-discharge SSIs have been included. The collection of post-discharge SSI data was not mandatory resulting in variable collection of those data. In addition, it is known that it can be difficult to detect post-discharge superficial SSI data accurately (Whitby and colleagues). These difficulties may account for much of the variability. In addition, tables like Table 2.4

can have a large number of cells if data from every institution are included making them too cluttered for display in a report. For reporting, it will often be best to concentrate on a subset of institutions of interest and use only most recent data. We include some scripts in the internet code file for additional tabulations.

```
# table 2.2 data by hospitals
ssi0506adj<-ssi0506adj[,c(1,3,5,6,7)]
a<-as.data.frame(xtabs(ssi0506adj[,3]~ ssi0506adj[,1]))
b1<-as.data.frame(xtabs(ssi0506adj[,4]~ ssi0506adj[,1]))
b2<-as.data.frame(xtabs(ssi0506adj[,5]~ ssi0506adj [,1]))
b3<-tapply(ssi0506adj[,1], ssi0506adj[,1],length)
Table<-data.frame(a,b3,round(b1[,2],1),round(b2[2],1))
names(Table)<-c("Hospital","SSIs","Procedures","StratExp","LogisExp")
row.names(Table)<-1:length(Table[,1])
TB<-data.frame("Total",sum(Table[,2]),sum(Table[,3]),round(sum(Table[,4])),
round(sum(Table[,5])))
names(TB)<-c("Hospital","SSIs","Procedures","StratExp","LogisExp")
Table<-rbind(Table,TB)
Table
```

	Hospital	SSIs	Procedures	StratExp	LogisExp
			Table 2.2		
1	A	20	242	10.0	10.0
2	B	13	391	16.0	16.0
3	C	6	279	10.8	10.9
4	D	9	285	11.8	11.8
5	E	22	416	16.5	16.5
6	F	11	178	7.2	7.2
7	G	33	1008	39.4	39.4
8	H	5	121	4.9	4.8
9	I	25	365	15.9	15.8
10	J	15	303	12.0	12.0
11	K	12	245	10.0	10.0
12	L	1	108	4.4	4.4
13	M	2	26	1.0	1.0
14	N	17	283	11.8	11.8
15	O	1	170	6.9	7.0
16	P	4	41	1.6	1.6
17	Q	25	949	38.0	38.0
18	R	6	212	8.6	8.6
19	Total	227	5622	227.0	227.0

```
# table 2.3, data aggregated by quarters
library(chron)
d<-chron(as.character(ssi0506adj[,2]),format="dd-mmm-yyyy",out.format=
"dd-mmm-yyyy")
# date format is for eg 31-Dec-2006
Year<-years(d)
m<-as.numeric(months(d))
Qtrs<-rep(0,length(m))
Qtrs[m>=1&m<=3]<-1
Qtrs[m>=4&m<=6]<-2
Qtrs[m>=7&m<=9]<-3
```

```
Qtrs[m>=10&m<=12]<-4
Table3a<-as.data.frame(xtabs(ssi0506adj[,3]~Qtrs+Year))
Table3b<-as.data.frame(xtabs(ssi0506adj[,4]~Qtrs+Year))
Q<-rep(1,length(ssi0506adj[,1]))
Table3c<-as.data.frame(xtabs(Q~Qtrs+Year))
Table<-data.frame(Table3a[,2],Table3a[,1],Table3a[,3],Table3c[,3],
round(Table3b[,3],1))
names(Table)<-c("Years","Quarters","SSIs","Procedures","Expected")
TB<-data.frame("0506","All",sum(Table[,3]),sum(Table[,4]),round(sum
(Table[,5])))
names(TB)<-c("Years","Quarters","SSIs","Procedures","Expected")
Table<-rbind(Table,TB)
Table
```

	Years	Quarters	SSIs	Procedures	Expected
			Table 2.3		
1	2005	1	31	668	26.8
2	2005	2	38	759	30.6
3	2005	3	28	682	27.5
4	2005	4	26	664	26.8
5	2006	1	24	585	23.6
6	2006	2	20	740	30.0
7	2006	3	30	786	32.0
8	2006	4	30	738	29.8
9	0506	All	227	5622	227.0

```
#Table 2.4 for selected hospitals in 2006
library(chron)
h<-ssi0506adj[,1]
d<-chron(as.character(ssi0506adj[,2]),format="dd-mmm-yyyy",out.format=
"dd-mmm-yyyy")
f<-ssi0506adj[,3]
e<-ssi0506adj[,4]
h06<-h[years(d)==2006]
d06<-d[years(d)==2006]
f06<-f[years(d)==2006]
e06<-e[years(d)==2006]
m<-as.numeric(months(d06))
Qtrs<-rep(0,length(m))
Qtrs[m>=1&m<=3]<-1
Qtrs[m>=4&m<=6]<-2
Qtrs[m>=7&m<=9]<-3
Qtrs[m>=10&m<=12]<-4
Table4a<-as.data.frame(xtabs(f06~Qtrs+h06))
Table4b<-as.data.frame(xtabs(e06~Qtrs+h06))
n06<-rep(1,length(h06))
Table4c<-as.data.frame(xtabs(n06~Qtrs+h06))
Table4d<-data.frame(Table4a,Table4c[,3],round(Table4b[,3],1))
Table<-Table4d[Table4d[,2]=="A"|Table4d[,2]=="E"|Table4d[,2]=="F"|Table4d
[,2]=="I"|Table4d[,2]=="N",]
names(Table)<-c("Quarters","Hospital","SSIs","Procedures","Expected")
Table<-Table[,c(2,1,3,4,5)]
TB<-data.frame("Selected","Totals",sum(Table[,3]),sum(Table[,4]),round(sum
(Table[,5])))
```

```
names(TB)<-c("Hospital","Quarters","SSIs","Procedures","Expected")
Table<-rbind(Table,TB)
row.names(Table)<-1: length(Table[,1])
Table #2006 data selected hospitals
```

	Hospital	Quarters	SSIs	Procedures	Expected
			Table 2.4		
1	A	1	0	0	0.0
2	A	2	2	31	1.3
3	A	3	4	40	1.7
4	A	4	0	36	1.4
5	E	1	3	37	1.5
6	E	2	0	37	1.5
7	E	3	3	50	2.0
8	E	4	5	51	2.0
9	F	1	0	19	0.8
10	F	2	3	20	0.8
11	F	3	1	20	0.8
12	F	4	2	27	1.1
13	I	1	5	50	2.2
14	I	2	0	54	2.4
15	I	3	3	39	1.8
16	I	4	4	42	1.9
17	N	1	2	28	1.1
18	N	2	0	39	1.6
19	N	3	2	45	1.9
20	N	4	4	45	1.9
21	Selected	Totals	43	710	30.0

2.3.2.1 Tables in wide format, using the reshape() command

Tabular data may be exported to office software for formatting via the clipboard using s.d().
However, it may be useful to display them in R in wide format using the reshape() and stack()
commands.

```
#wide format using reshape() and stack() commands
Tables<-Table[-length(Table[,1]),] # removes Totals row
names(Tables)<-c("Hosp","Quarter","AE","Ops","Exp")
d<-data.frame(rep(Tables[,1],3),rep(Tables[,2],3))
s<-stack(Tables[,c(3,4,5)])
e<-data.frame(d,s)
names(e)<-c("Hosp","Qtr","Dta","Cat")
f<-reshape(e,direction="wide",timevar="Qtr",idvar=c("Cat","Hosp"))
a<-f[f[,1]==f[1,1],]
for (i in 2:5){a<-rbind(a,f[f[,1]==f[i,1],])}
a[,3:6]<-round(a[,3:6],0)
row.names(a)<-NULL
names(a)<-c("Hosp","Cat","Qtr1","Qtr2","Qtr3","Qtr4")
Tot<-0
for (i in 1:15){Tot[i]<-sum(a[i,3:6])}
Tbl<-data.frame(a,Tot)
Tbl # the expected values are rounded, may not add up exactly
```

	Hosp	Cat	Qtr1	Qtr2	Qtr3	Qtr4	Tot
1	A	AE	0	2	4	0	6
2	A	Ops	0	31	40	36	107
3	A	Exp	0	1	2	1	4
4	E	AE	3	0	3	5	11
5	E	Ops	37	37	50	51	175
6	E	Exp	2	2	2	2	8
7	F	AE	0	3	1	2	6
8	F	Ops	19	20	20	27	86
9	F	Exp	1	1	1	1	4
10	I	AE	5	0	3	4	12
11	I	Ops	50	54	39	42	185
12	I	Exp	2	2	2	2	8
13	N	AE	2	0	2	4	8
14	N	Ops	28	39	45	45	157
15	N	Exp	1	2	2	2	7

2.3.2.2 Adding Z-scores

As discussed above, it is often useful when undertaking preliminary analysis of aggregated among institution data to display Z-scores (observed/expected differences converted to standard normal deviates). Differences that exceed the equivalent of two SD or runs of positive observed minus expected differences may indicate where more detailed data analysis should be concentrated. It is also worthwhile to scrutinise the data when the observed count is substantially below the expected count as this may be due to under-reporting. We repeat the analysis for Table 2.2 but add Z-scores. As described below, an adjustment for multiple comparisons, for example, using a Benjamini-Hochberg procedure, may be added when there are many institutions (Jones and colleagues). We note in Chapter 1 that comparisons of hospitals are frequently advocated. Since they are frequently members of a group of hospitals, consideration should be given to adjustments for multiple significance testing, for example, by using the Benjamini-Hochberg procedure.

```
# including Z-scores
library(exactci)
a<-as.data.frame(xtabs(ssi0506adj[,3]~ssi0506adj[,1]))
b1<-as.data.frame(xtabs(ssi0506adj[,4]~ssi0506adj[,1]))
b2<-tapply(ssi0506adj[,1],ssi0506adj[,1],length)
Table<-data.frame(a,b2,b1[,2])
Rate<-Table[,2]/Table[,3]
Expected<-Table[,4]/Table[,3]
Z<-0;p<-0
for (i in 1:length(Table[,1])){p[i]<-binom.exact(Table[i,2],Table[i,3],
Expected[i])$p.value;if(Rate[i]>Expected[i]){Z[i]<--
qnorm(p[i]/2)}else{Z[i]<-qnorm(p[i]/2)}}
Table<-data.frame(Table,round(Rate,4),round(Expected,4),round(p,3),
round(Z,2))
names(Table)<-c("Hospital","SSIs","Procedures","StratExp","ObsRate",
"ExpRate","P-Value","Z-Score")
row.names(Table)<-1:length(Table[,1])
Table
```

	Hospital	SSIs	Procedures	StratExp	ObsRate	ExpRate	P-Value	Z-Score
1	A	20	242	10.0220	0.0826	0.0414	0.006	2.76
2	B	13	391	15.9669	0.0332	0.0408	0.544	−0.61
3	C	6	279	10.8378	0.0215	0.0388	0.163	−1.40
4	D	9	285	11.8021	0.0316	0.0414	0.509	−0.66
5	E	22	416	16.4898	0.0529	0.0396	0.214	1.24
6	F	11	178	7.2150	0.0618	0.0405	0.220	1.23
7	G	33	1008	39.3593	0.0327	0.0390	0.342	−0.95
8	H	5	121	4.8719	0.0413	0.0403	1.000	0.00
9	I	25	365	15.9136	0.0685	0.0436	0.037	2.08
10	J	15	303	12.0453	0.0495	0.0398	0.457	0.74
11	K	12	245	10.0189	0.0490	0.0409	0.606	0.52
12	L	1	108	4.3759	0.0093	0.0405	0.128	−1.52
13	M	2	26	1.0121	0.0769	0.0389	0.537	0.62
14	N	17	283	11.8290	0.0601	0.0418	0.175	1.35
15	O	1	170	6.8974	0.0059	0.0406	0.014	−2.45
16	P	4	41	1.6281	0.0976	0.0397	0.158	1.41
17	Q	25	949	37.9675	0.0263	0.0400	0.030	−2.16
18	R	6	212	8.5756	0.0283	0.0405	0.485	−0.70

Further examples are provided in Appendix 1. These will often produce tables that are too large for publication in a report but may prove useful for deciding which data should be selected for further analysis, for example, by employing a cumulative observed minus expected plus CUSUM chart described in Chapter 3. Although too large for publication, they can be scrolled through on the computer screen to search for high Z-scores or runs of positive observed minus expected values in time series data (i.e. sequences of positive Z-scores).

2.3.3   Funnel plot and plot of multiple confidence intervals

Multiple confidence intervals are often employed, for example, in league tables. Although we have noted that this method of display is open to misinterpretation through inappropriate multiple comparisons (Adap and colleagues) we include an example (Figure 2.4).

```
# Figure 2.4, mltiple confidence intervals
ssi<-tapply(ssi0506adj[,3],ssi0506adj[,1],sum)
proc<-tapply(ssi0506adj[,3],ssi0506adj[,1],length)
exp<-tapply(ssi0506adj[,4],ssi0506adj[,1],sum)
```

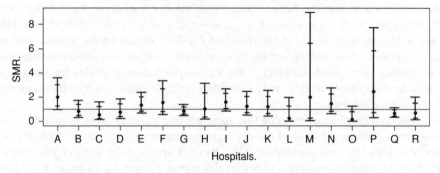

Figure 2.4   Chart employing multiple confidence intervals.

```
orthssi<-data.frame(names(ssi),as.numeric(ssi),as.numeric(proc),as.numeric
(exp))
names(orthssi)<-c("Hospital","SSI","Procedures","Expected")
a<- orthssi[,2]
b<- orthssi[,3]
x<-length(a)
s<-0;l<-0;u<-0
ll<-0;uu<-0
for (i in 1:x){s[i]<-binom.test(a[i],b[i])$estimate
l[i]<-binom.test(a[i],b[i])$conf.int[1]
u[i]<-binom.test(a[i],b[i])$conf.int[2]
ll[i]<-binom.test(a[i],b[i],conf.level=.997)$conf.int[1]
uu[i]<-binom.test(a[i],b[i],conf.level=.997)$conf.int[2]
}
ss<-data.frame(s,l,ll,u,uu)
oe<-orthssi[,2]/orthssi[,4]
u95<-orthssi[,3]*ss[,4]/orthssi[,4]
u997<-orthssi[,3]*ss[,5]/orthssi[,4]
l95<-orthssi[,3]*ss[,2]/orthssi[,4]
l997<-orthssi[,3]*ss[,3]/orthssi[,4]
mi<-min(c(oe,l997))
ma<-max(c(oe,u997))
n<-orthssi[,1]
par(xaxs="r")
plot(oe,axes=F,col="blue",pch=19,ylim=c(mi,ma),xlab="Hospitals.",
ylab="SMR.",main="Orthopaedic SSI SMR Multiple Confidence Limits.")
box()
abline(h=1)
axis(side=1,labels=n,at=1:length(n))
axis(side=c(2,3,4))
arrows(1:length(n),as.numeric(l95),1:length(n),as.numeric(u95),angle=90,
code=3,col="blue",lwd=2,length=.05)
arrows(1:length(n),as.numeric(l997),1:length(n),as.numeric(u997),angle=90,
code=3,col="blue",lwd=2,length=.1)
```

2.3.3.1 Funnel plot

Currently, the funnel plot is one of the preferred methods for the display of binary data from multiple institutions, ideal for initial screening of among hospital or unit data. These data are increasingly risk-adjusted. The binary data funnel plot is simply a Shewhart type control chart that has the institutions on the horizontal axis instead of times. These are sorted from smallest to largest to give the funnel effect as the smaller institutions have wider control limits. When the data are risk-adjusted, it is convenient to employ risk-adjusted rates. Hart[A] and her colleagues suggest that the mid-line of the chart should be the weighted average of the risk-adjusted rates and we employ this approach. Comparisons with the standard rate may sometimes be required. However, when the weighted average differs from a standard rate, consideration should be given to re-calibrating the risk-adjustment data for the group of institutions being studied.

An important consideration is that this approach uses the equivalent of indirectly standardised rates. These may be biased when risk groups among the institutions of interest differ markedly in both size and expectation. This does not appear to be a major problem with binary data but it can cause serious bias with risk adjusted count, for example, bacteraemia data (Morton[E] and colleagues). When binary data are grouped, for example by hospital, it is possible that this problem could occur if there are markedly differing sized groups and institutions that treat patients with very different risk profiles.

2.3.3.2   Using indirect standardisation

Indirect standardisation proceeds by calculating the observed (O) and expected (E) outcome numbers and determining a SMR (O/E) for each hospital. This is then multiplied by an overall average value to obtain a risk-adjusted rate that is then plotted for the hospital concerned. If E for any institution is very small, for example less than one, the O/E ratio may become very large and produce a spurious result; if this should occur, the analysis should be repeated with this institution's data removed and subjected to audit. The centre line of the chart is the weighted average of the risk-adjusted rates. Exact binomial control limits for the weighted average of the risk-adjusted rates are calculated for each hospital's procedure numbers using the pbeta() function in R. Control (prediction) limits and not confidence (precision) limits are used and this requires the implementation of a simple numerical search. If π_i is the expected outcome probability for the ith subject, these limits are often calculated from the variance obtained when the $\sum \pi_i \times (1-\pi_i)$ values for each institution are added. However, Hart[A] and colleagues have indicated that this may give limits that are too narrow. The method described by those authors appears to give satisfactory approximations.

If O_i is the outcome for the ith subject, E_i is the expected outcome probability for that subject and Ebar is an overall average outcome rate, the value for institution J is $A_J = (\sum_J O_i / \sum_J E_i) \times Ebar$ and the centre line is either $CL = \sum (n_J \times A_J) / \sum n_J$ (weighted average) or CL=Ebar (standard), where n_J is the sample size for institution J. The 2 sigma equivalent control limits are calculated for institution J by finding the values of x_J such that pbeta(CL,x_J,n_J-x_{J+1})=.02275 for the upper limit and 1-pbeta(CL,x_{J+1},n_J-x_J)=.02275 for the lower limit using the weighted average centre line. These must be found by trial and error or by implementing a simple numerical search, for example, for the upper limit x_j is increased progressively by one starting at x_j=round(CL×n_J) until pbeta(CL,x_J,n_J-x_{J+1})<.02275, and then decreased by .001 until pbeta(CL,x_J,n_J-x_{J+1})>=.02275. The required limit is then x_J/n_J. The process is repeated for the three sigma equivalent limits.

Figures 2.5 and 2.6 are funnel plots for the orthopaedic SSI data for 2005–06 with the weighted average as the midline and Figure 2.4 is a plot in which multiple confidence intervals

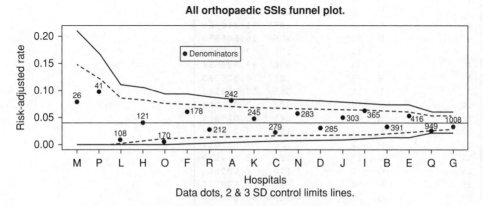

Figure 2.5   RAR funnel plot, hospitals on horizontal axis.

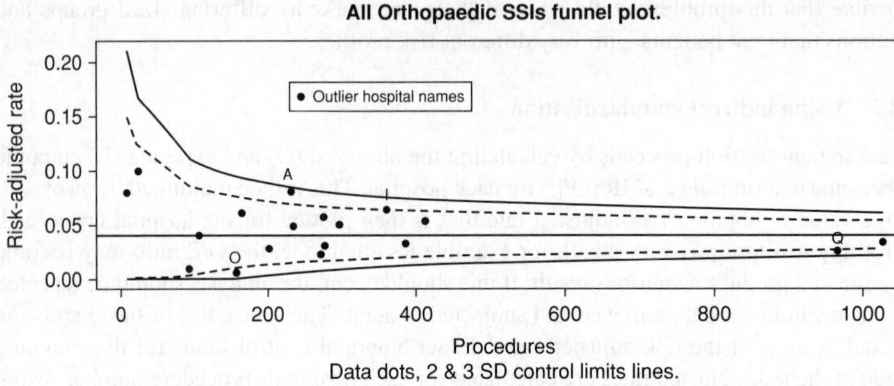

All Orthopaedic SSIs funnel plot.

Procedures
Data dots, 2 & 3 SD control limits lines.

Figure 2.6   RAR funnel plot, procedure numbers on horizontal axis.

(CIs) have been employed. Figures 2.4 and 2.5 have the individual units or hospitals on the horizontal axis. Figure 2.6 has the procedure denominators on the horizontal axis and the outlier hospital identifiers as labels. There are two possible high outliers. To perform the analysis, we use the data in ssi0506adj.csv. These data are copied to the clipboard and transferred to R. The functions bgroupfunnelinstitution() and bgroupfunnelprocedure() perform the analyses with individual units or hospitals, and with procedure denominators on the horizontal axis respectively. Since bgroupfunnelinstitution() and bgroupfunnelprocedure() are unwieldy words, it may be useful to type ls() and RETURN/ENTER at the R prompt, select bgroupfunnelinstitution() or bgroupfunnelprocedure() without the quotes with the mouse and employ Edit and then Copy and Paste to get bgroupfunnelinstitution() or bgroupfunnelprocedure() to the R prompt.

```
# Figure 2.5, using function bgroupfunnelinstitution()
bgroupfunnelinstitution(ssi0506adj[,c(1,3,4)])

# Do you have risk-adjusted data (Y/N) y
```

	Institution	AE	Procedures	Expected
1	A	20	242	10.029302
2	B	13	391	15.977033
3	C	6	279	10.847761
4	D	9	285	11.810966
5	E	22	416	16.503550
6	F	11	178	7.220485
7	G	33	1008	39.394534
8	H	5	121	4.875080
9	I	25	365	15.918948
10	J	15	303	12.056249
11	K	12	245	10.025868
12	L	1	108	4.378924
13	M	2	26	1.013034
14	N	17	283	11.834979
15	O	1	170	6.900853
16	P	4	41	1.629746
17	Q	25	949	38.000904
18	R	6	212	8.581781

```
Chart heading.
Enter heading for chart All Orthopaedic SSIs
X-axis heading.
Enter an X-axis heading Hospitals
```

Place the locator() cross on a clear part of the chart and press the left mouse button.

```
#Figure 2.6, procedure numbers on horizontal axis
bgroupfunnelprocedure(ssi0506adj[,c(1,3,4)])
#
# Do you have risk-adjusted data (Y/N) y
```

```
Chart heading.
Enter heading for chart All Orthopaedic SSIs
X-axis heading.
Enter an X-axis heading Procedures
```

Place the locator() cross on a clear area of the chart and press the left mouse button.

Funnel plots can be used for screening institutions to detect those requiring more rigorous study, for example, by audit. A difficulty is that when data from a number of institutions undergo analysis by a central authority, the possibility of data error is increased. In addition, it should be noted that it is possible to have a run of unsatisfactory outcomes that require investigation and that do not show up in funnel plots, especially if outcomes are otherwise good. The longer the period of observation, the greater the possibility of this occurring, hence the desirability of concomitant tabulations and control charts. Another problem with this chart is that, by the time the often yearly data are analysed and the result disseminated, any revealed problem may have occurred so long ago that finding its causes may be impossible. Finally, when data are employed in a judgemental way by central authorities, gaming can make them useless for learning how to improve.

Funnel plots should be based on the most recent data possible. Unfortunately, with many outcomes, all but the largest hospitals may have an insufficient volume of relevant subjects for funnel plots to be based only on the very recent data. In spite of the difficulties we describe, transparency and accountability are essential for satisfactory patient care and public reporting of hospital AE data provides a needed discipline. Funnel plots are useful for the display of these data.

It is imperative that suitable tables and charts that display monthly or quarterly data accompany funnel plots. Preferably, these should be performed by the staff of the individual institutions if the necessary expertise exists locally and there should be a determined focus on using data sequentially to learn how to improve. Changes will then be detected more promptly and local ownership should ensure accuracy.

Ownership is a powerful motivating force; it is preferable especially in larger institutions that whenever possible, sequential data analysis is performed locally. It is therefore important to train institution staff to undertake their own sequential within institution analysis, for example with tabulations and CUSUM and cumulative observed minus expected (O-E) charts. Institutions could then be subject to disciplinary action if (1) tabulations and charts were not maintained and aberrant results were not reported, (2) signals occurred that were not investigated or (3) systems problems that were revealed by an investigation were not dealt with. However, the emphasis should always be on using data to learn how to do better and central authorities should make every effort to act as coaches helping institution staff to improve rather than adopting the role of judges of performance.

Among institution funnel plots may tell us that there may be a problem; they do not tell us there definitely is a problem nor do they give any indication of the cause of a possible problem. These questions can only be answered by undertaking an analysis of the underlying system. Lilford and colleagues and Mohammed[B] and colleagues provide a template for investigating outliers: these workers recommend that we should first look for data or analysis error, then problems with risk adjustment, followed by system errors, and finally for problems involving staff. In addition, funnel plots may miss a problem completely or detect it at a time that is too late to identify causes if sequential methods are not also employed.

The funnel plot described above that employs indirect standardisation is a multiplicative plot. Hart[A] and colleagues also describe an additive plot for the observed and expected differences. However, the multiplicative plot in various forms is in wide use so we do not describe the additive plot. It is desirable to use the minimum number of plots that analyze the data clearly as the use of many charts increases the likelihood of false positive signals.

Overdispersion can be an issue with funnel plots, especially for very large data sets like those involving many hospitals, because risk-adjustment cannot deal with all between-patient heterogeneity. Spiegelhalter[B,C,D] and Mohammed[A] and Laney have described methods to deal with this problem. We illustrate Laney's method together with winsorising in Chapters 5 and 6. Examination of funnel and shrinkage plots (section 2.3.3.5 of this chapter) enables heterogeneity, especially in the former, to be studied more closely. We believe that it should be investigated. Approaches to investigating heterogeneity are described by Mohammed[B] and colleagues and Spiegelhalter[B,C,D]. We do not routinely include adjustments for overdispersion in binary data funnel plots.

2.3.3.3   False discovery

Jones and colleagues address the issue of false discovery. Figure 2.7 is a chart of Z-scores adjusted using the Benjamini-Hochberg procedure (see section 5.1 of Chapter 5 and Figure 5.10 for a funnel plot that incorporates an adjustment for false discovery). Risk adjusted rates and their weighted average were employed to obtain the P-values and Z-scores for Figure 2.7.

```
# Figure 2.7, dealing with false discovery
#using indirectly standardized rates
```

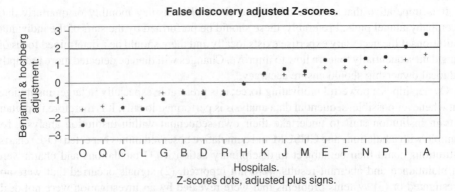

Figure 2.7   False-discovery adjusted Z-scores.

```
ssi<-tapply(ssi0506adj[,3], ssi0506adj[,1],sum)
proc<-tapply(ssi0506adj[,3], ssi0506adj[,1],length)
exp<-tapply(ssi0506adj[,4], ssi0506adj[,1],sum)
orthssi<-data.frame(names(ssi),as.numeric(ssi),as.numeric(proc),as.numeric
(exp))
names(orthssi)<-c("Hospital","SSI","Procedures","Expected")
hosp<-orthssi[,1]
ssi<-orthssi[,2]
proc<-orthssi[,3]
exp<-orthssi[,4]
oe<-ssi/exp
mrar<-sum(exp)/sum(proc)
rar<-oe*mrar
raravg<-sum(rar*proc)/sum(proc)
k<-0
for (i in 1:length(proc)){if (rar[i]>raravg){k[i]<-
pbeta(raravg,proc[i]*rar[i],proc[i]-proc[i]*rar[i]+1)}else{k[i]<-1-
pbeta(raravg,proc[i]*rar[i]+1,proc[i]-proc[i]*rar[i])}}
k<-2*k #two-sided P-values
padj<-p.adjust(k,"BH") # adjusted P-values
q<-0;qq<-0
for (i in 1:length(proc)){if (rar[i]>raravg){q[i]<--
qnorm(padj[i]/2); qq[i]<--qnorm(k[i]/2)}else{q[i]<-qnorm(padj[i]/2);qq[i]<-
qnorm(k[i]/2)}} #Z-scores for adjusted P-values
o<-order(q)
q0<-q[o]
hosp0<-hosp[o]
ko<-qq[o]
plot(q0,type="p",lwd=2,pch=19,col="dark blue",axes=F,ylim=c(-3,3),
xlab="Z-scores red, Adjusted blue.",
ylab="Benjamini & Hochberg Adjustment.",
main="False Discovery Adjusted Z-scores.")
box()
axis(side=1,tick=T,labels=hosp0,at=1:length(hosp0))
axis(side=c(2,3,4))
points(ko,lwd=2,col="red")
abline(h=0)
abline(h=1.96,lwd=2,col="black")
abline(h=-1.96,lwd=2,col="black")
mtext(side=1,line=2,"Hospitals.")
```

2.3.3.4 Using an SMR

Occasionally institutions of interest may have both markedly differing sample sizes and differing risk profiles (Morton[E] and colleagues). When this occurs, it is important to ensure that the analysis employing indirect standardisation is not biased. Analysis of the SMRs can be performed as a check. The R commands are shown below and the figures that correspond to Figure 2.5 and Figure 2.6 are 2.8 and 2.9. In this case there is no suggestion that the analysis using indirect standardisation might be biased.

```
#SMR funnel plots
#institutions on the horizontal axis
graphics.off()
library(chron)
```

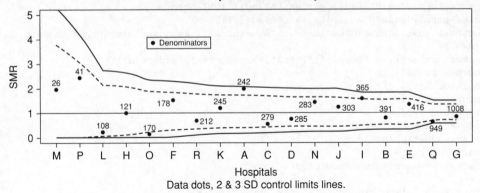

Figure 2.8 SMR funnel plot, hospitals on horizontal axis.

```
datain1<-ssi0506adj[,-c(2,5)]
hosp<-datain1[,1];outc<-datain1[,2];expect<-datain1[,3]
a<-as.data.frame(xtabs(outc~hosp))
b<-as.numeric(table(hosp))
d<-as.numeric(xtabs(expect~hosp))
dataout<-cbind(a,b,d)
names(dataout)<-c("hosp","outc","tot","exp")
d1<-dataout[,2]
d2<-dataout[,3]
d3<-dataout[,4]
da<-dataout[,1]
lda<-1:length(d1)
d<-d1/d3
p<-d3/d2
n<-d2
#finding lower limits
L1<-0;L2<-0
```

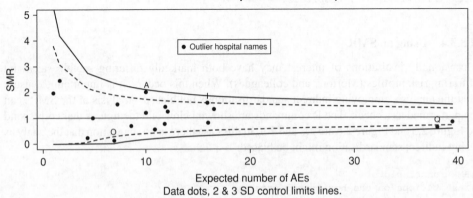

Figure 2.9 SMR funnel plot, expected AE numbers on horizontal axis.

```
for (I in 1:2){
if (I==1){Z<-.02275}
if (I==2){Z<-.00135}
L0<-0
for (i in 1:length(n)){
P<-p[i];N<-n[i]
X<-0
if (1-pbeta(P,X+1,N-X)>=Z){X<-0}else{
X<-P*N
A<-1
bl<-F
while (bl==F){
X<-X-A
K<-1-pbeta(P,X+1,N-X)
if (K<=Z){bl<-T}
}
A<-.001
bl<-F
while (bl==F){
X<-X+A
K<-1-pbeta(P,X+1,N-X)
if (K>=Z){bl<-T}
}
}
L0[i]<-X/n[i]
}
if (I==1){12<-L0}
if (I==2){l13<-L0}
}
#finding upper limits
U1<-0;U2<-0
for (I in 1:2){
if (I==1){Z<-.02275}
if (I==2){Z<-.00135}
U0<-0
for (i in 1:length(n)){
P<-p[i];N<-n[i]
X<-N
if (pbeta(P,X,N-X+1)>=Z){X<-N}else{
X<-N*P
A<-1
bl<-F
while (bl==F){
X<-X+A
K<-pbeta(P,X,N-X+1)
if (K<Z){bl<-T}
}
A<-.001
bl<-F
while (bl==F){
X<-X-A
K<-pbeta(P,X,N-X+1)
if (K>=Z){bl<-T}
}
}
U0[i]<-X/n[i]
```

```
}
if (I==1){u2<-U0;u2[u2==0]<-1}
if (I==2){uu3<-U0;uu3[uu3==0]<-1}
}
l2a<-l2*n;l2a<-l2a/d3
ll3a<-ll3*n;ll3a<-ll3a/d3
u2a<-u2*n;u2a<-u2a/d3
uu3a<-uu3*n;uu3a<-uu3a/d3
o<-order(uu3a,decreasing=T)
u2o<-u2a[o];l2o<-l2a[o];dno<-d[o];dao<-da[o];d2o<-d2[o];d3o<-d3[o]
uu3o<-uu3a[o];ll3o<-ll3a[o]
l2o[l2o<0]<-0
ll3o[ll3o<0]<-0
eh<-"All Orthopaedic SSIs"
eh<-paste(eh," funnel plot.",sep="")
ej<-"SMR"
eq<-paste("Data blue, 2 & 3 SD control limits red.")
minn<-min(c(ll3o,dno));maxx<-max(c(uu3o,dno))
minn<-0;maxx<-5
par(xaxs="r")
plot(dno,type="p",lwd=2,col="dark blue",ylim=c(minn,maxx),xlab=eq,ylab=ej,
main=eh,axes=F)
box()
par(cex=.8)
axis(side=1,labels=dao,at=lda)
axis(side=c(2,3,4))
par(cex=1)
abline(h=1,lwd=2,col="black")
lines(u2o,lwd=2,lty=2,col="red")
lines(l2o,lwd=2,lty=2,col="red")
lines(uu3o,lwd=2,lty=1,col="red")
lines(ll3o,lwd=2,lty=1,col="red")
mtext("Hospitals.",side=1,line=2)
par(font=2)
text(dno,labels=as.character(d2o),pos=3,offset=.3,cex=.8,lwd=3,col="brown4")
par(font=1)
legend(locator(1),legend="Denominators Brown",pch=19,col="brown4",cex=.8)

#Figure 2.9, expected values on the horizontal axis
graphics.off()
library(chron)
datain1<-ssi0506adj[,-c(2,5)]
hosp<-datain1[,1];outc<-datain1[,2];expect<-datain1[,3]
a<-as.data.frame(xtabs(outc~hosp))
b<-as.numeric(table(hosp))
d<-as.numeric(xtabs(expect~hosp))
dataout<-cbind(a,b,d)
names(dataout)<-c("hosp","outc","tot","exp")
d1<-dataout[,2]
d2<-dataout[,3]
d3<-dataout[,4]
da<-dataout[,1]
lda<-1:length(d1)
d<-d1/d2
p<-d3/d2
n<-d2
```

```
#finding lower limits
L1<-0;L2<-0
for (I in 1:2){
if (I==1){Z<-.02275}
if (I==2){Z<-.00135}
L0<-0
for (i in 1:length(n)){
P<-p[i];N<-n[i]
X<-0
if (1-pbeta(P,X+1,N-X)>=Z){X<-0}else{
X<-P*N
A<-1
bl<-F
while (bl==F){
X<-X-A
K<-1-pbeta(P,X+1,N-X)
if (K<=Z){bl<-T}
}
A<-.001
bl<-F
while (bl==F){
X<-X+A
K<-1-pbeta(P,X+1,N-X)
if (K>=Z){bl<-T}
}
}
L0[i]<-X/n[i]
}
if (I==1){l2<-L0}
if (I==2){l13<-L0}
}
#finding upper limits
U1<-0;U2<-0
for (I in 1:2){
if (I==1){Z<-.02275}
if (I==2){Z<-.00135}
U0<-0
for (i in 1:length(n)){
P<-p[i];N<-n[i]
X<-N
if (pbeta(P,X,N-X+1)>=Z){X<-N}else{
X<-N*P
A<-1
bl<-F
while (bl==F){
X<-X+A
K<-pbeta(P,X,N-X+1)
if (K<Z){bl<-T}
}
A<-.001
bl<-F
while (bl==F){
X<-X-A
K<-pbeta(P,X,N-X+1)
if (K>=Z){bl<-T}
}
```

```
}
U0[i]<-X/n[i]
}
if (I==1){u2<-U0;u2[u2==0]<-1}
if (I==2){uu3<-U0;uu3[uu3==0]<-1}
}
dn<-d1/d3
l2a<-l2*n;l2a<-l2a/d3
l13a<-l13*n;l13a<-l13a/d3
u2a<-u2*n;u2a<-u2a/d3
uu3a<-uu3*n;uu3a<-uu3a/d3
o<-order(uu3a,decreasing=T)
u2o<-u2a[o];l2o<-l2a[o];dno<-dn[o];dao<-da[o];d2o<-d2[o];d3o<-d3[o]
uu3o<-uu3a[o];l13o<-l13a[o];ldao<-lda[o]
l2o[l2o<0]<-0
l13o[l13o<0]<-0
eh<-"All Orthopaedic SSIs"
eh<-paste(eh," funnel plot",sep="")
ej<-"SMR"
eq<-paste("Data blue, 2 & 3 SD control limits red.")
minn<-min(c(l13o,dno));maxx<-max(c(uu3o,dno))
minn<-0;maxx<-5
par(xaxs="r")
plot(dno~d3o,type="p",lwd=2,col="dark blue",ylim=c(minn,maxx),xlab=eq,
ylab=ej,main=eh)
abline(h=1,lwd=2,col="black")
lines(u2o~d3o,lwd=2,lty=2,col="red")
lines(l2o~d3o,lwd=2,lty=2,col="red")
lines(uu3o~d3o,lwd=2,lty=1,col="red")
lines(l13o~d3o,lwd=2,lty=1,col="red")
mtext("Expected Number of AEs",side=1,line=2)
par(font=2)
oe2<-rep("",length(dno))
for (i in 1:length(oe2)){if (dno[i]>u2o[i]){oe2[i]<-as.character(dao[i])}}
text(dno~d3o,labels=oe2,pos=3,offset=.3,cex=.8,lwd=3,col="brown4")
oe2<-rep("",length(dno))
for (i in 1:length(oe2)){if (dno[i]<l2o[i]){oe2[i]<-as.character(dao[i])}}
text(dno~d3o,labels=oe2,pos=3,offset=.3,cex=.8,lwd=3,col="brown4")
par(font=1)
legend(locator(1),legend="Outlier Hospital Names Brown",pch=19,col="brown4",
cex=.8)
```

2.3.3.5   Shrinkage analysis

A further limitation of the funnel plot is that smaller institutions may be shown in an unfavourable light due to random variation from effects related to regression to the mean that can be important for these institutions. Thus a small institution may have a favourable report one year and an unfavourable one the next or vice versa without any change in its systems. Reward or disciplinary action can then depend on random variation, a situation that is very bad for morale. To deal with this problem, Bayesian shrinkage (random effects) methods are advocated; here the institutions are assumed collectively to have their own distribution. Unfortunately, in the process of improving precision, shrinkage can occasionally increase bias. The result is that, while better control of random variation can reduce the likelihood of a false positive result, shrinkage may rarely suggest that a performance is satisfactory when it may not be; the possibility of false negative error may thus be slightly increased. One approach is to perform the analysis with a funnel plot and then employ shrinkage if one or more results are outside the two sigma equivalent limits. If a result without shrinkage suggests the presence of a problem, the staff in the institution of interest should still study the relevant systems of their institution. If no cause for the aberrant result is found and the predicted shrinkage value suggests acceptable performance, confidence that the result was due to predictable variation is then increased.

The function lmer in the lme4 and arm libraries or hglm in the hglm library of R can be used to perform random-effects logistic regression to provide a shrinkage analysis. These packages employ an empirical Bayes approach in which some parameters are first estimated and then plugged in as values in the analysis. The shrinkage analysis can also be performed using the software program OpenBUGS (mathstat.helsinki.fi/openbugs/). When expected outcome rates are less than about 10%, random-effects Poisson regression can be employed with aggregated data. Higher rates (e.g. intensive and coronary care mortality) can be analysed using lmer or hglm. In most practical situations, rates will be sufficiently low for the OpenBUGS approach to be employed. It appears to be superior to the empirical Bayes methods since it avoids plug-in values and takes into account the variability in all of the estimates.

2.3.3.6 Using OpenBUGS Gamma-Poisson Hierarchical Model

OpenBUGS is specialised software and its use is generally beyond the scope of these notes. However, we describe here the very useful gamma-Poisson hierarchical model. First, the program gammapoisson.odc is loaded into OpenBUGS. The code for the gamma-Poisson hierarchical model is in Examples Volume 1. Since there are 18 hospitals, data list(n=18) must be set. Next, use File New. Select the observed and expected SSI columns in the data.frame orthssi in R and copy to the clipboard.

```
#in R, ensure the hospitals are in alphabetical order
s.d(orthssi[,-c(1,3)])
#Use clipboard (c) or a data file (d) c
```

In the new OpenBUGS window select Edit Paste Special and Plain Text. At the bottom of the first column type END and at the top of this column change the heading to x[] and change the heading of the second column to t[].

```
OpenBUGS (count.odc).

# program window
model
{
for (i in 1:n)
{
theta[i]~dgamma(alpha,beta)
lamda[i]<-theta[i]*t[i]
x[i]~dpois(lamda[i])
}
alpha~dexp(1)
beta~dgamma(.1,.1)
}
data
```

```
list(n = 18)
inits
list(alpha = 1, beta = 1)

# data window
x[]    t[]
20     10.0293023734598
13     15.9770327972534
6      10.8477612083708
9      11.810966418767
22     16.5035503772056
11     7.22048488132029
33     39.3945341959009
5      4.87507975860748
25     15.9189482969966
15     12.056248752296
12     10.0258679125789
1      4.37892427060518
2      1.0130340607886
17     11.8349791810765
1      6.90085331220496
4      1.62974645057201
25     38.0009044493425
6      8.58178130265702
END
```

Now return to the program window. Click somewhere around theta and Select Model and Specification from the drop-down Menu and select Check Model. The program reports Syntactically Correct. Double click on List below Data to select it and then on Load Data; Data Loaded appears. Select the Window containing the data (eg untitled1), double click on the x at the top of the first column and repeat Load Data and Data Loaded again appears. Next, return to the program window, click again near theta and select Compile; Model Compiled is reported. Now double click on the List below Inits and select Load Inits. It may then be necessary to select Gen Inits to set up the analysis (initial values generated, model initialised).

Select Inference and Samples from the drop-down Menu. Type theta in Node and click Set. Now select Model again and Update. In Updates type 41000 and click on Update. This number is employed as it provides stable three sigma equivalent credible limits.

When the update is complete, select Samples again from the Inference Menu. Click on the arrow beside Node and select theta. Change the 1 in Beg to 1001 to discard the first 1000 updates for each hospital. Click on Coda, Select All & Copy to get the required output. The above steps are described at www.divms.uiowa.edu/~gwoodwor/. Select Woodworth's Website for Biostatistics: A Bayesian Introduction and Appendix B. The next steps can be performed in R and the result is in Figure 2.10. The credible (confidence) limit calculations can be performed using shrink(datain, number of institutions, number of updates minus number discarded that is typically 1000).

```
g.d() # data from OpenBUGS via clipboard
# no headings, no dates in first column
#
# using the function shrink()
shrink(datain,18,40000) # data in data.frame d
#
#get the aggregated data into datain
```

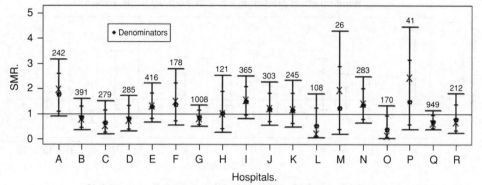

Figure 2.10   OpenBUGS shrinkage plot.

```
datain<-orthssi

#Figure 2.10, random-effects (shrinkage) chart
d1<-d
o<-order(datain[,1])
datain1<-datain[o,]
d1<-d1[o,]
nn1<-datain1[,1]
P1<-datain1[,2]/datain1[,4]
mn<-0;mx<-ceiling(max(d1$u))+.1
par(xaxs="r")
z1<-"Shrinkage prediction with 2 & 3 SD "
z2<-"equivalent limits blue, data red."
z3<-paste(z1,z2,sep="")
plot(P1,col="red",pch=19,ylim=c(mn,mx),axes=F,lwd=3,
main="BUGS Shrinkage Plot All Orthopaedic SSIs.",
xlab=z3,ylab="SMR.")
box()
points(d1$m,col="blue",lwd=3)
abline(h=1)
par(cex=.7)
axis(side=1,tick=T,nn1,at=1:length(nn1))
axis(side=c(2,3,4))
par(cex=1)
points(d1$ll,pch="-",lwd=3,col="blue",cex=1.5)
points(d1$ul,pch="-",lwd=3,col="blue",cex=1.5)
arrows(1:length(d1$m),d1$l,1:length(d1$m),d1$u,angle=90,code=3,lwd=2,col=
"blue",length=.15)
mtext("Hospitals.",side=1,line=2)
par(font=2)
text(d1$u,labels=as.character(datain1[,3]),pos=3,offset=.3,cex=.8,lwd=3,
col="brown4")
par(font=1)
legend(locator(n=1),legend="Denominators Brown",
pch=19,col="brown4",cex=.8)
```

Clinical staff may wish to know the principle of the shrinkage analysis. Although it applies to the case where different (e.g. empirical Bayes) software is employed, the following approximate explanation due to Simpson and colleagues is useful and is illustrated as follows.

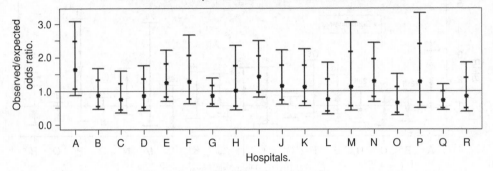

Figure 2.11   Shrinkage plot using lmer().

If a unit has an observed number of complications (O) and an expected number (E) and O/E (shrink) is sO/E, then sO/E is approximately (O+1/V)/(E+1/V) where V is the among units variance. Suppose that for one unit O=10, E=5 and the among unit variance V=.05, so O/E=2. Then, sO/E≈(10+20)/(5+20)=1.2. However, if O=100, E=50 and V=.25, then sO/E≈(100+4)/(50+4)=1.93. When samples are small or variation among them is not large, the predicted estimate is drawn towards the average value. This is likely to give a truer picture than other approaches such as multiple confidence intervals that are often employed in league tables.

An important issue for shrinkage analysis is exchangeability. This is discussed in section 2.3.1 of this chapter.

As an alternative to conventional use of measures of precision to detect outlying observations, it has been recommended that clinically important thresholds should be established and the probability of an observation exceeding the threshold reported. For example, if a surgical site infection rate of 3% is expected for a particular procedure and rates below 5% are considered attainable, a shrinkage-adjusted SSI rate with a probability of 50% of exceeding 5% is considered to be a possible outlier (Christiansen and Morris). We have not implemented this approach.

2.3.3.7   Using lmer and hglm

We mentioned above that the analysis can be performed with standard statistical software employing a method called empirical Bayes. This provides an alternative to the OpenBUGS Gamma-Poisson Hierarchical Model described above. When the expected proportions exceed about 10%, the use of lmer or hglm would be satisfactory. The chart produced by lmer is Figure 2.11.

```
#Figure 2.11, shrinkage plot using lmer in function ebshrinkageb()
ebshrinkageb(ssi0506adj[,-c(2,5)])
```

```
Do you have risk-adjusted data (Y/N) y
Enter a chart heading All Orthopaedic SSIs 2005-06
Enter horizontal axis heading Hospitals
Enter vertical axis heading O/E OR
The data are in chartout
```

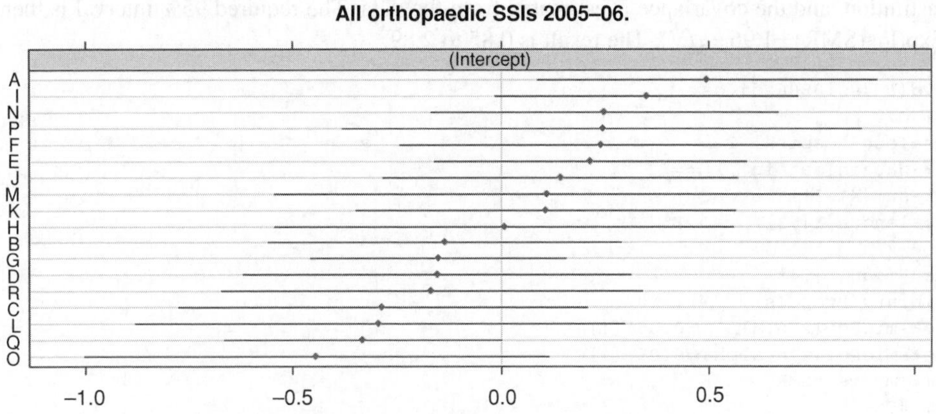

All orthopaedic SSIs 2005–06.

Figure 2.12   Plot using dotplot() function.

Figure 2.12 is a caterpillar plot produced by lmer using postVar=T in ranef that displays the random effects. It employs a log scale and 95% CIs using the built-in dotplot function. The object produced by the ebshrinkageb analysis is lout and it is in the workspace as is ranf produced by ranef with postVar=T.

```
dotplot(ranf,main="All Orthopaedic SSIs 2005-06.")
```

2.3.3.8   Using bootstrap for SMR intervals

Use of the bootstrap to obtain SMR intervals is illustrated in the internet code file. This is very time consuming and does not add substantially to the analysis.

2.4   When the Es are not fixed

This issue is discussed in section 2.3.1 of this chapter. In some cases the data used to calculate the expected values (Es) come from relatively small local samples involving uncommon AEs. Moreover, the institution whose SMR is being investigated may have contributed data for this purpose. Silcocks, and Faris and colleagues discuss the problem of the uncertainty of the Es. With count data or binary data with rare AEs it is usual to employ a standard Poisson-based approach or a binomial approach for AEs that are not so rare. The Es are often regarded as fixed. Ng and colleagues have described a risk-adjusted observed versus expected (ROVE) plot in which both the observed number of AEs (O) and the expected number (E) are plotted with their confidence intervals and there is considered to be an abnormal result if these do not overlap. The ROVE plot can be extended using Newcombe's method described in Chapter 1.

Hospital I had 25 SSIs and 15.9 were predicted (SMR=1.57). It performed 365 procedures in 2005–06 out of a total of 5622 performed by the 18 hospitals. Conventional confidence limits were 1.06 to 2.24 implying that it may differ from one.

The approximate delta variance of log(O/E) is $V=V(O)/O^2+V(E)/E^2-2\times$covariance $(O,E)/(O\times E)$, where $V(O)=O\times(N-O)/N$ is the variance of O, $V(E)=\sum_N(e_i\times(1-e_i))$ is the variance of E, N is the number of procedures each with prediction e_i performed by the institution, and the covariance is estimated from the data. The required 95% interval is then $Exp(\log(SMR)\pm1.96\times\sqrt{V})$. The result is 0.85 to 2.89.

```
g.d() #ssi0506adj.csv

#select hospital I
X<-datain[datain[,1]=="I",]
x<-sum(X[,3])
n<-length(X[,3])
mo<-x/n
me<-mean(X[,4])
library(PropCIs)
lo<-midPci(x,n,alpha=0.05)[1]
uo<-midPci(x,n,alpha=0.05)[2]
sm<-mo/me #SMR
sm #SMR
#[1] 1.571
#SMR limits using binomial limits around O, E assumed fixed
#suggests SMR may differ from one
SMRl<-lo/me;SMRl # [1] 1.057366
SMRu<-uo/me;SMRu # [1] 2.2378

#Newcombe modification of ROVE method
#variance of Es
v<-sum(X[,4]*(1-X[,4]))/length(X[,4])^2
s<-v^.5
#CIs of Es
ue<-me+1.96*s
le<-me-1.96*s
#difference between Os and Es
d<-mo-me
#CIs for difference with covariance ignored
dl<-d-((mo-lo)^2+(ue-me)^2)^.5
du<-d+((me-le)^2+(uo-mo)^2)^.5
d # [1] 0.0248795 (O-E)
dl # [1] -0.005782446 (lower confidence limit)
du # 1] 0.06073927 (upper confidence limit)

#adding estimated covariance
cv<-cov(X[,3],X[,4])
dlcv<-d-((mo-lo)^2-2*cv*(mo-lo)*(ue-me)+(ue-me)^2)^.5
ducv<-d+((me-le)^2-2*cv*(me-le)*(uo-mo)+(uo-mo)^2)^.5
dlcv #[1] -0.0057828 (lower confidence limit with covariance)
ducv #[1] [1] 0.06074 (upper confidence limit with covariance)
#approximate CI for SMR using method of Altman and Bland
SED<-abs((0.06074--0.0057828)/(2*1.96))
Z<-0.02489425/SED
SESMR<-abs(log(sm)/Z)
U<-exp(log(sm)+1.96*SESMR)
U #[1] 2.8704
L<-exp(log(sm)-1.96*SESMR)
L #[1] 0.85924

# using delta variance method
O<-x
E<-me*n
```

```
VO<-O*(n-O)/n
VE<-sum(X[,4]*(1-X[,4]))
V<-VO/O^2+VE/E^2-2*cv/(O*E)
L<-exp(log(sm)-1.96*V^.5)
U<-exp(log(sm)+1.96*V^.5)
L;U
#
#[1]  0.85214
#[1]  2.8943
```

The first method described by Silcocks gives 95% confidence limits of 0.81 to 3.15. This method assumes that there is zero covariation. Using the beta distribution, the following are required –

beta(P_L,O,N-O+1)=0.025 and beta(P_U,O+1,N-O)=0.975, where N=O+E.

P_L=qbeta(.025,O,N-O+1)

P_L=0.446

P_U=qbeta(.975,O+1,N-O)

P_U=0.759

U=P_U/(1-P_U)

L=P_L/(1-P_L)

Assuming the presence of covariation, Silcocks describes the following method. In the following formula, q is the covariation. Its estimated value is cv=-2.3374e-05 that is in this case insignificant. Nevertheless, we include it for illustration. Then, using a Fieller-based approach that assumes the Os and Es are sufficiently large for normal approximations to be used $X^2 \times A + X \times B + C = 0$, where, for a 95% interval, A=E×(E-3.8614), B=-2×O×(E-q×3.8614), C=O×(O-3.8614), and X=(B±(B^2-4×A×C)$^{0.5}$)/(2×A). The required limits are the two solutions for X (L=0.83 and U=3.31).

An alternative is to employ a bootstrap analysis. This suggests that the SMR may in fact differ from one (CI 1.06 to 2.26 using the BCa bootstrap). The calculations are very time-consuming and they appear to add little to the analysis. See also section 2.3.3.8.

It seems desirable that further work be performed to clarify the calculation of SMR CIs and particularly the observed/expected covariance. It is possible that the latter is typically small and can usually be ignored. However, there can be hospital groups that are dominated by one or two very large institutions, in which case the covariance may be important.

Another alternative is to exclude the data from the hospital of interest and calculate its risk adjustment scores from the remaining data, thus eliminating the need to adjust for covariation. This approach may be a problem when the hospital of interest provides a large proportion of the patients. However, in the present case, hospital I provided only 6.5% of the 2005–06 data. Using this approach, the CI was 0.88 to 3. This analysis is further illustrated in Appendix 2 of this chapter.

In practice, when calculating SMR confidence intervals and using them in, for example, a chart like Figure 2.4, the variation of the Es is usually ignored. It is important to realise that this will frequently result in limits that are too narrow. However, it is worth repeating Nelson's observation: statistical quality control is meant to be a practically useful process-improvement tool, not an exact statistical method. If, with our aggregated data, we concentrate on the 2.5 (99% approximately) or 3 (99.7%) SD equivalent limits and use the analysis to learn how to practice more safely, the slightly narrow confidence and control limits should not be a serious problem.

2.5   Complex Surgical Site Infections

A difficulty occurs with SSIs due to early discharge of patients after surgery. Many superficial post-discharge SSIs are relatively minor and their ascertainment is imperfect (Whitby and colleagues). For example, a lymph fistula with some redness can be counted erroneously as a superficial SSI. This difficulty has led to suggestions by Anderson and colleagues that complex SSIs be counted. Complex SSIs are deep or organ space infections and, as patients require readmission, they can be counted accurately. Although not all SSIs are then counted, rates of complex SSIs and changes in their rates can be used for monitoring. These infections should also be the subject of morbidity and mortality (M&M) audits as described by Singer. Their analysis is illustrated using the data in ssiorthcomplx.csv.

2.5.1   Funnel plot analysis

The funnel plot analysis is repeated using the complex SSI data.

```
g.d() # ssiorthcomplx.csv, first column is not a date column

#using function bgroupfunnelinstitution(), Figure 2.13
#copy and paste long name to R prompt
bgroupfunnelinstitution(datain[,-2])

#Do you have risk-adjusted data (Y/N) y
```

	Institution	AE	Procedures	Expected
1	A	27	865	11.277718
2	B	9	1069	12.170602
3	C	8	796	7.283942
4	D	10	891	10.593548
5	E	3	997	11.036592
6	F	6	550	6.636854
7	G	30	2598	21.704200
8	H	7	373	4.240971
9	I	21	1079	15.545339
10	J	2	714	7.555217
11	K	6	477	5.414240
12	L	0	227	2.307229
13	M	0	125	1.252000
14	N	4	589	7.524477
15	O	1	292	2.855033
16	P	0	149	1.273060
17	Q	16	1984	20.554258
18	R	3	351	3.774722

```
Chart heading.
Enter heading for chart Complex Orthopaedic SSIs
X-axis heading.
Enter an X-axis heading Hospitals
```

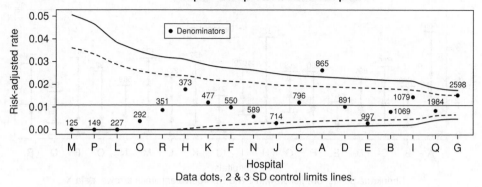

Figure 2.13 RAR funnel plot of complex SSIs, hospitals on horizontal axis.

Place the locator() cross at a suitable clear area on the chart and press the left mouse button.

```
#using function bgroupfunnelprocedure(), Figure 2.14
#copy long function name and paste at R prompt
bgroupfunnelprocedure(datain[,-2])

#Do you have risk-adjusted data (Y/N) y
```

```
Chart heading.
Enter heading for chart Complex Orthopaedic SSIs
X-axis heading.
Enter an X-axis heading Procedures
```

Place the locator() cross at a suitable clear area on the chart and press the left mouse button.

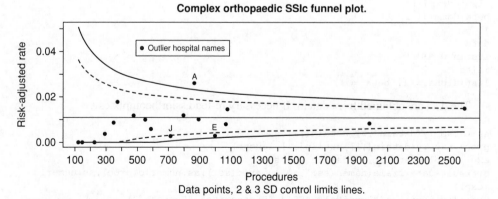

Figure 2.14 RAR funnel plot of complex SSIs, procedures on horizontal axis.

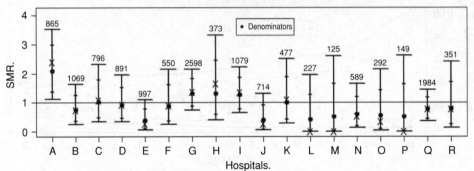

Figure 2.15 OpenBUGS shrinkage plot, complex SSIs.

2.5.2 Shrinkage analysis

Shrinkage analysis can be used with complex SSI and other binary data such as surgical mortality data. With these relatively uncommon AEs, empirical Bayes random-effects logistic regression appears to be inferior to the OpenBUGS gamma-Poisson method and use of lmer() and hglm() are not described here.

```
#Figure 2.15. OpenBUGS Shrinkage Plot.
#load OpenBUGS and count.odc
#set data list(n=18)
#
model
{
for (i in 1:n)
{
theta[i]~dgamma(alpha,beta)
lamda[i]<-theta[i]*t[i]
x[i]~dpois(lamda[i])
}
alpha~dexp(1)
beta~dgamma(.1,.1)
}
data
list(n = 18)
inits
list(alpha = 1, beta = 1)
```

The data are obtained from datain. If necessary re-load ssiorthcomplx.csv.

```
ssi<-tapply(datain[,3],datain[,1],sum)
proc<-tapply(datain[,3],datain[,1],length)
exp<-tapply(datain[,4],datain[,1],sum)
orthssi<-data.frame(names(ssi),as.numeric(ssi),as.numeric(proc),as.numeric
(exp))
names(orthssi)<-c("Hospital","SSI","Procedures","Expected")
# check that the hospital names are in alphabetical order
```

```
s.d(orthssi[,c(2,4)]) # export to OpenBUGS

# Use clipboard (c) or a data file (f) c
```

Returning to OpenBUGS, select File New. In the data window use Edit Paste Special Plain Text, add END at the bottom of the first column and change the headings to x[] and t[] at the top of the two columns. The data appear as follows.

```
x[]     t[]
27      11.277718049004
9       12.1706019874657
8       7.28394160485425
10      10.5935480676423
3       11.0365918725718
6       6.63685427962406
30      21.704199943734
7       4.24097077438927
21      15.5453389230668
2       7.55521658276885
6       5.41423999532935
0       2.30722858168556
0       1.2519996761201
4       7.52447698710421
1       2.85503250309017
0       1.27305982632053
16      20.5542582142914
3       3.77472213093781
END
```

Now click somewhere around theta and Select Model and Specification from the drop-down Menu and select Check Model. The program reports Syntactically Correct. Double click on List below Data to select it and then on Load Data; Data Loaded appears. Select the Window () containing the data. Now double click on the x at the top of the first column and repeat Load Data and Data Loaded again appears. Next, return to the count Window, click again near theta and select Compile; Model Compiled is reported. Now double click on the List below Inits and select Load Inits. It may then be necessary to select Gen Inits to set up the analysis (initial values generated, model initialised).

Select Inference and Samples from the drop-down Menu. Type theta in Node and click Set. Now select Model again and Update. In Updates type 41000 and click on Update. This number is employed as it provides stable three sigma equivalent credible limits.

When the update is complete, select Samples again from the Inference Menu. Click on the arrow beside Node and select theta. Change the 1 in Beg to 1001 to discard the first 1000 updates for each institution. Click on Coda, Select All & Copy to get the required output. The above steps are described in www.divms.uiowa.edu/~gwoodwor/. Select Professor Wood-worth's Website for Biostatistics: A Bayesian Introduction and Appendix B (with clearer screenshots). The next steps are in R and the result is in Figure 2.15.

```
g.d() # data from OpenBUGS via clipboard

#no headings, first column not a date column
# data in datain
shrink(datain,18,40000) # data in data.frame d
```

```
#getting the aggregated data into datain
datain<-orthssi

#Figure 2.15, shrinkage plot
d1<-d
o<-order(datain[,1])
datain1<-datain[o,]
d1<-d1[o,]
nn1<-datain1[,1]
P1<-datain1[,2]/datain1[,4]
mn<-0;mx<-ceiling(max(d1$u))+.1
z1<-"Shrinkage prediction with 2 & 3 SD "
z2<-"equivalent limits blue, data red."
z3<-paste(z1,z2,sep="")
plot(P1,col="red",pch=19,ylim=c(mn,mx),axes=F,lwd=3,
main="BUGS Shrinkage Plot Complex Orthopaedic SSIs.",
xlab=z3,ylab="SMR.")
box()
points(d1$m,col="blue",lwd=3)
abline(h=1)
par(cex=.7)
axis(side=1,tick=T,nn1,at=1:length(nn1))
axis(side=c(2,3,4))
par(cex=1)
points(d1$ll,pch="-",lwd=3,col="blue",cex=1.5)
points(d1$ul,pch="-",lwd=3,col="blue",cex=1.5)
arrows(1:length(d1$m),d1$l,1:length(d1$m),d1$u,angle=90,code=3,lwd=2,col=
"blue",length=.15)
mtext("Hospitals.",side=1,line=2)
par(font=2)
text(d1$u,labels=as.character(datain1[,3]),pos=3,offset=.3,cex=.8,lwd=3,
col="brown4")
par(font=1)
legend(locator(1),legend="Denominators Brown",pch=19,col="brown4",cex=.8)
```

2.6   Complex SSI risk-adjustment discrimination

Finally, the discriminative ability of the complex SSI risk-adjustment is shown in Figure 2.16. At 0.62 it is better than for the all SSI data. We have employed the rocchart() function.

```
g.d() # ssiorthcomplx.csv, first column does not contain dates

rocchart(data.frame(datain[,3],datain[,4]))

#Enter a name for the ROC chart Complex Orthopaedic SSI
```

2.7   Appendix 1 – Further tabulation methods

Tabulations can be required by institutions and by weeks, months, quarters, half-years or years. We illustrate some further methods for accomplishing these tables and, where required, we show time periods in a format suitable either for placing in a report or for producing a chart using a suitable R function.

Weekly binary data will often have insufficient numbers for weekly tabulations to be useful although weekly count data are occasionally useful. Because of the sparseness of the

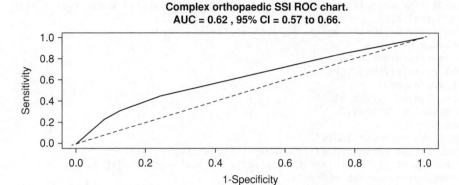

Figure 2.16   AUC chart complex SSI data.

data, it will usually be impractical to include Z-scores. In addition, there will often be too many rows so it is only practicable to scroll down through the data. However, data for a particular institution, years or institutions within years can be obtained. When binary data are sufficiently numerous, for example, a large ICU may have as many as 100 discharges per month, tabulating and displaying them by months can be useful. When they are too few for monthly tabulation, displaying them by quarters may be worthwhile, especially for clinical staff who may wish to know the current rate. Variable life-adjusted (VLAD) and similar displays (Lovegrove and colleagues) show cumulative data, not current rates. These issues are discussed further in Chapter 3. Half yearly and yearly tabulations are less likely to be useful. We illustrate with quarterly data.

```
g.d()   # ssi0506adj.csv
```

```
Loading data.
Data from clipboard (C) or file (F) c
Do data column(s) have heading(s) (Y/N) y
Is column 1 a date column (Y/N) n
```

```
#data for institutions and quarters with risk-adjustment
library(chron)
d<-chron(as.character(datain[,2]),format="dd-mmm-yyyy",out.format=
"dd-mmm-yyyy")
# date format is for eg 31-Dec-2006
H<-datain[,1]
Year<-years(d)
m<-as.numeric(months(d))
Qtrs<-rep(0,length(m))
Qtrs[m>=1&m<=3]<-1
Qtrs[m>=4&m<=6]<-2
Qtrs[m>=7&m<=9]<-3
Qtrs[m>=10&m<=12]<-4
Table3a<-as.data.frame(xtabs(datain[,3]~Qtrs+Year+H))
Table3b<-as.data.frame(xtabs(datain[,4]~Qtrs+Year+H))
Q<-rep(1,length(datain[,1]))
Table3c<-as.data.frame(xtabs(Q~Qtrs+Year+H))
Table<-data.frame(Table3a[,3],Table3a[,1],Table3a[,2],Table3a[,4],Table3c
[,4],Table3b[,4])
names(Table)<-c("Inst","Qtrs","Yrs","AEs","Proc","Exp")
```

```
TB<-data.frame("AllInst","AllQtrs","AllYrs",sum(Table[,4]),sum(Table[,5]),
sum(Table[,6]))
names(TB)<-c("Inst","Qtrs","Yrs","AEs","Proc","Exp")
TableChart<-Table
Table<-rbind(Table,TB)
Table<-Table[Table[,5]!=0,]
library(exactci)
Rate<-Table[,4]/Table[,5]
d<-Table[,6]/Table[,5]
Z<-0;p<-0
for (i in 1:length(Table[,1]))
{p[i]<-binom.exact(Table[i,4],Table[i,5],d[i])$p.value;
if(Rate[i]>d[i]){Z[i]<--qnorm(p[i]/2)}else{Z[i]<-qnorm(p[i]/2)}}
Table$Exp<-round(Table$Exp,1)
Z<-round(Z,1)
Table<-data.frame(Table,Z)

#re-formatting years and quarters
Tbl<-Table[-length(Table[,1]),]
Q<-paste(Tbl[,3],"Q",Tbl[,2],sep="")
Tbl<-data.frame(Tbl[,1],Q,Tbl[,-(1:3)])
names(Tbl)<-c("Inst","Qtrs","AEs","Proc","Exp","Z-score")
TB1<-data.frame(TB[,-3],0)
names(TB1)<- c("Inst","Qtrs","AEs","Proc","Exp","Z-score")
Tbl<-rbind(Tbl,TB1)
row.names(Tbl)<-1:length(Tbl[,1])

# Hospital A
HospA<-Tbl[Tbl$Inst=="A",]
HospA
```

	Inst	Qtrs	AEs	Proc	Exp	Z-score
1	A	2005Q1	3	25	1.0	1.4
2	A	2005Q2	5	45	1.8	1.8
3	A	2005Q3	5	35	1.5	2.2
4	A	2005Q4	1	30	1.3	0.0
5	A	2006Q2	2	31	1.3	0.3
6	A	2006Q3	4	40	1.7	1.4
7	A	2006Q4	0	36	1.4	−0.7

```
# Hospitals A and Q in 2005
Tbl2005<-Tbl[substr(Tbl$Qtrs,4,4)=="5",]
Tbl2005AQ<-Tbl2005[Tbl2005$Inst=="A"|Tbl2005$Inst=="Q",]
row.names(Tbl2005AQ)<-1:length(Tbl2005AQ[,1])
Tbl2005AQ
```

	Inst	Qtrs	AEs	Proc	Exp	Z-score
1	A	2005Q1	3	25	1.0	1.4
2	A	2005Q2	5	45	1.8	1.8
3	A	2005Q3	5	35	1.5	2.2
4	A	2005Q4	1	30	1.3	0.0
5	Q	2005Q1	0	105	4.2	−2.2
6	Q	2005Q2	4	131	5.2	−0.3
7	Q	2005Q3	1	131	5.2	−1.9
8	Q	2005Q4	5	110	4.4	0.1

```
# wide format using stack and reshape
d<-data.frame(rep(Tbl2005AQ[,1],4),rep(Tbl2005AQ[,2],4))
s<-stack(Tbl2005AQ[,c(3,4,5,6),])
e<-data.frame(d,s)
names(e)<-c("Hosp","Qtr","Dta","Cat")
f<-reshape(e,direction="wide",timevar="Qtr",idvar=c("Cat","Hosp"))
a<-f[f[,1]==f[1,1],]
b<-f[f[,1]==f[2,1],]
a<-rbind(a,b)
Tot<-0
for (i in 1:8){Tot[i]<-sum(a[i,3:6])}
# when adding Z-scores, divide by square root of number
Tot[c(4,8)]<-Tot[c(4,8)]/4^.5
Tbl2005AQW<-data.frame(a,Tot)
names(Tbl2005AQW)<-c("Hosp","Cat","Qtr1","Qtr2","Qtr3","Qtr4","Tot")
Tbl2005AQW
```

	Hosp	Cat	Qtr1	Qtr2	Qtr3	Qtr4	Tot
1	A	AEs	3.0	5.0	5.0	1.0	14.00
9	A	Proc	25.0	45.0	35.0	30.0	135.00
17	A	Exp	1.0	1.8	1.5	1.3	5.60
25	A	Z-score	1.4	1.8	2.2	0.0	2.70
5	Q	AEs	0.0	4.0	1.0	5.0	10.00
13	Q	Proc	105.0	131.0	131.0	110.0	477.00
21	Q	Exp	4.2	5.2	5.2	4.4	19.00
29	Q	Z-score	-2.2	-0.3	-1.9	0.1	-2.15

2.8   Appendix 2 – SMR CIs and tests, further scripts. Hospital expected values from other hospitals in group

Calculating an interval for an SMR for a particular hospital when risk-adjustment is obtained from local data may involve determining the variation in the expected count for that hospital derived from the summation of its risk-adjustment values. For the hospital of interest there may also be observed/expected covariation. This has been discussed in section 2.4 of this chapter. An alternative approach that may be employed provided the hospital of interest does not furnish a large proportion of the local data, is to determine its expected count from the local data with its data excluded. When this is feasible, observed/expected covariation should be eliminated. An approach is now illustrated. Hospital I provides 7.6% of the data in orth0106.csv and we use it for illustration.

```
# SMR for hospital using risk adjustment scores
# calculated from other hospitals' data
g.d() # orth0106.csv, first column is not a date column

tbl<-table(datain[,1])
tbl
```

A	B	C	D	E	F	G	H	I	J	K	L	M	N	O	P	Q	R
865	1069	796	891	997	550	2598	373	1079	714	477	227	125	589	292	149	1984	351

```
I<-as.numeric(tb1[9])
I
#[1] 1079
L<-length(datain[,1])
I/L #Hospital I proportion of 2001-2006 data
#[1] 0.07638397
datainall<-datain #hold data when Hospital I data removed
datain<-datain[datain[,1]!="I",] #hospital I removed
tb2<-table(datain[,1])
tb2
```

A	B	C	D	E	F	G	H	I	J	K	L	M	N	O	P	Q	R
865	1069	796	891	997	550	2598	373	0	714	477	227	125	589	292	149	1984	351

```
#stratify data
a<-rep(1,length(datain[,1]))
d<-data.frame(datain,a)
a<-as.data.frame(xtabs(d[,5]~d[,4]+d[,2]))
b<-as.data.frame(xtabs(d[,6]~d[,4]+d[,2]))
ab<-data.frame(a,b[,3])
e<-ab[,3]/ab[,4]
ssi<-data.frame(ab,e)
names(ssi)<-c("RIs","Procedure","SSI","Procedures","Proportion")
ssi
```

	RIs	Procedure	SSI	Procedures	Proportion
1	0	PHR	4	79	0.05063291
2	1	PHR	12	133	0.09022556
3	2	PHR	3	25	0.12000000
4	0	RTHR	20	330	0.06060606
5	1	RTHR	13	178	0.07303371
6	2	RTHR	3	37	0.08108108
7	0	RTKR	14	204	0.06862745
8	1	RTKR	12	125	0.09600000
9	2	RTKR	2	22	0.09090909
10	0	THR	121	3429	0.03528726
11	1	THR	71	1512	0.04695767
12	2	THR	17	178	0.09550562
13	0	TKR	184	4565	0.04030668
14	1	TKR	89	2000	0.04450000
15	2	TKR	19	230	0.08260870

```
# amalgamate similar risk categories, small counts of SSIs
Expected<-ssi[,5]
Expected[2:3]<-sum(ssi[2:3,3])/sum(ssi[2:3,4])
Expected[5:6]<-sum(ssi[5:6,3])/sum(ssi[5:6,4])
Expected[8:9]<-sum(ssi[8:9,3])/sum(ssi[8:9,4])
ssi<-data.frame(ssi[,-5],Expected)
ssi
```

	RIs	Procedure	SSI	Procedures	Expected
1	0	PHR	4	79	0.05063291
2	1	PHR	12	133	0.09493671
3	2	PHR	3	25	0.09493671
4	0	RTHR	20	330	0.06060606
5	1	RTHR	13	178	0.07441860
6	2	RTHR	3	37	0.07441860
7	0	RTKR	14	204	0.06862745
8	1	RTKR	12	125	0.09523810
9	2	RTKR	2	22	0.09523810
10	0	THR	121	3429	0.03528726
11	1	THR	71	1512	0.04695767
12	2	THR	17	178	0.09550562
13	0	TKR	184	4565	0.04030668
14	1	TKR	89	2000	0.04450000
15	2	TKR	19	230	0.08260870

```
Rate<-ssi[,3]/ssi[,4]
Table1<-data.frame(ssi[,2],ssi[,1],ssi[,3:4],Rate,ssi[,5])
names(Table1)<-c("Procedure","RiskIndex","SSIs","Procedures","ObservedRate",
"StratumRate")
Table1
```

	Procedure	RiskIndex	SSIs	Procedures	ObservedRate	StratumRate
1	PHR	0	4	79	0.05063291	0.05063291
2	PHR	1	12	133	0.09022556	0.09493671
3	PHR	2	3	25	0.12000000	0.09493671
4	RTHR	0	20	330	0.06060606	0.06060606
5	RTHR	1	13	178	0.07303371	0.07441860
6	RTHR	2	3	37	0.08108108	0.07441860
7	RTKR	0	14	204	0.06862745	0.06862745
8	RTKR	1	12	125	0.09600000	0.09523810
9	RTKR	2	2	22	0.09090909	0.09523810
10	THR	0	121	3429	0.03528726	0.03528726
11	THR	1	71	1512	0.04695767	0.04695767
12	THR	2	17	178	0.09550562	0.09550562
13	TKR	0	184	4565	0.04030668	0.04030668
14	TKR	1	89	2000	0.04450000	0.04450000
15	TKR	2	19	230	0.08260870	0.08260870

```
#add RI to orth0106 data (minus Hospital I) in datain
e<-ssi[,5]
RI<-rep(0,length(datain[,1]))
for (i in 1:length(datain[,1])){
if (datain[i,2]=="PHR"&datain[i,4]==0){RI[i]<-e[1]}
if (datain[i,2]=="PHR"&(datain[i,4]==1|datain[i,4]==2)){RI[i]<-e[2]}
if (datain[i,2]=="RTHR"&datain[i,4]==0){RI[i]<-e[4]}
if (datain[i,2]=="RTHR"&(datain[i,4]==1|datain[i,4]==2)){RI[i]<-e[5]}
if (datain[i,2]=="RTKR"&datain[i,4]==0){RI[i]<-e[7]}
if (datain[i,2]=="RTKR"&(datain[i,4]==1|datain[i,4]==2)){RI[i]<-e[8]}
if (datain[i,2]=="THR"&datain[i,4]==0){RI[i]<-e[10]}
if (datain[i,2]=="THR"&datain[i,4]==1){RI[i]<-e[11]}
if (datain[i,2]=="THR"&datain[i,4]==2){RI[i]<-e[12]}
if (datain[i,2]=="TKR"&datain[i,4]==0){RI[i]<-e[13]}
if (datain[i,2]=="TKR"&datain[i,4]==1){RI[i]<-e[14]}
```

```
if (datain[i,2]=="TKR"&datain[i,4]==2){RI[i]<-e[15]}
}
ssi0106<-data.frame(datain,RI)
head(ssi0106)
```

	Hospital	Procedure	ProcedureDate	RiskIndex	SSI	RI
1	A	TKR	1-Feb-01	0	0	0.04030668
2	A	PHR	5-Feb-01	1	0	0.09493671
3	A	TKR	7-Feb-01	1	0	0.04450000
4	A	TKR	8-Feb-01	1	0	0.04450000
5	A	THR	12-Feb-01	0	0	0.03528726
6	A	TKR	14-Feb-01	1	0	0.04450000

```
#change date column data from factors to dates
#select 2005-2006 data
ssi0106a<-ssi0106
d<-ssi0106a[,3]
d<-chron(as.character(d),format="dd-mmm-yy",out.format="dd-mmm-yyyy")
ssi0506<-ssi0106a[d>="01-Jan-2005",]
names(ssi0506)<-c("Hospital","Procedure","ProcedureDate","RiskIndex","SSI",
"StratRI")
head(ssi0506)
```

	Hospital	Procedure	ProcedureDate	RiskIndex	SSI	StratRI
624	A	THR	13-Jan-05	0	0	0.03528726
625	A	TKR	21-Jan-05	0	0	0.04030668
626	A	TKR	24-Jan-05	1	1	0.04450000
627	A	TKR	25-Jan-05	0	0	0.04030668
628	A	THR	28-Jan-05	1	0	0.04695767
629	A	THR	1-Feb-05	0	0	0.03528726

```
#check risk adjustment (RA) fit to SSI data
length(ssi0506[,1]) #number of procedures
#[1] 5257
sum(ssi0506[,5]) #number of SSIs
#[1] 202
sum(ssi0506[,6]) #expected from stratification risk scores
#[1] 219.8718


#recalibration of stratification risk scores
g<-glm(ssi0506[,5]~ssi0506[,6],family=binomial)
StratRiskAdj<-g$fitted
ssi0506adj<-data.frame(ssi0506[,-c(6,7)],StratRiskAdj)
head(ssi0506adj)
```

	Hospital	Procedure	ProcedureDate	RiskIndex	SSI	StratRiskAdj
624	A	THR	13-Jan-05	0	0	0.03632020
625	A	TKR	21-Jan-05	0	0	0.03785181
626	A	TKR	24-Jan-05	1	1	0.03917874
627	A	TKR	25-Jan-05	0	0	0.03785181
628	A	THR	28-Jan-05	1	0	0.03997706
629	A	THR	1-Feb-05	0	0	0.03632020

```
#tabulate RA
a<-as.data.frame(xtabs(ssi0506adj[,6]~ssi0506adj[,4]+ssi0506adj[,2]))
x<-rep(1,length(ssi0506adj[,1]))
```

```
b<-as.data.frame(xtabs(x~ssi0506adj[,4]+ssi0506adj[,2]))
RI<-data.frame(a[,-3],a[,3]/b[,3])
names(RI)<-c("RI","Ptocedure","RiskScore")
RI
```

	RI	Ptocedure	RiskScore
1	0	PHR	0.04120004
2	1	PHR	0.05904313
3	0	RTHR	0.04470162
4	1	RTHR	0.05002209
5	0	RTKR	0.04772200
6	1	RTKR	0.05918638
7	0	THR	0.03632020
8	1	THR	0.03997706
9	0	TKR	0.03785181
10	1	TKR	0.03917874

```
#extract Hospital I data for 2005-2006
d<-datainall[,3] #convert factors to dates
d<-chron(as.character(d),format="d-mmm-yy",out.format="dd-mmm-yyyy")
hospitali<-datainall[datainall[,1]=="I"&d>"31-Dec-2004",]
length(hospitali[,1]) #number of procedures for Hospital I in 2005-2006

#[1] 365

#expected values to Hospital I data in vector EE
EE<-0
for (i in 1:length(hospitali[,1])){
if (hospitali[i,2]=="THR"&hospitali[i,4]==0){EE[i]<-0.03632020}
if (hospitali[i,2]=="THR"&hospitali[i,4]==1){EE[i]<-0.03997706}
if (hospitali[i,2]=="PHR"&hospitali[i,4]==0){EE[i]<-0.04120004}
if (hospitali[i,2]=="PHR"&hospitali[i,4]==1){EE[i]<-0.05904313}
if (hospitali[i,2]=="RTHR"&hospitali[i,4]==0){EE[i]<-0.04470162}
if (hospitali[i,2]=="RTHR"&hospitali[i,4]==1){EE[i]<-0.05002209}
if (hospitali[i,2]=="RTKR"&hospitali[i,4]==0){EE[i]<-0.04772200}
if (hospitali[i,2]=="RTKR"&hospitali[i,4]==1){EE[i]<-0.05918638}
if (hospitali[i,2]=="TKR"&hospitali[i,4]==0){EE[i]<-0.03785181}
if (hospitali[i,2]=="TKR"&hospitali[i,4]==1){EE[i]<-0.03917874}
}

#expected number of SSIs for Hospital I in 2005-2006
#obtained with hospital I data excluded
E<-sum(EE)
E
#[1] 15.34367
sum(hospitali[,5]) #observed number of SSIs for Hospital I in 2005-2006
#[1] 25
25*(365-25)/365 #variance of the observed number
#[1] 23.28767
sum(EE*(1-EE)) #variance of the expected number
#[1] 14.68348
#SMR and CIs
O<-25;E<-15.34;VO<-23.29;VE<-14.68
#approximate delta method variance of log SMR (O/E)
V<-VO/O^2+VE/E^2
V
```

```
#[1] 0.099648
SMR<-O/E
L<-exp(log(SMR)-1.96*V^.5)
L #lower confidence limit
#[1] 0.87783
U<-exp(log(SMR)+1.96*V^.5)
U #upper confidence limit
#[1] 3.0257
SMR
#[1] 1.6297
#
#approximate Z-score and P-value (Bland and Altman)
Z<-log(SMR)/V^.5
Z
#[1] 1.5472
P<-exp(-0.717*Z-0.416*Z^2)
P
#[1] 0.12182

# extending the ROVE procedure
#using difference and Miettinen's test-based method
D<-O-E
VD<-23.28767+14.68348
Z<-D/VD^.5
Z
#[1] 1.5677
P<-exp(-0.717*Z-0.416*Z^2)
P
#[1] 0.11691
L<-SMR^(1-1.96/Z)
L
#[1] 0.88494
U<-SMR^(1+1.96/Z)
U
#[1] 3.0013

#observed-expected difference using Newcombe's method
OL<-O-1.96*VO^.5
OU<-O+1.96*VO^.5
EU<-E+1.96*VE^.5
EL<-E-1.96*VE^.5
L<-D-((O-OL)^2+(EU-E)^2)^.5
U<-D+((E-EL)^2+(OU-O)^2)^.5
D;L;U
#[1] 9.66 (Difference)
#[1] -2.4175 (Lower limit)
#[1] 21.737 (Upper limit)

#observed-expected ratio using Newcombe's method
LO<-log(O)
LE<-log(E)
LD<-LO-LE
LOL<-LO-1.96*(VO/O^2)^.5
LOU<-LO+1.96*(VO/O^2)^.5
LEU<-LE+1.96*(VE/E^2)^.5
```

```
LEL<-LE-1.96*(VE/E^2)^.5
LL<-exp(LD-((LO-LOL)^2+(LEU-LE)^2)^.5)
UU<-exp(LD+((LE-LEL)^2+(LOU-LO)^2)^.5)
LD<-exp(LD)
LD;LL;UU
#[1] 1.6297 (SMR)
#[1] 0.87783 (Lower limit)
#[1] 3.0257) (Upper limit)

#Silcock's method
Nn<-O+E
PL<-qbeta(.025,O,Nn-O+1)
PU<-qbeta(.975,O+1,Nn-O)
U<-PU/(1-PU)
L<-PL/(1-PL)
L #lower confidence limit for SMR
#[1] 0.82989
U #upper confidence limit for SMR
#[1] 3.3042
SMR<-O/E
SMR
#[1] 1.6297
SE<-(U-L)/(2*1.96)/SMR #Taylor series approximation for log(SMR)
Z<-log(SMR)/SE
Z
#[1] 1.261
P<-exp(-0.717*Z-0.416*Z^2)
P
#[1] 0.20894

# usual SMR CI
library(PropCIs)
lo<-midPci(25,365,alpha=0.05)[1]
uo<-midPci(25,365,alpha=0.05)[2]
L95<-lo*365/E
U95<-uo*365/E
L95;U95
#[1] 1.0969
#[1] 2.3223
```

3

Sequential binary data

Although examining aggregated data is important, it is by analysing sequentially accumulating data that we can get timely warning of system changes or unforeseen problems. There is often some delay in acquiring these data (for example, a microbiology specimen is collected, it must be processed and then the result reported). Complications like postoperative mortality are frequently counted if they occur within 30 days. Thus an early death may be followed by a later one in the same time interval. However, although potentially preventable serious adverse events (AEs) require prompt attention, for many practical purposes monthly data analysis will suffice. Sequential analysis also has the ability to help staff resist tampering with systems in the face of events that are predictable and often random in nature. However, a single case of an unusual AE or an unusually serious AE should be dealt with immediately using, for example, morbidity and mortality (M&M) audit and systems analysis as described by Singer and by Taylor-Adams and Vincent.

We describe the following methods.

```
1. CUSUM (cumulative sum charts),
2. Cumulative observed minus expected (O-E) charts,
3. Combined CUSUM and O-E charts,
4. Risk adjustment,
5. Shewhart charts for binary data,
6. Exponentially Weighted Moving Average (EWMA) charts,
7. Combined Shewhart/EWMA charts for binary data,
8. Run-sums,
9. Generalized Additive Model (GAM) charts.
```

To aid in the selection of a suitable method, there is an appendix entitled Control Chart Menu at the end of the introductory chapter. In addition, there is a corresponding function CCMenu() in rprogs.

Statistical Methods for Hospital Monitoring with R, First Edition. Anthony Morton, Kerrie Mengersen, Michael Whitby and George Playford.
© 2013 John Wiley & Sons, Ltd. Published 2013 by John Wiley & Sons, Ltd.

3.1   CUSUM and related charts for binary data

Cumulative sum (CUSUM) analysis is widely employed for detecting small process shifts in production lines (Montgomery). In the hospital, it can be adapted to detect runs of adverse events (AEs).

The CUSUM method we employ is the sequential probability ratio CUSUM for binary data described by Steiner and colleagues. This CUSUM, which we label the Steiner CUSUM or CUSUM Test, is based on odds and likelihood. It is designed to deal with risk adjusted binary data but it can also be employed with proportion data that have a single expected outcome probability. We also discuss a Bernoulli CUSUM, for which a risk adjustment method has recently been proposed by Rossi and colleagues, later in the chapter.

Each new patient or procedure is allocated a score (S) of 1 if the AE of interest occurs and zero if it does not. These scores are then converted to weights (W) by employing the formulas: $W=\log_e[OR/(1-P+OR\times P)]$ if $S=1$ and $W=\log_e[1/(1-P+OR\times P)]$ if $S=0$. OR is the increase in the odds of $S=1$ occurring that one wishes to detect and P is the probability of $S=1$ taking place for each patient or procedure. It is frequently practically useful with hospital AE data to set $OR=2$ and then the formulas simplify to $\log((1+S)/(1+P))$. The contiguous Ws are accumulated.

If the accumulated value falls below zero and monitoring is being performed to detect increases in the numbers of AEs, the accumulated value is set to zero. Detecting an increase is required most commonly. Steiner and colleagues describe using the CUSUM to detect decreasing numbers of AEs.

If the accumulated weights reach a decision value, commonly labeled h, a signal is said to occur indicating that there is a high probability that the odds of the AE occurring have increased to the level to be detected (i.e. there has been a run of the AEs). Therefore there should be a search for assignable causes. As discussed in Chapter 1 and again in Chapter 2, this does not mean that there is a problem as false positive signals can occur and the analysis described by Mohammed[B] and his colleagues should be employed: look first for data or analysis error, then for problems with risk adjustment if used, then for system (structure and process) errors, and finally for problems involving staff. However, a signal does mean that the probability of a problem being present has become sufficiently high for a search for one to be required. The CUSUM should be re-set to zero and monitoring should resume.

The value for h is selected so that recognition of the occurrence of runs of AEs is prompt with a low probability of false positive signals occurring. The former requires a sensitive analysis and the latter a specific one. It is usually not possible to have both high sensitivity and high specificity simultaneously and a balance must be found. Undetected problems are of particular concern with hospital AE data. Conversely, too frequent false positive signals may induce tampering with satisfactory systems of patient care and this can increase the probability of an AE occurring. Alternatively, potentially important signals may be ignored.

Provided the hospital environment is not excessively judgemental, it will usually not be difficult for specialist staff to detect false positive signals. However, this will usually not be the case with community public health data where the status of apparent disease clusters may be difficult to determine. Thus, occasional false positive signals can be tolerated in the hospital environment to ensure that sensitivity is kept sufficiently high to minimise the probability of a genuine problem being missed or detected only after an excessive delay. If with uncommon AEs h is kept high, for example $h=5$, the probability of a false positive signal will be very low. However, if there is a genuine increase in the odds of the AE of interest, the CUSUM may fail to detect it or take too long to do so. If h is low, for example h=2, the CUSUM will respond quickly to changes, but there may be too frequent false positive signals that may induce tampering or tuning out.

Use of the Steiner CUSUM when AE rates are very low (e.g. below about 5%) has been criticised (Webster). In addition, doubling of the odds ratio is thought to be an unrealistically small change to detect, especially in the presence of risk-adjustment with its attendant increase in variation. Exponentially weighted moving average (EWMA) charts have been suggested as alternatives (Cook[A,B] and colleagues describe one version of the method although they illustrate it with intensive care and myocardial infarction mortality data that have a higher expected AE rate than 5%). It has been our experience that in practice the CUSUM usually performs well even when rates are low. However, it is wise to bear this reservation in mind. The simultaneous use of a cumulative observed minus expected (O-E) chart is of additional value (Grunkemeier and colleagues).

The value for h is usually determined by calculating the average run length to a signal (ARL). If the AE rate is not increasing, the ARL should be as long as possible. False positive signals should then be infrequent. However, if the AE rate has increased, the ARL should be as short as possible so that a signal occurs promptly. There must be a compromise between these two objectives. Simulation or the employment of a Markov chain method can be used to select the most suitable value for h.

Hospital X had $100 \times 45/286 = 15.7\%$ of its patients in then Australian National Diagnosis Related Group 252 (ANDRG 252), heart failure and shock, exceeding the 90th percentile for length of stay (LOS) in 1994–95, calculated from the state reference database. The 90th percentile value in the reference database was 16.4 days and for Hospital X it was 21.4 days. Since this was a relatively common DRG and patient stays can easily become long term if careful discharge planning is not practiced, the administration of a hospital faced with this proportion of long stay patients would need to revise its discharge planning system and processes.

Suppose that the hospital staff reviewed and implemented a sound evidence-based system of discharge planning and the proportion of lengths of stay of 17 or more days was then reduced to 7.5% [Odds=$0.075/(1-0.075) \approx 0.08$]. The staff would wish to monitor LOS for this DRG continuously and have an efficient warning mechanism if the odds for 17 or more days were again to double to 0.16 [proportion=$0.16/(1+0.16) \approx 0.14$]. Suppose that the following sequence was obtained at this stage.

$$1\,0\,0\,0\,1\,0\,1\,0\,0\,1\,0\,0\,1\,0\,0\,0\,1\,1\,0$$

where 0 represents an LOS of 16 days or less and 1 an LOS of 17 or more days; for these hypothetical data the rate exceeding the overall 90th percentile would have been $100 \times 7/19 = .37$ or 37%. Since the rate may increase for a brief period due to predictable variation, a statistical test is required to distinguish increases in the proportion of LOS of 17 or more days that are sufficiently large for predictable variation to be an improbable reason for their occurrence. The CUSUM test performs this function (Figure 3.1).

```
# basic CUSUM
los90<-c(1,0,0,0,1,0,1,0,0,1,0,0,1,0,0,0,1,1,0)
d<-los90
```

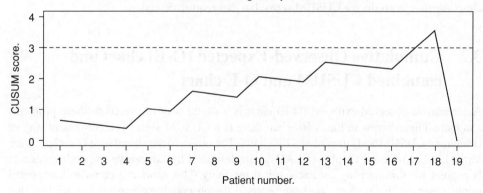

Figure 3.1   Basic CUSUM.

```
a<-.075;h<-3 # Expected rate=.075, note that h has been set to 3
x<-log((d+1)/(1+a)) # simplified formula for W when OR=2
b<-x[1]
for (i in 2:length(x)){if (b[i-1]>=h){b[i]<-max(c(x[i],0))}else{b[i]<-
max(c(b[i-1]+x[i],0))}}
l<-1:length(d)
par(lab=c(length(l),5,7))
plot(b,type="l",col="blue",axes=F,main="LOS values exceeding 90th per-
centile for DRG.",ylab="",xlab="Patient number.",ylim=c(0,4),lwd=3)
mtext(text="CUSUM score.",side=2,line=2)
axis(side=1,tick=T,labels(as.character(l)),at=l)
box()
abline(h=3,col="red",lwd=2)
axis(side=c(2,3,4))
```

Simulations show that, when h=3, the ARL, when the adverse event rate of 7.5% [odds=0.075/(1-0.075)=0.08] does not increase, is about 1000 and it is approximately 90 when the odds double to give a rate of 14% (0.16/(1+0.16)=0.14). This appears to be a satisfactory compromise for sensitivity and specificity. The function binarl() performs the simulations.

```
#to use the ARL function for binary data without risk-adjustment
binarl()
```

```
Enter expected value .075
Enter significance level 3
Enter ARL for observed rate (1) or double odds (2) 2
[1] 97.26
```

The Steiner CUSUM has wide potential application for monitoring outcomes that are either a success or a failure, or satisfactory or unsatisfactory. Examples include discharge summaries and other documentation, allocation of patients to DRGs, procedures such as successfully completed endoscopies, and compliance with treatment guidelines and evidence based bundles. In general, it is an excellent way to analyse sequential binary data. However, as it is only capable of displaying a signal, it does not give the user a good feel for the data.

In addition, there are occasions when there are increased AEs that may not occur sufficiently close together to produce a CUSUM signal but that require detection.

3.2   Cumulative Observed-Expected (O-E) chart and combined CUSUM and O-E chart

A cumulative observed-expected (O-E) chart is a useful way to overcome these problems and including an arrow in the chart when there is a CUSUM signal is a convenient way of combining CUSUM and cumulative O-E charts. The origin of the cumulative O-E chart is the Variable Life Adjusted Display (VLAD) chart described by Lovegrove and colleagues that is popular for summarising cardiac surgical mortality. This chart is a cumulative expected minus observed (E-O) chart. We have reversed the observed and expected as we find that staff are more used to charts that show increased AE rates as an upward deflection. The two sigma equivalent limits shown for this chart are prediction (control) limits calculated using a simple search with the R pbeta() function. Since this involves multiple significance testing, a signal in either the CUSUM or cumulative O-E does not prove that a problem exists but it does indicate that the probability of one having occurred has become sufficiently high for it to be investigated further, for example, by M&M audit. As we have indicated, it is important to adhere to the method described by Mohammed and colleagues.

This combined chart is an excellent representation of the process being examined. The cumulative O-E chart may sometimes identify an unsatisfactory process that the CUSUM test chart fails to recognise, for example when the overall process is unsatisfactory but there is no definite run of adverse outcomes to cause the CUSUM to signal. In addition, it indicates how many more or less adverse outcomes have occurred than expected at any time. This can be a valuable resource when presenting outcome data to management. Clinical staff also like to know the current AE rate and the EWMA chart described by Cook[A,B] and colleagues has this advantage. However, when AE rates are low, for example, below about 5%, a useful alternative may be to provide quarterly rates. This issue is dealt with in more detail in section 3.20.3 of this chapter.

An issue that requires attention is when to set the cumulative O-E chart back to zero and re-commence its monitoring. It would seem that when either of the control limit lines is crossed or there is a CUSUM signal, an examination of the underlying system should occur. This would seem to be a good place to re-start the cumulative O-E chart. In addition, if the chart is not re-started periodically the control limits become increasingly wide and this should prompt consideration for re-starting. In this situation it would seem desirable to select a time when the cumulative O-E line is approximately horizontal suggesting a stable process. The new chart may be difficult to implement to begin with and for the first few observations it may be better to rely on tabulations.

3.3   Cumulative funnel plot and combined CUSUM and funnel plot

The cumulative funnel plot is an alternative to the O-E chart that has become popular in cardiology. When the data are not risk-adjusted, the centre line of the chart is the overall

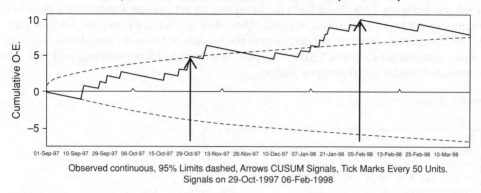

Figure 3.2   Cumulative Observed minus Expected plus CUSUM chart (O-E/CUSUM).

expected AE rate and as the outcome of each new procedure becomes available, the average of the accumulated observed outcomes is calculated and displayed. We find that this plot is less useful than the cumulative O-E chart. The two sigma equivalent limits shown for this chart are prediction (control) limits also calculated using a simple search with pbeta(). If the upper control limit is breached, the recommendations of Lilford and colleagues and Mohammed[B] and colleagues should again be followed.

3.4   Example

A series of lower limb vascular operations was performed in 1997 and 1998. There were 240 operations with 20 SSIs, giving a rate of 8.3%. The expected SSI rate was 5%. Surgical site infections occurred at the following operations: 21, 22, 31, 35, 43, 68, 76, 81, 82, 90, 91, 130, 144, 150, 155, 158, 160, 172, 178, and 211. Figures 3.2 and 3.3 are the cumulative O-E and CUSUM charts and Figure 3.4 is the cumulative funnel plot and CUSUM chart. It can be seen

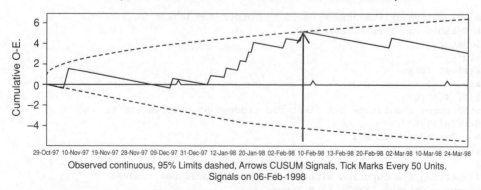

Figure 3.3   O-E CUSUM, re-setting to baseline with CUSUM signal.

that there were two occasions when the CUSUM test signaled. These occurred in October 1977 and February 1998. In addition the upper two sigma equivalent cumulative observed minus expected (O-E) limit was exceeded. These data are in file ssi.csv. The function g.d() is used to enter the data in R and the function boecusum() performs the cumulative observed minus expected (O-E) plus CUSUM analysis. The function bfunnelcusum() performs the combined CUSUM and funnel plot analysis.

```
g.d() # ssi.csv
```

```
Loading data.
Data from clipboard (C) or file (F) c
Do data column(s) have heading(s) (Y/N) y
Is column 1 a date column (Y/N) y
Date format.
 1-Sep-97
Date format.
Enter the required date format d-mmm-yy
```

```
#using  the cumulative O-E/CUSUM function
boecusum(datain) # Figure 3.2
```

```
Date format.
 01-Sep-1997
Date format.
Enter the required date format dd-mmm-yyyy
Do you have risk-adjusted data (Y/N) n
The mean outcome rate is  0.083
Do you wish to enter another value (Y/N) y
Enter the required value .05
Cumulative sum alert.
Enter the Cumulative sum (CUSUM) alert value 3
Chart heading.
Enter heading for chart Orthopaedic SSI Cumulative O - E chart
Cusum h = 3
Cusum signals on
[1] 29-Oct-1997 06-Feb-1998
```

```
# using locator()to detect where the upper cumulative O-
# E limit was first crossed
locator()
#$x
#[1] 81.76695
#$y
#[1] 4.877028
#the upper cumulative O-E limit was crossed at observation 82
datain[82,]
#    ProcedureDate SSI
#82    29-Oct-1997   1
#
#repeating the function with the first 82 procedures removed
boecusum(datain[-(1:82),]) # Figure 3.3
```

```
Date format.
 29-Oct-1997
Date format.
Enter the required date format dd-mmm-yyyy
Do you have risk-adjusted data (Y/N) n
The mean outcome rate is  0.07
Do you wish to enter another value (Y/N) y
Enter the required value .05
Cumulative sum alert.
Enter the Cumulative sum (CUSUM) alert value 3
Chart heading.
Enter heading for chart Orthopaedic SSI Cumulative O - E chart
Cusum h = 3
Cusum signals on
[1] 06-Feb-1998
```

```
locator() #to determine position of remaining signal
#$x
#[1] 95.81143
#$y
#[1] 5.220153
#signal occurred at 96+82=178th observation
datain[178,]
#      ProcedureDate SSI
#178   06-Feb-1998    1
length(datain[-(1:179),1]) # remaining observations after second signal
#[1] 61
sum(datain[-(1:178),2]) #only one ssi following second signal
#[1] 1

#using the bfunnelcusum function
bfunnelcusum(datain)# Figure 3.4
```

```
Date format.
 01-Sep-1997
Date format.
Enter the required date format dd-mmm-yyyy
Do you have risk-adjusted data (Y/N) n
The mean outcome rate is  0.083
Do you wish to enter another value (Y/N) y
Enter the required value .05
Cumulative sum alert.
Enter the Cumulative sum (CUSUM) alert value 3
Chart heading.
Enter heading for chart Cumulative Funnel Plot
The funnel plot Y axis limits are 0 and 1
Do you wish to change the upper limit (Y/N) y
Enter the new value .2 (may need to repeat function for best result)
Do you wish to change the lower limit (Y/N) n
Cusum h = 3
Cusum signals on
[1] 29-Oct-1997 06-Feb-1998
```

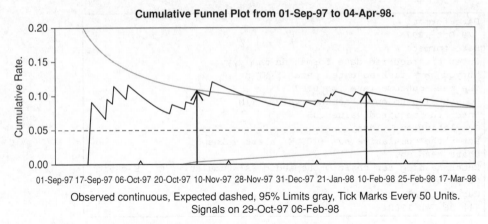

Figure 3.4   Cumulative funnel plot plus CUSUM chart.

3.5   Including risk adjustment

As discussed in Chapters 1 and 2, risk-adjusted binary data are becoming increasingly available. The CDC National Nosocomial Infection Surveillance (NNIS) surgical risk index allocates probabilities of SSIs occurring by considering the procedure involved, the wound class, the length of the surgical procedure and the patient's ASA score (Horan and colleagues). Also, superior SSI risk scores for particular procedures are becoming available, for example, diabetes, obesity, female gender, number of coronary arteries affected and use of bilateral internal thoracic arteries for coronary artery bypass surgery (Farsky and colleagues). Risk-adjustment formulas are now available for in-hospital AEs complicating a wide variety of procedures and diagnoses, for example death following cardiac surgery, aortic aneurysm surgery, myocardial infarction, intensive care, general surgery and pneumonia.

An important characteristic of the Steiner CUSUM is that its ARL is relatively long for a given h value when the average expected probability of the adverse outcome (AE) is very low, for example following coronary artery surgery (typically below 2%). When the average expected probability of the adverse outcome is higher as it is for ICU or CCU mortality (typically around 10% to 15%), the ARL at any h value is much shorter. In addition, when risk scores either do not vary or vary very little as with most NNIS risk-adjusted surgical site infections (SSIs), ARL values for any average risk score and h value are shorter than ARL values for similar average scores when there is a large spread of risk scores as there is with predicted ICU mortality. This has two consequences. First, ARL values need to be determined for each situation, for example by simulation. Secondly, if there is an apparent run of adverse events associated with a run of high expected outcome probabilities within a low average expected outcome probability procedure, it may be due to an increase in the probability of a false positive signal. A consequence of using this CUSUM is that there can be serious delay in detecting a subtle change when the expected outcome rate is very low. When adverse outcomes are rare, it is preferable to rely foremost on systems analysis and M&M audit. However, it is still desirable to employ, for example, a CUSUM analysis, especially in a judgemental environment, to minimise the risk of tampering with sound systems when occasional AEs are occurring at a predictable rate.

For a particular surgical procedure AE, the CUSUM ARL for the consultant who takes the difficult cases may differ from the ARL for the advanced trainee who on average operates on better risk patients. In addition, a surgeon who treats a lot of both high and low risk patients will have a different ARL value for a particular level of h than one who treats mostly patients with an average expected outcome probability. ARL values should be determined separately for each situation. In addition, when a signal occurs, the approach of Mohammed and his colleagues should be followed: first, check the data and its analysis; next check the risk adjustment; then the system; finally for problems involving staff. If no assignable causes can be found, a chart of the expected outcome probabilities can be examined to see if there has been any change in the average expected outcome rate or its variation. These difficulties should be remembered when a signal occurs and there appears to be no assignable cause. As with the SSI data described above, the cumulative observed minus expected chart is useful for presenting these data and the presence of a CUSUM signal can be indicated with an arrow. The funnel plot is preferred in some departments, for example in cardiology.

We emphasise that the Pareto idea of concentrating on the few prominent potential causative agents when a signal occurs should be applied with some caution. The emergent behaviour of complex systems depends on the interactions of many agents and, cumulatively, seemingly minor difficulties with several interacting agents may cause the behaviour of a complex system to become unpredictable (Johnson). This can be demonstrated, for example, by employing a Bayesian network (Waterhouse and colleagues).

When AEs that are uncommon occur it is important, in order to avoid delay, to concentrate first on systems analysis. We need to ask: has the best currently available evidence, increasingly embodied in bundles and checklists, been followed? Use M&M audits and then employ the cumulative observed minus expected chart, including CUSUM signals if present, for data presentation and to guard against making system changes when occasional events occur in a predictable system.

Root cause analysis is a popular approach. However, as we discuss in several places in these notes, AEs may represent the emergent bahaviour of an unfavourable state of a complex system. There may be no root cause; instead there may be multiple interacting agents, none of which taken singly may appear seriously at fault. We discuss this further in Chapter 8.

3.6   CUSUM chart

The data in aaamort.csv are amalgamated postoperative abdominal aortic aneurysm surgery mortality data from a group of hospitals so that any signal has no significance for any particular hospital (we are grateful to Mr Barry Beiles for these data). There were 1235 procedures and 106 deaths occurred (8.6%). ARL with h=3.5 is approximately 2500 when the rate does not change and about 150 when the odds double. The CUSUM chart (Beiles and Morton) is combined with a cumulative observed minus expected chart.

3.7   Cumulative observed minus expected (O-E) chart

The cumulative O-E chart may also be used with risk-adjusted data. This chart is an excellent semi-quantitative representation of the process being examined. However, it should be reset to zero at regular intervals as the cumulative O-E control limits continue to diverge as the procedures accumulate and older data become less relevant; a suggested approach is to

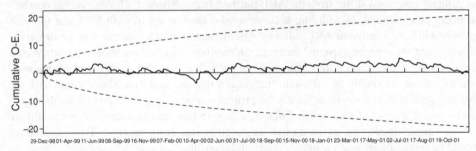

AAA Mortality Cumulative O-E and CUSUM chart from 29-Dec-98 to 06-Jan-02.

Observed continuous, 95% Limits dashed, Arrows CUSUM Signals, Tick Marks Every 50 Units.

Figure 3.5   O-E/CUSUM with risk adjustment.

include the 100 to 200 most recent observations but to endeavour to re-set at a time when the cumulative O-E line is approximately horizontal (i.e. the AE rate is predictable). A further reason for resetting may be the occurrence of a CUSUM signal or the cumulative O-E line going outside the control limits provided there are sufficient data after the signal for the new chart to be feasible (in the interim, the process can be followed with tabulations). Since an audit should occur at this time followed by system changes, if needed, it is a sensible time to consider re-setting the charts. Clearly these issues can require some judgement.

The cumulative O-E chart may identify an unsatisfactory process that the CUSUM test chart fails to recognise, for example when the overall process is unsatisfactory but there is no definite run of adverse outcomes to cause the CUSUM to signal. Figure 3.5 is the chart for the abdominal aortic aneurysm mortality data; there is no CUSUM signal.

```
g.d() # aaamort.csv
```

```
Loading data.
Data from clipboard (C) or file (F) c
Do data column(s) have heading(s) (Y/N) y
Is column 1 a date column (Y/N) y
Date format.
 3-Feb-99
Date format.
Enter the required date format d-mmm-yy
```

```
# O-E/CUSUM Chart Figure 3.5
boecusum(datain)
```

```
Date format.
 03-Feb-1999
Date format.
Enter the required date format dd-mmm-yyyy
Do you have risk-adjusted data (Y/N) y
Cumulative sum alert.
Enter the Cumulative sum (CUSUM) alert value 3.5
Chart heading.
Enter heading for chart AAA Mortality
```

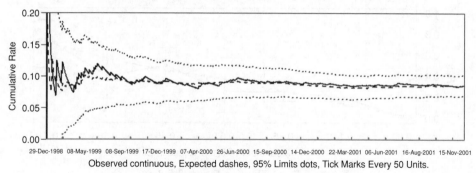

AAA Mortality Cumulative Funnel Plot from 29-Dec-98 to 06-Jan-02.

Observed continuous, Expected dashes, 95% Limits dots, Tick Marks Every 50 Units.

Figure 3.6   Cumulative funnel plot with risk adjustment.

A fast initial response (FIR) feature is described by Lucas and Crosier. When a CUSUM is re-set following a signal it can be re-started halfway between zero and h. If the process has become predictable the CUSUM quickly falls to zero. However, if the process remains in an unpredictable state, a further CUSUM signal will occur promptly. We do not employ the FIR feature at this time.

3.8   Funnel plot

This plot is preferred by some workers, particularly in interventional cardiology (Kunadian and colleagues, Morton[F] and colleagues). While the cumulative O-E chart displays the cumulative number of AEs that are more or less than expected, the cumulative funnel plot displays the corresponding risk-adjusted rates. It is illustrated in Figure 3.6. This plot is more useful when the vertical axis limits are selected manually. It can be untidy when the baseline mean rate is changing as data accumulate and the cumulative expected rate changes.

```
#using the bfunnelcusum() function, Figure 3.6
bfunnelcusum(datain)
```

```
Date format.
 01-Jan-1995
Date format.
Enter the required date format dd-mmm-yyyy
Do you have risk-adjusted data (Y/N) y
Cumulative sum alert.
Enter the Cumulative sum (CUSUM) alert value 3.5
Chart heading.
Enter heading for chart AAA Mortality
The funnel plot Y axis limits are 0 and 1
Do you wish to change the upper limit (Y/N) y
Enter the new value .2
Do you wish to change the lower limit (Y/N) n
```

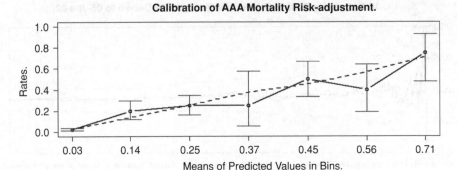

Figure 3.7 Calibration Figure 3.5 data.

When a signal occurs in one or more control charts, staff should examine their system and, if a problem is found it is important that it be dealt with. However, it is important to realise that a signal does not prove that there is a problem; it shows that the probability of a problem being present is sufficiently high to require investigation. The method proposed by Mohammed and his colleagues should be followed: look first for data error, then problems with risk adjustment, analytical errors, system errors, and finally for problems involving staff.

If there are repeated signals, the probability of a problem being present is increased. However, occasional false positive signals will inevitably ultimately occur. Fortunately, with hospital data (but frequently not with community public health data), it is usually not difficult for knowledgeable clinicians to determine when a signal is a false positive one.

3.9   Discrimination and calibration of risk adjustment

It is important to consider the discrimination and calibration of the risk-adjustment method. Figure 3.7 shows the calibration for the AAA mortality data and Figure 3.8 its discrimination. If the calibration systematically under or over-estimates outcome probabilities, it may indicate that the risk-adjustment method requires re-calibration. For example, a risk-adjustment

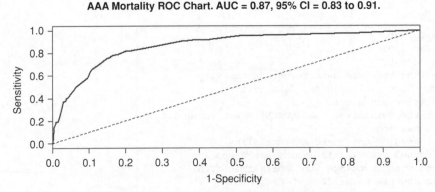

Figure 3.8 Discrimination Figure 3.5 data.

formula developed in one centre may not be optimal for another especially if they come from different countries with differing hospital systems.

```
g.d() # aaamort.csv
```

```
Loading data.
Data from clipboard (C) or file (F) c
Do data column(s) have heading(s) (Y/N) y
Is column 1 a date column (Y/N) y
Date format.
 3-Feb-99
Date format.
Enter the required date format d-mmm-yy
```

```
# AAA data calibration, Figure 3.7
# requires some trial and error to get number of categories
a<-datain[,2];b<-datain[,3]
k<-c(0,.1,.2,.3,.4,.5,.6,1)
q<-mean(b[b<=k[2]])
for (i in 2:(length(k)-1)){q[i]<-mean(b[b>k[i]&b<=k[i+1]])}
p<-mean(a[b<=k[2]])
for (i in 2:(length(k)-1)){p[i]<-mean(a[b>k[i]&b<=k[i+1]])}
l<-length(a[b<=k[2]])
for (i in 2:(length(k)-1)){l[i]<-length(a[b>k[i]&b<=k[i+1]])}
n<-l*p
n<-n[l!=0]
p<-p[l!=0]
q<-q[l!=0]
l<-l[l!=0]
library(exactci)
lo<-0
for (i in 1:length(l)){if (n[i]==0){lo[i]<-0}else{lo[i]<-
binom.exact(n[i],l[i])$conf[1]}}
up<-0
for (i in 1:length(l)){if (n[i]==l[i]){up[i]<-1}else{up[i]<-
binom.exact(n[i],l[i])$conf[2]}}
lk<-1:length(q)
par(lab=c(length(q),5,7));par(xaxs="r")
plot(p,type="b",col="blue",lwd=2,axes=F,main="Calibration of AAA Mortality
Risk-adjustment.",xlab="Means of Predicted Values in Bins.",
ylab="Rates.",ylim=c(0,1))
box()
axis(side=1,tick=T,labels=as.character(round(q,2)),at=lk);axis(side=
c(2,3,4))
arrows(lk,lo,lk,up,angle=90,code=3,col="red")
lines(q,col="black",lwd=2)

# goodness of fit
Pval<-0
for(i in 1:length(lk)){Pval[i]<-binom.exact(n[i],l[i],q[i])$p.value}
Z<--0.862+(0.743-2.404*log(Pval))^.5
ch<-sum(Z^2)
ch
#[1] 4.158933
df<-length(Z)-1
```

**Complex SSIs Cumulative O-E and CUSUM chart
from 05-Jan-05 to 28-Dec-05.**

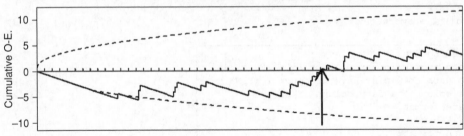

Observed continuous, 95% Limits dashed, Arrows CUSUM Signals, Tick Marks every 50 Units.
Signals on 26-Aug-05

Figure 3.9   Cumulative O-E CUSUM, low rate data with risk adjustment.

```
1-pchisq(ch,df)
#[1] 0.6551783
rm(df) # df is an F distribution function

# Hosmer-Lemmeshow goodness of fit
library(MKmisc)
HLgof.test(datain[,3],datain[,2])$C
```

```
Hosmer-Lemeshow C statistic
X-squared = 4.0711, df = 5, p-value = 0.5392
```

```
#using rocchart for discrimination
rocchart(datain[,-1]) # Figure 3.8

#Enter a name for the ROC chart AAA Mortality
```

Figures 3.9 and 3.10 are cumulative O-E/CUSUM and cumulative funnel plot/CUSUM charts for complex SSIs during 2005. They are from a number of hospitals so, while useful

Complex SSI Cumulative Funnel Plot from 05-Jan-05 to 28-Dec-05.

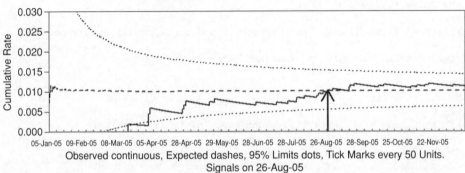

Observed continuous, Expected dashes, 95% Limits dots, Tick Marks every 50 Units.
Signals on 26-Aug-05

Figure 3.10   Cumulative funnel plot plus CUSUM low rate data with risk adjustment.

to illustrate methods, the chart signal has no significance for any hospital. Early on the rate was very low. Might there have been some under-reporting?

```
g.d() # allssicomplx.csv
```

```
Loading data.
Data from clipboard (C) or file (F) c
Do data column(s) have heading(s) (Y/N) y
Is column 1 a date column (Y/N) y
Date format.
 1-Feb-01
Date format.
Enter the required date format d-mmm-yy
```

```
# get 2005 data
ssicomplx<-datain[years(datain[,1])==2005,]
```

```
# save data in a file
s.d(ssicomplx)
```

```
Use clipboard (c) or a data file (f) f
Enter a file name d:/ssicomplx2005
```

```
# check ARL values
binarladj(ssicomplx[,3])
```

```
Select baseline OR (B) or double OR (D) b
Significance level (h) 2.75
Enter the number of trials 100
[1] 4177.9
```

```
binarladj(ssicomplx[,3])
```

```
Select baseline OR (B) or double OR (D) d
Significance level (h) 2.75
Enter the number of trials 100
[1] 561.59
```

Since there are nearly 2800 rows in ssicomplx, these h values should be suitable. Individual institutions with fewer data annually may find a lower value is needed but much lower h values may result in excessive numbers of signals.

```
# cumulative O-E/CUSUM
boecusum(ssicomplx) # Figure 3.9
```

```
Date format.
 13-Jan-2005
Date format.
Enter the required date format dd-mmm-yyyy
Do you have risk-adjusted data (Y/N) y
Cumulative sum alert.
Enter the Cumulative sum (CUSUM) alert value 2.75
Chart heading.
```

```
Enter heading for chart Complex SSIs in 2005
Cusum h = 2.75
Cusum signals on
[1] 26-Aug-2005
```

```
# cumulative funnel plot/CUSUM
bfunnelcusum(ssicomplx) # Figure 3.10
```

```
Do you have risk-adjusted data (Y/N) y
Cumulative sum alert.
Enter the Cumulative sum (CUSUM) alert value 2.75
Chart heading.
Enter heading for chart Complex SSIs in 2005
The funnel plot Y axis limits are 0 and 1
Do you wish to change the upper limit (Y/N) y
Enter the new value .03
Do you wish to change the lower limit (Y/N) n
Cusum h = 2.75
Cusum signals on
[1] 26-Aug-2005
```

3.10   Shewhart P chart and EWMA chart

These charts may be used to analyse binary data when the data are sufficiently numerous to enable them to be grouped, for example, by months (Hart[A] and colleagues). Examples include the proportion of patients each month for whom LOS exceeds a certain percentile for a particular DRG, the proportion of surgical patients receiving appropriate prophylactic antibiotics and the proportion of antibiotic prescriptions that comply with antibiotic guidelines. Many documentation functions could also be analysed with these charts. Examples include the proportion of patients correctly classified by DRG, the proportion of patients discharged within a particular time-frame, the proportion of admission records correctly documented, the proportion of patients whose discharge planning is performed correctly, or the proportion of discharge summaries that are incomplete.

These charts may also be used with risk-adjusted data, for example monthly intensive care unit (ICU) mortality, where indirect standardisation may be employed. If O_i is the observed count for time i and E_i is the corresponding expected value, $O_{adj}=ebar \times O_i/E_i$, where ebar is an overall average. Although these data may not be binomially distributed, approximate limits based on the binomial distribution are frequently employed. Also, it must be kept in mind that indirect standardisation can be biased when denominators and risk profiles differ markedly. As far as we are aware, this is unlikely to be a serious problem with binary data in control charts but it has been demonstrated to be so with some risk-adjusted count data (Morton[D] and colleagues), so the possibility of bias should be kept in mind. Count data risk-adjustment employs the characteristics of the institutions of interest and is described in Chapter 5.

As illustration, the clinicians of a small teaching hospital were concerned at the low autopsy rate which they considered to be due to the pathologists' unwillingness to perform autopsies. However, the pathologists believed that the problem was an administrative one over which they had little control. In order to understand the problem better, data were collected for 12 consecutive months on the number of deaths and autopsies. These data are in the file autopsy.csv. Although control charts are ideally based on at least 20 time periods during which the process being monitored is in a predictable state, we proceed with this analysis that involves just 12.

The overall autopsy rate was $P=82/418=19.6\%$ and this could be considered inadequate for a teaching hospital. For these data the standard deviation (SD) for each month can be calculated using the large sample normal approximation. The formula is $SD=\sqrt{[P\times(1-P)/N_i]}$, where $P=0.196$ is the overall autopsy rate and N_i is the number of deaths for the ith month. Thus for the first month it is $SD=\sqrt{[0.196\times(1-0.196)/52]}=0.055$, so that the upper 2 SD control limit is $U_2=0.196+2\times0.055=0.306$. Three SD limits are calculated in a similar way. In addition, the one standard deviation limits are frequently calculated. It may be especially useful to record the latter when an EWMA chart is not employed, as they can be used in run-sum tests that add an approximate CUSUM analysis (Champ and Rigdon). Run-sum analysis is described in section 3.11 of this chapter.

Samples available in hospitals for study are frequently small and the large sample normal approximation may be unreliable with small samples. Following from Chapter 1, we prefer to determine control limits by employing the beta distribution. This requires a simple search using the R pbeta() function as described in section 2.3.3.2 of Chapter 2.

It is often useful first to examine these data in a table and barchart (bbar()). It is also valuable to perform a trend test using the MannKendall seasonal trend test. A Shewhart chart (bshew()) may then be employed.

```
g.d() # autopsy.csv
```

```
Loading data.
Data from clipboard (C) or file (F) c
Do data column(s) have heading(s) (Y/N) y
Is column 1 a date column (Y/N) y
Date format.
1-Jan-85
Date format.
Enter the required date format d-mmm-yy
```

```
#using bbar() function, Figure 3.11
bbar(datain)
```

```
#Chart heading.
Enter heading for chart Autopsies Performed in 1985.
```

```
#using the binomial shewhart chart bshew(), Figure 3.12
bshew(datain)
```

```
Date format.
 01-Jan-1985
Date format.
Enter the required date format dd-mmm-yyyy
Do you have risk-adjusted data (Y/N) n
The mean outcome rate is  0.196
Do you wish to enter another value (Y/N) n
Chart heading.
Enter heading for the chart Autopsies
```

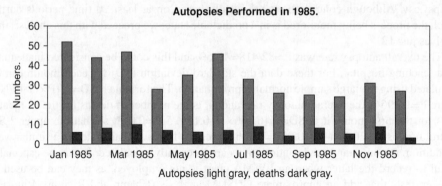

Figure 3.11   Bar chart binomial data.

The chart is in control so there was no evidence of unpredictable work among the pathologists.

```
# trend test
library(Kendall)
MannKendall(datain[,2]/datain[,3])

# tau = 0.152, 2-sided pvalue =0.53713

MannKendall(datain[,2]) # count of autopsies

#tau = -0.188, 2-sided pvalue =0.446

MannKendall(datain[,3]) # count of deaths

#tau = -0.606, 2-sided pvalue =0.00749

# no trend in the autopsies or the autopsy rate although a down trend in
# deaths
```

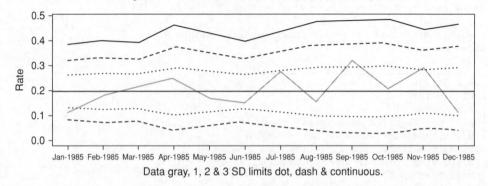

Figure 3.12   Shewhart chart binomial data.

3.11 Note on the Run-sum chart

The Run-sum CUSUM is a simple addition to the Shewhart chart. It is able to provide excellent supplementary run rules for Shewhart charts, but appears to be under-utilised for this purpose (Champ and Rigdon).

When a result is outside the U_2 or L_2 limits or their percentile equivalents, a score of ± 2 is assigned, and ± 1 is assigned when it is between the U_1 and U_2 or L_1 and L_2 limits. If the data point is between the U_1 and the centre line (CL) or CL and L_1, the score is 0. The scores are accumulated. If the data points X_{i-1} and X_i are on different sides of the CL, the accumulated score is re-set to zero and then recommenced with the X_i score. Results outside U_3 or L_3 are considered significant without summation. There is an example in section 6.5 of Chapter 6.

By employing additional lines at $U_{0.5}$ and $L_{0.5}$, $U_{1.5}$ and $L_{1.5}$ and $U_{2.5}$ and $L_{2.5}$ extra zones can be created with scores of 0.5, 1.5 and 2.5 respectively which may increase the power of the test. Some authors use other scoring systems, for example two consecutive values above $U_{1.5}$.

A significant shift in the mean should be suspected if the cumulative run-sum score reaches 4 or more. If there is a signal, the run-sum is re-commenced at zero. By adding supplementary rules to the Shewhart chart, it improves the ability of the latter to detect changes in the mean value, thus making it better for detecting unpredictable variation. However, when multiple rules are applied to data in control charts, the probability of false positive signals increases. This must be borne in mind when using run-sum and other supplementary run rules, such as seven consecutive points on one side of the midline or six consecutive points increasing or decreasing, with Shewhart charts.

3.12 The EWMA chart

EWMA charts are generally superior to Shewhart charts for displaying smaller persistent changes in the mean count or rate. Figure 3.13 is a combined Shewhart/EWMA chart for the data in ssis.csv that have been aggregated by quarters (we refer to quarterly data and data without a date column in section 3.16 of this chapter). The EWMA chart displays clearly the

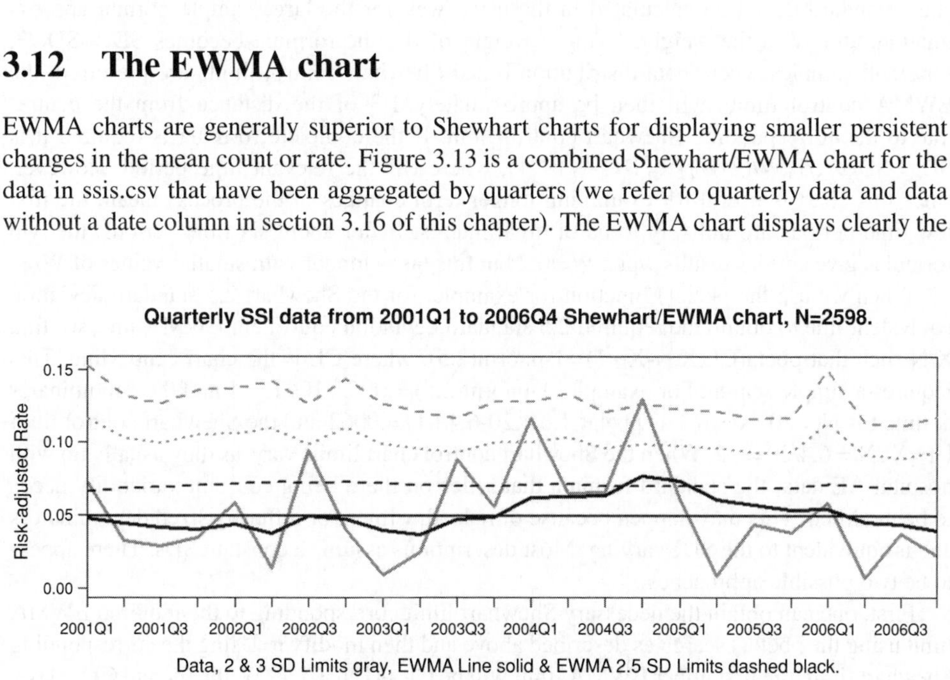
Quarterly SSI data from 2001Q1 to 2006Q4 Shewhart/EWMA chart, N=2598.
Risk-adjusted Rate
0.15
0.10
0.05
0.00
2001Q1
2001Q3
2002Q1
2002Q3
2003Q1
2003Q3
2004Q1
2004Q3
2005Q1
2005Q3
2006Q1
2006Q3
Data, 2 & 3 SD Limits gray, EWMA Line solid & EWMA 2.5 SD Limits dashed black.

Figure 3.13 Shewhart/EWMA chart quarterly risk adjusted binary data.

changes in the mean value. When used with large sample normal approximations, the EWMA chart is much less sensitive than the Shewhart chart to the requirement for block data means to be approximately normally distributed; it has been described as an almost nonparametric chart (Montgomery).

To construct an EWMA chart a weight W has to be selected. Although different weights can give slightly better performance for false negative and false positive errors in different situations, or equivalently better run lengths when the process is in control and when it is out of control (i.e. in a predictable or unpredictable state), W=0.2 is a suitable general purpose weight for aggregated binary data when numerators and denominators are sufficiently large (technically the optimum weight minimises the squared forecast errors). When very variable or trended data are being analysed, a larger weight such as 0.4 or 0.5 will fit the data better. Use of spline smooth (see below) or loess smooth methods may be more valuable in the latter situation. This may be so especially when the data display autocorrelation that is encountered rarely with AE binary data aggregated by months.

The chart begins at zero time. We employ loess smoothing using the R function lowess() to determine a suitable starting value. At the first time that data become available, this value is multiplied by 1-W=0.8 and the first data value is multiplied by the weight W=0.2 and the results are added. Thus the EWMA at the first data period is $EWMA=0.2 \times Y_1 + 0.8 \times E$, where E is the starting value and Y_1 is the observed value. Thereafter each new value is multiplied by W=0.2 and added to 1-W=0.8 times the previous EWMA value to give the current EWMA value.

Calculation of the standard deviation for the EWMA chart is complicated for approximately the first six values when W=0.2 but thereafter it is straightforward: $SD_E = SD_S \times \sqrt{[W/(2-W)]}$, where SD_E is the EWMA standard deviation, SD_S is the Shewhart chart standard deviation calculated in the usual way for the large sample normal approximation, and W is the weight. Using a weight of 0.2 the formula becomes $SD_E = SD_S/3$; for small samples where beta distribution based Shewhart control limits are preferred, the EWMA control limits will then be approximately 1/3 of the distance from the centreline to the corresponding Shewhart control limit. If the complete formula is required it is $SD_E = SD_S \times \sqrt{[\{W/(2-W)\} \times \{1-(1-W)^{2 \times t}\}]}$, where t is the relevant time period. However, since this chart is useful for examining longer term changes in the process mean, the first few time periods are unlikely to be of great interest. After about six time periods, the two formulas give similar results when W=0.2 but this takes longer with smaller values of W.

When we use the pbeta() function for example, for the Shewhart 2.5 standard deviation equivalent line to obtain the required 2.5 standard deviation equivalent EWMA line, we find X/N such that pbeta(CL,X,N-X+1)=1-pnorm(2.5), where CL is the chart centre line. This requires a simple search. For example, 1-pnorm(2.5)=.0062. If CL=.1 and the denominator at time t is Nt=20, Xt=6.4 as pbeta(.1,6.4,20-6.4+1)=.0062 and the Shewhart control limit Ut=Xt/Nt=6.4/20=.32. When the Shewhart control chart limits vary, as they usually do with hospital AE data, the standard formula that relies on there being constant variability needs to be modified. This may happen because of risk adjustment or differing sized denominators and is equivalent to the SD_S varying. Most descriptions assume a constant SDs. There appear to be two possible approaches.

First, one can obtain the necessary Shewhart limit corresponding to the required EWMA limit using the pbeta() search as described above and then modify it. Using the corresponding Shewhart limit, the first upper EWMA limit will be $CL+(Us_1-CL) \times W$, the second $CL+(Us_2-CL) \times \sqrt{(W^2+W^2 \times (1-W)^2)}$, the third $CL+(Us_3-CL) \times \sqrt{(W^2+W^2 \times (1-W)^2+W^2 \times (1-W)^4)}$,

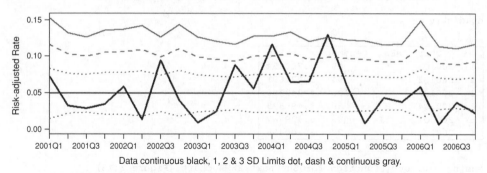

Figure 3.14   Shewhart chart quarterly risk adjusted binary data.

and so on, where the Us values constitute the Shewhart values corresponding to the required EWMA limit. This approach results in slightly unsmooth EWMA limits but appears to be satisfactory with monthly attribute data.

The second approach appears to be necessary when variance-based limits are employed and these may vary substantially, for example with the EWMA described by Cook[A,B] and colleagues mentioned above and that we return to in the Appendix (section 3.22). Assuming a constant variance V_0, the EWMA variance for time t can be expressed as $V_3=V_0\times W^2\times(1-W)^{(2\times0)}+V_0\times W^2\times(1-W)^{(2\times1)}+V_0\times W^2\times(1-W)^{(2\times2)}\ldots$. When the variance is calculated from individual risk adjusted values, for example, $\pi_i\times(1-\pi_i)$ for the ith subject, as in the method described by Cook[A,B] and colleagues, one can use $V=V_1\times W^2\times(1-W)^{(2\times0)}+V_2\times W^2\times(1-W)^{(2\times1)}+V_3\times W^2\times(1-W)^{(2\times2)}\ldots$. We mention this further in the Appendix (section 3.22) and illustrate in the internet code file.

The first few time periods have narrower EWMA control limits because the expected value employed in the calculation of the starting value is not considered to be a variable. A simple way to incorporate this difference in the control chart when the Shewhart control limit is the pbeta equivalent of $CL+Z\times SDs$ with $W=0.2$ so that $SDs\approx(U-CL)/Z$, and the control limits do not vary, is to use the formula $SD_E=k\times SD_S/3$ ($\sqrt{[W/(2-W)]}=1/3$ when $W=.2$) and for the first six time periods k is 0.6, 0.77, 0.86, 0.91, 0.94, and 0.97 respectively. Thereafter, $k\approx1$.

It is incorrect to include multiple control limits in EWMA charts because of the correlation between the successive data points, so a single control limit is employed, for example 2.5 has an ARL of approximately 100 when $W=0.2$ and this will often be suitable with monthly or quarterly proportion and count data. The function bewmaqtr() produces the Shewhart/EWMA chart (Figure 3.13). A Shewhart chart for these risk-adjusted data (Figure 3.14) is also illustrated using bshewqtr(). Data may be aggregated by months using binmonths() for data that are not risk-adjusted or binmonthsra() for risk-adjusted data or binqtrs() and binqtrsra() for quarterly data or ordered data with a first column that is not a date. Monthly data are in the data.frame dataout and quarterly data are in qtrs.

```
g.d() # ssis.csv, Figure 3.13
```

```
#using functions binqtrs() and binqtrsra() to aggregate by quarters
#binqtrs(datain[,-3]) will aggregate the data without risk-adjustment
```

```
binqtrsra(datain) #quarterly data in qtrs

head(qtrs)
```

	Qtrs	AEs	Denoms	Exp
1	2001Q1	5	65	2.780354
2	2001Q2	3	94	3.774691
3	2001Q3	3	106	4.242300
4	2001Q4	3	88	3.495525
5	2002Q1	5	86	3.439767
6	2002Q2	1	78	3.100495

```
#using bewmaqtr()function for Shewhart/EWMA chart (Figure 3.13)
bewmaqtr(qtrs)
```

```
Do you have risk-adjusted data (Y/N) y
EWMA weight.
Enter weight between 0.2 & 0.6 .2
EWMA control limit.
Enter limit 2, 2.5 or 3 SD 2.5
Chart heading.
Enter heading for the chart Quarterly SSI data
```

```
#using bshewqtr() function for Shewhart chart
bshewqtr(qtrs) # Figure 3.14
```

```
Do you have risk-adjusted data (Y/N) y
Chart heading.
Enter heading for the chart Quarterly SSI data
```

3.13   Plotting the expected values

Systematic changes in expected values can influence risk-adjusted charts. In the absence of obvious assignable causes for a chart signal, it is useful to examine a plot of the expected values as runs of higher expected values may have contributed to the signal. In this case there is no reason to suspect that changing risk scores contributed to the elevated quarterly rates in 2004.

```
# plot of risk scores, Figure 3.15
library(chron)
da<-qtrs[,1]
d1<-qtrs[,2]
d2<-qtrs[,3]
d3<-qtrs[,4]
s1<-da[1]
s2<-da[length(da)]
lda<-1:length(da)
d4<-sum(d3)/sum(d2)
low<-lowess(d3/d2,f=1/3)
N<-sum(d2)
```

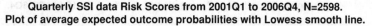

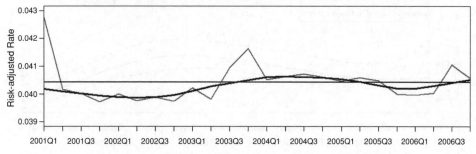

Figure 3.15 Plot of risk scores.

```
eha<-paste("Quarterly SSI Data Risk Scores from ",s1," to ",s2,", N=",N,".",
sep="")
maa0<-"\nPlot of average expected outcome probabilities with "
maa1<-"Lowess smooth line."
maa<-paste(eha,maa0,maa1,sep="")
plot(d3/d2,type="l",lwd=2,col="dark blue",axes=F,xlab="",ylab="Expected
values",main=maa,ylim=c(0.039,0.043))
box()
axis(side=1,tick=T,labels=as.character(da),at=lda)
axis(side=c(2,3,4))
abline(h=d4,lwd=2,col="black")
lines(low,lwd=2,col="dark green")
```

3.14   Using a spline or generalised additive model (GAM) chart

When the data of interest lack a predictable mean value conventional control charts can mislead (Morton[B] and colleagues). This may be less of a problem with risk-adjusted binary data than with count data described in Chapters 6 and 7. However, we use the quarterly ssi data to illustrate the use of spline regression with risk-adjusted binary data. The chart displays the time series data, the predicted smoothed mean value and its confidence interval, and an upper two sigma equivalent control limit line. The confidence limits describe the precision of the predicted smoothed mean and do not refer to the individual monthly values. The upper two sigma equivalent control limit line may help determine which, if any, monthly values vary significantly from the overall time series (this needs to be the subject of further study, see for example, the note on Poisson outbreak detection in the paper by Pelecanos and colleagues). When the data are risk-adjusted, indirect standardisation is employed. Note that with the default spline 3 degrees of freedom the deviance is reduced from 58.734 on 23 degrees of freedom to 44.373 on 20 degrees of freedom, 1-pchisq(58.734-44.373,3)=0.00245. This suggests that significant changes in the mean rate were predicted by the analysis. The rate for the fourth quarter of 2004 appears to be an outlier (Figure 3.16). The MannKendall trend test is not significant but the rate declines in 2005 and 2006. The bgamqtr() function is used to provide the GAM chart.

The presence of nonlinear changes in the SSI rate suggest that it may be useful to repeat the analysis using for example 5 degrees of freedom for the spline to reduce the extent of the

Spline Smooth Plot of quarterly SSI data from 2001Q1 to 2006Q4.

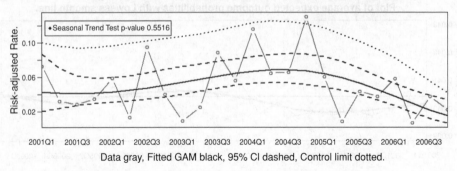

Data gray, Fitted GAM black, 95% CI dashed, Control limit dotted.

Figure 3.16   GAM chart quarterly risk adjusted binary data (3 DF).

smoothing. The result is in Figure 3.17 that has a better appearance than Figure 3.16 although the anova test result is marginal (1-pchisq(5.1757,2)=0.075).

```
#using the bgamqtr() function, Figure 3.16
bgamqtr(qtrs) # Quarterly SSI data
```

```
Do you have risk-adjusted data (Y/N) y
Change degrees of freedom (Y/N) n
Chart heading.
Enter heading for the chart Quarterly SSI data

The model is in mmg.
Type summary(mmg)/predict(mmg,se=T) to see.
tau = -0.087, 2-sided pvalue =0.55164

Coefficients:
                Estimate Std. Error z value Pr(>|z|)
(Intercept)      -3.1045     0.3833  -8.099 5.56e-16 ***
(Dispersion parameter for binomial family taken to be 1)
    Null deviance: 58.734  on 23   degrees of freedom
Residual deviance: 44.373  on 20   degrees of freedom
AIC: 131.08
```

Quarterly SSI data from 2001Q1 to 2006Q4, N=2598.

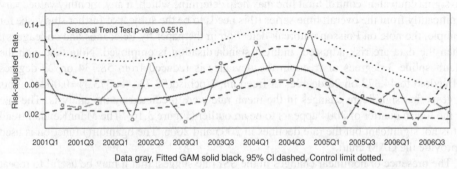

Data gray, Fitted GAM solid black, 95% CI dashed, Control limit dotted.

Figure 3.17   GAM chart quarterly risk adjusted binary data (5 DF).

```
mmg0<-mmg # save object for anova with 5 DF GAM

bgamqtr(qtrs) # repeat with 5 DF (Figure 3.17)
```

```
Do you have risk-adjusted data (Y/N) y
Change degrees of freedom (Y/N) y
Enter degrees of freedom 5
Chart heading.
Enter heading for the chart Quarterly SSI data

The model is in mmg.
Type summary(mmg)/predict(mmg,se=T) to see.
tau = -0.087, 2-sided pvalue =0.55164

Coefficients:
                Estimate Std. Error z value Pr(>|z|)
(Intercept)      -2.8991     0.4696  -6.174 6.66e-10 ***
    Null deviance: 58.734  on 23  degrees of freedom
Residual deviance: 39.198  on 18  degrees of freedom
AIC: 129.48
Warning message:
In eval(expr, envir, enclos) : non-integer #successes in a
binomial glm!
```

An abbreviated summary of the GAM analysis is shown above. The noninteger warning occurs because the numerators of risk-adjusted rates are usually not integers. Use locator() to position the trend test result in a clear area of the chart.

```
anova(mmg0,mmg)# comparing GAM with 3 and 5 DF
```

```
Analysis of Deviance Table
Model 1: a/d2 ~ bs(id, df = df1)
Model 2: a/d2 ~ bs(id, df = df1)
  Resid. Df Resid. Dev Df Deviance
1        20     44.373
2        18     39.198  2   5.1757
1-pchisq(5.1757,2)=0.075
```

3.15   When there are few time periods

Sometimes data involving few time periods are available, for example yearly data many be available for only five or six years. Often the best that can be done is to calculate confidence intervals for the data for each of the time periods. Because confidence intervals apply only to the immediate data, this has the disadvantage that the overall structure of the data is not utilised as it is in a control chart and, when risk adjustment is available, variability in expected values is often ignored. Thus, intervals may be too narrow. However, as Nelson has described, control charts are meant to be practically useful process-improvement tools, not exact statistical tests. If we concentrate on the 3 or 2.5 standard deviation (SD) equivalent limits (99.7% and approximately 99%) and use the analysis to learn how to practice more

Few Time Periods CI Demonstration.

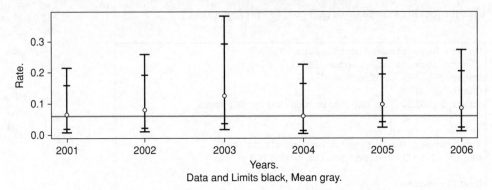

Figure 3.18 Few time periods confidence intervals chart.

safely, the slightly narrow limits should not be a serious problem. Figures 3.18 and 3.19 illustrate multiple CIs of short run data without and with risk adjustment.

```
#multiple CI illustration of short run data without risk adjustment
Year<-2001:2006 # Figure 3.18
SSI<-c(4,4,4,3,7,4)
Proc<-c(61,50,32,51,71,47)
ExpRate<-.0606
Exp<-ExpRate*Proc
M<-0;L95<-0;U95<-0;L997<-0;U997<-0
l<-1:length(Year)
for (i in 1:length(SSI)){M[i]<-SSI[i]/Proc[i]
if (SSI[i]==0){L95[i]<-0}else{L95[i]<-qbeta(.025,SSI[i],Proc[i]-SSI[i]+1)}
U95[i]<-qbeta(.975,SSI[i]+1,Proc[i]-SSI[i])
if (SSI[i]==0){L997[i]<-0}else{L997[i]<-qbeta(.0015,SSI[i],Proc[i]-
SSI[i]+1)}
```

Few Time Periods Risk-adjusted Rate (RAR) Demonstration.

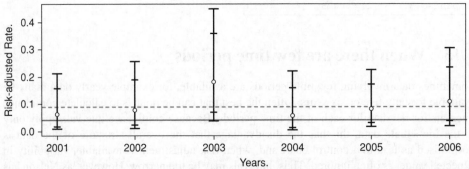

Figure 3.19 Few time periods risk adjusted rate confidence intervals chart showing weighted mean rate for the data and the mean rate of the risk adjustments.

```
U997[i]<-qbeta(.9985,SSI[i]+1,Proc[i]-SSI[i])
}
par(xaxs="r")
plot(M,ylim=c(min(L997),max(U997)),col="blue",axes=F,lwd=2,
main="Few Time Periods CI Demonstration.",ylab="Rate.",
xlab="Data and Limits Blue, Mean Red.")
box()
axis(side=1,labels=Year,at=l)
axis(side=c(2,3,4))
arrows(l,L95,l,U95,angle=90,code=3,length=.075,col="blue",lwd=2)
arrows(l,L997,l,U997,angle=90,code=3,length=.125,col="blue",lwd=2)
abline(h=ExpRate,lwd=2,col="red")
mtext("Years.",side=1,line=2)

# multiple CI illustration of short run data with risk-adjustment
Year<-2001:2006 # Figure 3.19
SSI<-c(4,4,4,3,7,4)
Proc<-c(61,50,32,51,71,47)
Exp<-c(2.6,2.1,.9,2.2,3.5,1.5)
ebar<-sum(Exp)/sum(Proc)
SSIAdj<-SSI*ebar/Exp
SSIAdj1<-SSIAdj*Proc
M<-0;L95<-0;U95<-0;L997<-0;U997<-0
l<-1:length(Year)
for (i in 1:length(SSIAdj)){M[i]<-SSIAdj[i]
if (SSIAdj1[i]==0){L95[i]<-0}else{L95[i]<-qbeta(.025,SSIAdj1[i],Proc[i]-
SSIAdj1[i]+1)}
U95[i]<-qbeta(.975,SSIAdj1[i]+1,Proc[i]-SSIAdj1[i])
if (SSIAdj1[i]==0){L997[i]<-0}else{L997[i]<-qbeta(.0015,SSIAdj1[i],Proc[i]-
SSIAdj1[i]+1)}
U997[i]<-qbeta(.9985,SSIAdj1[i]+1,Proc[i]-SSIAdj1[i])
}
par(xaxs="r")
plot(M,ylim=c(min(L997),max(U997)),col="blue",axes=F,lwd=2,
main="Few Time Period Risk-adjusted Rate (RAR) Demonstration.",
ylab="Risk-adjusted Rate.",
xlab="Data and Limits Blue, Ebar Red, Weighted Mean of RARs Green.")
box()
axis(side=1,labels=Year,at=l)
axis(side=c(2,3,4))
arrows(l,L95,l,U95,angle=90,code=3,length=.075,col="blue",lwd=2)
arrows(l,L997,l,U997,angle=90,code=3,length=.125,col="blue",lwd=2)
abline(h=ebar,lwd=2,col="red")
abline(h=sum(M*Proc)/sum(Proc),lwd=2,col="green4")
mtext("Years.",side=1,line=2)
```

3.16   Charts for quarterly data and data without a first date column

In some cases, as with Figures 3.13 to 3.17, there are insufficient numbers of AEs for monthly display in a control chart and quarterly data may be used provided there are sufficient quarters of data available (preferably 20 or more). In other cases there may not be a first column of dates available for example for monthly or quarterly data. In this case it is important that the data are suitably sorted by time and a first column may need to be added such as 1 to 20 for 20 ordered monthly or quarterly (or other time period) rows of data. There are three functions: bshewqtr() for a Shewhart chart, bewmaqtr() for an Shewhart/EWMA chart and bgamqtr() for a spline (GAM) chart. The latter is used to illustrate this additional analysis using data in ssi0106.xls.

```
g.d()  # ssi0106.xls, Figure 3.20

# data for all hospitals
# first, data must be placed e.g. in quarters
# or use function binqtrsra() output data in data.frame qtrs
library(chron)
d<-datain[,3]
a<-datain[,5]
b<-datain[,6]
d<-chron(as.character(d),format="dd-mmm-yy",out.format="dd-mmm-yyyy")
o<-order(d)
d<-d[o]
a<-a[o]
b<-b[o]
y<-years(d)
m<-months(d)
dates<-paste(m,y)
aes<-tapply(a,dates,sum)
totals<-tapply(a,dates,length)
expecteds<-tapply(b,dates,sum)
month<-names(aes)
month<-paste("1",month)
month<-chron(as.character(month),format="dd mmm yyyy",out.format=
"dd-mmm-yyyy")
o<-order(month)
Month<-month[o]
aes<-as.numeric(aes)
totals<-as.numeric(totals)
expecteds<-as.numeric(expecteds)
AEs<-aes[o]
Totals<-totals[o]
Expecteds<-expecteds[o]
Table<-data.frame(Month,AEs,Totals,Expecteds)
dataout<-Table
d<-chron(as.character(dataout[,1]),format="dd-mmm-yyyy",out.format=
"dd-mmm-yyyy")
f<-dataout[,2]
n<-dataout[,3]
e<-dataout[,4]
Y<-years(d)
m<-as.numeric(months(d))
Q<-rep(0,length(m))
Q[m>=1&m<=3]<--1
Q[m>=4&m<=6]<--2
Q[m>=7&m<=9]<--3
Q[m>=10&m<=12]<--4
Tablea<-as.data.frame(xtabs(f~Q+Y))
Tableb<-as.data.frame(xtabs(n~Q+Y))
Tablec<-as.data.frame(xtabs(e~Q+Y))
```

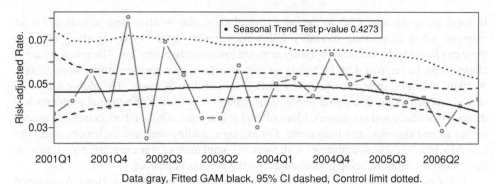

Figure 3.20 shows Quarterly SSI data. GAM chart, quarterly data.

Quarterly SSI data.

Data gray, Fitted GAM black, 95% CI dashed, Control limit dotted.

Figure 3.20 GAM chart, quarterly data.

```
Qtrs<-paste(Tablea[,2],"Q",Tablea[,1],sep="")
Table1<-data.frame(Qtrs,Tablea[,3],Tableb[,3],Tablec[,3])
names(Table1)<-c("Qtrs","AEs","Denoms","Exp")
Table1<-Table1[Table1[,3]!=0,]
head(Table1)
```

```
    Qtrs   AEs   Denoms        Exp
1  2001Q1   11      274   14.05324
2  2001Q2   20      420   21.87518
3  2001Q3   25      410   20.73655
4  2001Q4   17      410   19.96599
5  2002Q1   28      330   16.08150
6  2002Q2   10      395   18.51788
```

```
#using function bgamqtr(), Figure 3.20
bgamqtr(Table1)
```

```
Do you have risk-adjusted data (Y/N) y
Change degrees of freedom (Y/N) n
Chart heading.
Enter heading for the chart Quarterly SSI data
```

An abbreviated summary of the GAM regression follows. Although the data appear more variable at the beginning of the series, there is very little evidence of change in the predicted mean (1-pchisq(43.65-39.88,23-20) = 0.287395).

```
Coefficients:
                 Estimate Std. Error z value Pr(>|z|)
(Intercept)     -3.031138    0.176215 -17.201   <2e-16 ***
  Null deviance: 43.650  on 23  degrees of freedom
Residual deviance: 39.879  on 20  degrees of freedom
AIC: 169.71
```

3.17   Charts for composite measures

In some cases we may wish to devise a control chart that involves several indicators, for example, when monitoring mortality following coronary artery bypass grafting (CABG) there can be difficulty because mortality rates are low, usually below 2%. The power to detect changes can be improved by including an indicator for major postoperative complications. A useful indicator appears to be a stay in ICU longer than 96 hours. By adding long ICU stay to mortality, rates rise to 4% or 5%. This makes the detection of potential problems less difficult (De Maria and colleagues, Morton[G] and colleagues). This method, called all-or-none by Nolan and Berwick, has limitations. For example, adding outcome indicators with rates less than 10% to process indicators with rates of compliance of, for example, 80% results in the composite measure being overwhelmed by the process indicators.

The American College of Cardiology Foundation and the American Heart Association (ACCF/AHA) have published guidelines for the use of composite measures and it is suggested that their recommendations be understood before composite measures are employed with clinical indicators. However, there exists considerable potential for their development, for example, track, trigger and report (TTR) systems for the early detection of acute deterioration may benefit from the development of a composite measure that encompasses changes in blood pressure, pulse rate, temperature, respiratory rate, oxygenation and level of consciousness (Mitchell and colleagues). Waterhouse and her colleagues report the use of a multivariate control chart for monitoring radiation during percutaneous coronary interventions.

3.18   Additional tabulations

Tabulations are important and underutilised approaches to understanding QI and IM data. Faced with data from several institutions or units within institutions over several time periods, it is useful to be able to pinpoint when AE rates may have been unusual. This involves multiple looks at the data so a result of two standard deviations or more above expected (Z-score>=2) or a contiguous series of positive Z-scores does not necessarily indicate any problem but it does indicate where to look for possible problems. We repeat that the method of Mohammed[B] and his colleagues should be followed: look first for data or analysis error, then problems with risk adjustment, system errors, and finally for problems involving staff. In addition, multiple significance testing will turn up occasional abnormal results by chance alone. It is very important to avoid condemning units for unusual outcome data that arise from predictable, often random, variation.

There are several issues with these data. If data are sparse, it may only be possible to tabulate by half years or years. If risk scores are available, expected outcome rates are of interest. With SSI data, classification may be by NNIS risk index if available. It is not possible to illustrate all the possible ways that tabulations can be used to help to understand these data so a selection illustrating particularly the use of the R xtabs(), stack() and reshape() functions appears in the code file.

We provide one example here to illustrate an important point. Data from the file orthssi0106.xls, a subset of the data in ssi0106.csv from which non-elective procedures have been removed, is employed. We select Hospital Q that reported many less SSIs than predicted. When these data were collected, it was optional to report post-discharge SSIs so this low count may indicate that Hospital Q did not collect these data. It is known that superficial post-discharge SSIs cannot be counted accurately using routine surveillance methods and this is another potential source of bias in these data (Whitby and colleagues). A further potential source of bias is the length of stay of these patients in hospital as very early discharge means that more superficial SSIs will appear after discharge. As Anderson and colleagues illustrate, surveillance of complex (deep and organ space) SSIs is more reliable as these patients require readmission. As we note the potential sources of bias in data aggregated from a number of institutions, we also note that individual institutions usually have much less variable data because between institution variability is eliminated. Thus these potential biases are minimised. Therefore sequential within hospital surveillance combined with audit of the hospital's compliance with evidence-based bundles is liable to be a superior approach to the among hospital analysis described in Chapter 2. It can give a much earlier and more reliable warning of unpredictable outcome rates. In addition, surveillance could concentrate on complex SSIs with their early referral to M&M audits as these more serious infections can be counted accurately and may indicate the need for system review.

```
#data from orthssi0106.xls
g.d() #orthssi0106.xls
```

```
Loading data.
Data from clipboard (C) or file (F) c
Do data column(s) have heading(s) (Y/N) y
Is column 1 a date column (Y/N) n
```

```
library(chron)
library(exactci)
library(Kendall)
AllSSI<-tapply(datain[,3],datain[,1],sum)
AllOps<-tapply(datain[,3],datain[,1],length)
AllExp<-tapply(datain[,4],datain[,1],sum)
All<-data.frame(AllSSI,AllOps,AllExp)
All
```

	AllSSI	AllOps	AllExp
A	60	747	36.019951
B	38	1040	48.514467
C	24	783	34.058310
D	33	854	38.928766
E	25	693	33.351792
F	25	519	24.777943
G	128	2575	101.977657
H	25	343	16.508235
I	58	823	39.887837
J	30	708	30.251686
K	30	462	22.208908
L	1	224	10.596107
M	6	125	5.860533
N	17	239	11.947792
O	3	257	11.531651
P	8	147	6.195912
Q	50	1956	85.052494
R	12	343	15.329957

```
# hospital Q
datain1<-datain # keep datain
datain1<-datain1[datain1[,1]=="Q",-1] #hospital Q data
d<-datain1[,1]
d<-chron(as.character(d),format="d-mmm-yy",out.format="dd-mmm-yyyy")
Comps<-datain1[,2]
Counts<-rep(1,length(d))
RI<-datain1[,3]
Years<-years(d)
Months<-as.numeric(months(d))
Qtrs<-rep(0,length(Months))
Qtrs[Months>=1&Months<=3]<-1
Qtrs[Months>=4&Months<=6]<-2
Qtrs[Months>=7&Months<=9]<-3
Qtrs[Months>=10&Months<=12]<-4
Tots<-as.data.frame(xtabs(Counts~Qtrs+Years))
AEs<-as.data.frame(xtabs(Comps~Qtrs+Years))
RIs<-as.data.frame(xtabs(RI~Qtrs+Years))
Ops<-Tots$Freq
RIs<-RIs$Freq
AEs<-data.frame(AEs,Ops,RIs)
AEs<-AEs[AEs$Ops!=0,]
names(AEs)<-c("Qtrs","Years","AEs","Ops","RIs")
Rate<-AEs[,3]/AEs[,4]
d<-AEs[,5]/AEs[,4]
Expected<-d
z<-0;p<-0
for (i in 1:length(AEs[,1]))
{p[i]<-binom.exact(AEs[i,3],AEs[i,4],d[i])$p.value;
if(Rate[i]>d[i]){z[i]<--qnorm(p[i]/2)}else{z[i]<-qnorm(p[i]/2)}}
Rate<-round(Rate,2)
Exp<-round(Expected*AEs[,4],2)
p<-round(p,2)
Z<-round(z,2)
Table<-data.frame(AEs[,-5],Exp,Z)
head(Table)
```

	Qtrs	Years	AEs	Ops	Exp	Z
3	3	2001	0	1	0.04	0.00
6	2	2002	1	27	1.14	0.00
7	3	2002	1	66	2.97	−0.86
8	4	2002	5	72	3.28	0.74
9	1	2003	2	88	4.00	−0.74
10	2	2003	1	108	4.81	−1.71

```
# Trend test
OE<-AEs[,3]/AEs[,5]
library(Kendall)
s<-SeasonalMannKendall(ts(OE))
s
#
#tau = 0.15, 2-sided pvalue =0.36145

# Z-score chart Figure 3.21
da<-paste(Table[,2],".",Table[,1],sep="") #z-score chart
ld<-1:length(da)
```

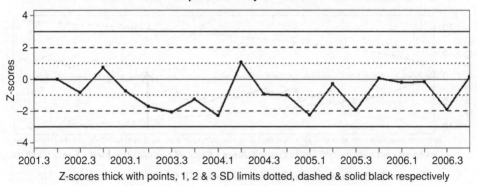

Figure 3.21   Z-score chart quarterly data.

```
d1<-OE
s1<-da[1]
s2<-da[length(da)]
spl<-"Z-scores"
mb<-paste("Z-score Chart Hospital Quarterly SSI data from ",s1," to ",s2,".",
sep="")
z[z<.01 & d1>1]<-.01
z[z>-.01 & d1<1]<--.01
par(xaxs="i")
plot(z,type="l",lwd=3,axes=F,xlab="Z-scores thick with points, 1, 2 & 3 SD
limits dotted, dashed & solid black respectively",ylab=spl,main=mb,ylim=
c(-4,4))
points(z,lwd=3,pch=20)
box()
par(cex=.8)
axis(side=1,tick=T,labels=da,at=ld)
axis(side=c(2,3,4))
abline(h=0)
abline(h=1,lwd=2,lty=3)
abline(h=2,lwd=2,lty=2)
abline(h=3,lwd=2)
abline(h=-1,lwd=2,lty=3)
abline(h=-2,lwd=2,lty=2)
abline(h=-3,lwd=2)
```

Section 3.11 of this chapter describes run-sum charts. There is a run-sum of six and one of four in the Z-score chart.

```
# yearly data
SSI<-tapply(Table[,3],Table[,2],sum)
n<-names(SSI)
Tot<-sum(SSI)
SSIs<-c(as.numeric(SSI),Tot)
names(SSIs)<-c(n,"Tot")
OPS<-tapply(Table[,4],Table[,2],sum)
n<-names(OPS)
Tot<-sum(OPS)
```

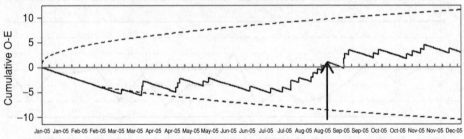

Cumulative O-E plus RA Bernoulli CUSUM from Jan-05 to Dec-05.

Observed continuous, 95% Limits dashed, Arrows CUSUM Signals, Tick Marks Every 50 Units.

Figure 3.22 Cumulative O – E with Bernoulli CUSUM, low rate data.

```
OPSs<-c(as.numeric(OPS),Tot)
names(OPSs)<-c(n,"Tot")
EXP<-tapply(Table[,5],Table[,2],sum)
n<-names(EXP)
Tot<-sum(EXP)
EXPs<-c(as.numeric(EXP),Tot)
names(EXPs)<-c(n,"Tot")
TABLE<-rbind(SSIs,OPSs,EXPs)
P<-0
for (i in 1:7){P[i]<-poisson.exact(TABLE[1,i],TABLE[2,i],TABLE[3,i]/
TABLE[2,i])$p.value}
Z<-0
for (i in 1:7){if (TABLE[1,i]>TABLE[3,i]){Z[i]<--qnorm(P[i]/2)}else{Z[i]<-
qnorm(P[i]/2)}}
TABLEQ<-data.frame(t(TABLE),round(Z,3))
names(TABLEQ)<-c("SSIs","OPS","EXPs","Z")
TABLEQ<-TABLEQ[-1,]
TABLEQ
```

	SSIs	OPS	EXPs	Z
2002	7	165	7.39	0.000
2003	5	392	17.83	−3.376
2004	15	475	21.45	−1.314
2005	10	475	19.55	−2.205
2006	13	448	18.79	−1.245
Tot	50	1956	85.05	−4.036

```
TABLEQ<-round(t(TABLEQ),1)
TABLEQ # cannot round to integers as Z-scores require reals
```

	2002	2003	2004	2005	2006	Tot
SSIs	7.0	5.0	15.0	10.0	13.0	50
OPS	165.0	392.0	475.0	475.0	448.0	1956
EXPs	7.4	17.8	21.4	19.6	18.8	85
Z	0.0	−3.4	−1.3	−2.2	−1.2	−4

3.19   The issue of under-reporting

As central authorities impose financial sanctions when certain AEs are reported, under-reporting may become a serious problem. The previous section highlighted potential sources of bias when data are obtained from a number of institutions. While it is certainly necessary for disciplinary action to be taken when a member of staff persistently fails to comply with evidence-based bundles, it is also unwise to penalise staff for occasional AEs that occur within a predictable system. Good systems work on trust, trust depends on justice and it is not just to admonish someone for the occurrence of an AE that they could not have prevented. Instead of using data to learn how to improve, in an overly judgemental environment data tend to be used to prove compliance with targets, and borderline cases are unlikely to be counted or used for learning. We should not underestimate the value of learning from near misses.

In addition to the above, it becomes necessary to be able to identify under-reporting. Alert surveillance staff may become suspicious and instigate an assessment. A cumulative observed minus expected chart that displays steadily decreasing numbers of AEs in the absence of a system overhaul should alert staff to the possibility that under reporting is occurring. As we discuss below, using a CUSUM to detect decreasing AE rates quickly when they are ordinarily very low is seldom successful; this may not be the case when the problem is under-reporting, and it is possible that other control chart methods may be used in a similar way. We have no experience with this aspect of monitoring. However, if hospitals are to be fined when AEs occur, it may become of increasing importance with potential methods requiring rigorous study. We know that optimum performance is dependent on trust that has its basis in justice. Disciplinary action is correct when it is just; it is not when an AE is part of a predictable system and not therefore potentially preventable.

3.20   New CUSUM and EWMA charts, low-rate data

The Steiner CUSUM is in regular use to monitor hospital adverse outcomes such as SSIs or other complications of surgery, and mortality following surgical procedures (Steiner and colleagues, Morton[F] and colleagues). However, there have been misgivings about its use with low-rate risk-adjusted binary data, especially when there is considerable variation in the risk scores. Several approaches have been suggested, for example, Webster, Gan and Tan and Loke and Gan, and Jones and Steiner. Very recently Rossi and colleagues have proposed a risk-adjusted Bernoulli CUSUM that employs corrected diffusion approximations. This excellent CUSUM was described in 1999 by Reynolds and Stoumbos and its use has been reported for monitoring liver transplant surgery by Leandro and colleagues. However, until the report by Rossi and colleagues, its use has been restricted because a mechanism for including risk-adjustment has been lacking. Although we illustrate this CUSUM in Figure 3.22, it needs to undergo further evaluation before its routine use can be recommended. Some preliminary calculations suggest that it may be valuable, for example, with risk-adjusted surgical mortality data having average expected rates between 1% and 5%.

However, the Steiner CUSUM remains useful in this situation (Morton[F] and colleagues) if used with careful checking of run lengths, for example, by simulation. Assessment of the possible practical superiority of the risk-adjusted Bernoulli CUSUM will require further work before it could be recommended for routine use. Early use suggests that it may take slightly longer to signal than the Steiner CUSUM, the calculation of its run length equivalent (ANOS) is more straightforward (as Webster has pointed out, there can be problems with the Markov chain approach with the Steiner CUSUM due to difficulties with matrices, and simulation may be preferable), it may be more stable than the Steiner CUSUM in the face of variable risk, but its calculation is more involved.

Mortality and morbidity (M&M) analyses and independent audits are being performed with increasing frequency and skill when monitoring low frequency, high impact adverse events (AEs). Statistical analysis can often most usefully act as an adjunct to the systems analysis that occurs at properly performed M&M analyses and independent audits. The function of the CUSUM in this situation will often be to minimise the risk of tampering when the occurrence of occasional adverse events in a judgemental environment encourages changing a system that is in fact performing predictably.

Another approach is to employ an exponentially weighted moving average (EWMA) chart (Cook[A,B] and colleagues, Pilcher and colleagues and Koetsier and colleagues). They point out that, unlike the CUSUM, it is not re-set when there is an out of control signal. In addition, it communicates approximate information about the current observed and expected rates whereas the VLAD, cumulative observed minus expected and cumulative funnel plot charts convey cumulative and not current information. This is important as clinicians prefer to know the current as well as the cumulative count or rate. The EWMA approach has been shown to be useful with ICU and CCU mortality that have higher average AE rates (typically 10% to 15%) but obtaining EWMA control limits for individual patients when expected rates are around 1% to 5% is currently the subject of evaluation. We describe the EWMA chart further in Chapter 6 where it is illustrated with count (e.g. bacteraemia) data. As indicated, this chart has the advantage that, unlike the cumulative O-E/CUSUM, it provides an estimate of the current mean count or rate. The CUSUM can be combined with a cumulative observed minus expected chart or funnel plot as described in the present chapter and Chapter 6 but this cumulative information differs from the current state of the process. For this reason, a combined EWMA and CUSUM chart is worth considering and is illustrated. As described by Cook[A,B] and colleagues the EWMA weight for low-rate individual patient data should be between 0.005 and 0.02. Providing quarterly rates is an alternative approach that we feel may be preferable for displaying ongoing as opposed to cumulative rates in low rate AE data.

There appears to be considerable interest in obtaining incremental improvements in the speed of response of control charts to a distribution change. However, other considerations are also important. For example, with 30-day AEs, one or more may occur soon after a procedure and there may be earlier patient procedures which may or may not be associated with the AE within an overlapping 30 day interval. With some AEs such as SSIs, there may be some delay in obtaining information, for example, some of these patients present at different hospitals from the one where their first procedure was performed. A further consideration is transparency: hospital scientists need to have a general understanding of the CUSUM or other monitoring process. The Steiner CUSUM appears to be conceptually simpler than the CUSUM proposed by Rossi and colleagues.

When AEs are uncommon it will rarely be useful to attempt to determine when a very low AE rate falls further although this may change if under-reporting becomes an issue. In this note, the CUSUM has been set to detect a doubling of the AEs odds. If required, a halving of the AE odds could be assessed by searching for a doubling of the non-AE odds.

3.20.1   The risk-adjusted Bernoulli CUSUM

For very low average expected AE rates, an increase in the observed AE rate will be of interest rather than a decrease. Let p0 be the average AE predicted rate and p1 be the change in p0 to be detected. It is convenient, as with the Steiner CUSUM, for p1 to be twice the odds of p0, for example, $p1 = 2 \times p0/(1+p0)$. Next, the level to which the CUSUM score must rise for there to be a signal is obtained; this is commonly called h. The value of h is determined by the desired average number of observations to signal (ANOS). CUSUMs will ultimately signal even when a process remains predictable and the objective is for this to occur rarely while at the same time for the CUSUM to signal promptly when the process changes. To identify the required value for h, it is necessary for it to be modified: $h1 = h + E \times \sqrt{(p0 \times (1-p0))}$, where E is calculated as follows –

if $p0 <= .01$ then $E = (\sqrt{((1-p0)/p0)} - \sqrt{(P0/(1-P0))})/3$;

if p0 is above .01 and less than or equal to .5 then $E = .41 - .0842 \times (\log(p0)) - .0391 \times (\log(p0))^3 - .00376 \times (\log(p0))^4 - .000008 \times (\log(p0))^7$;

if p0 is greater than .5 then $q0 = 1-p0$ and $E = (\sqrt{((1-P0)/P0)} - \sqrt{(p0/(1-p0))})/3 + (.41 - .0842 \times (\log(q0)) - .0391 \times (\log(q0))^3 - .00376 \times (\log(q0))^4 - .000008 \times (\log(q0))^7)$.

Next, the following are calculated:

$R1 = -\log((1-p1)/(1-p0))$;

$R2 = \log((p1 \times (1-p0))/(p0 \times (1-p1)))$; and $ANOS = (\exp(h1 \times R2) - h1 \times R2 - 1)/abs(R2 \times p0 - R1)$.

To obtain a suitable ANOS, several values for h may need to be tested.

For each successive observation i with predicted outcome probability $p0_i$, $k_i = R1_i/R2_i$. In addition, $h1_i$ is calculated as above for observation i and $S_i = \max(0, S_{i-1} + c_i \times (O_i - k_i))$, where $c_i = h/h1_i$ and O_i is one if the AE occurred at observation i, otherwise it is zero. The CUSUM signals if $S_i = h$. The chart is illustrated in Figure 3.22.

```
g.d() #ssicomplx2005.csv

# order data
library(chron)
n<-names(datain)
d<-datain[,1]
o<-order(d)
datain<-datain[o,]
names(datain)<-n

# RA Bernoulli CUSUM (Rossi)
# ARL (ANOS)
P0<-.01
OR<-2
H<-4
E<-0
P1<-OR*P0/(1+OR*P0-P0)
if (P0<.01){E<-(((1-P0)/P0)^.5-(P0/(1-P0))^.5)/3}
```

```
if (P0>.01&P0<=.5){E<-.41-.0842*(log(P0))-.0391*(log(P0))^3-
.00376*(log(P0))^4-.000008*(log(P0))^7}
if (P0>.5){Po<-1-P0;E<-(((1-P0)/P0)^.5-(P0/(1-P0))^.5)/3+(.41-
.0842*(log(Po))-.0391*(log(Po))^3-.00376*(log(Po))^4-.000008*(log(Po))^7)}
H1<-H+E*(P0*(1-P0))^.5
R1<--log((1-P1)/(1-P0))
R2<-log((P1*(1-P0))/(P0*(1-P1)))
A<-(exp(H1*R2)-H1*R2-1)/abs(R2*P0-R1)
A
#[1] 4050.342, suitable value so h=4


# RA Bernoulli CUSUM
library(chron)
d<-datain[,1]
a<-datain[,2]
p<-datain[,3]
d<-chron(as.character(d),format="dd-mmm-yyyy",out.format="dd-mmm-yyyy")
o<-order(d)
d<-d[o]
a<-a[o]
p<-p[o]
h<-4
p0<-.01
OR<-2
p1<-OR*p0/(1+OR*p0-p0)
r1<--log((1-p1)/(1-p0))
r2<-log((p1*(1-p0))/(p0*(1-p1)))
k<-0
for (i in 1:length(p)){p0[i]<-p[i]
p1[i]<-OR*p0[i]/(1+OR*p0[i]-p0[i])
r1[i]<--log((1-p1[i])/(1-p0[i]))
r2[i]<-log((p1[i]*(1-p0[i]))/(p0[i]*(1-p1[i])))
k[i]<-r1[i]/r2[i]
}
E<-0
p00<-p0
for (i in 1:length(p)){
if (p00[i]<=.01){E[i]<-(((1-p00[i])/p00[i])^.5-(p00[i]/(1-p00[i]))^.5)/3}
if (p00[i]>.01&p00[i]<=.5){E[i]<-.41-.0842*(log(p00[i]))-
.0391*(log(p00[i]))^3-.00376*(log(p00[i]))^4-.000008*(log(p00[i]))^7}
if (p00[i]>.5){poo<-1-p00[i];E[i]<-(((1-p00[i])/p00[i])^.5-(p00[i]/(1-
p00[i]))^.5)/3+(.41-.0842*(log(poo))-.0391*(log(poo))^3-.00376*(log(poo))^4-
.000008*(log(poo))^7)}
}
h1<-h+E*(p0*(1-p0))^.5
cu<-max(0,h*(a[1]-k[1])/h1[1])
for (i in 2:length(p)){if (cu[i-1]>h){cu[i]<-max(0,h*(a[i]-k[i])/h1[i])
}else{
cu[i]<-max(0,cu[i-1]+h*(a[i]-k[i])/h1[i])
}
}
cus<-which(cu>=h) # CUSUM signal procedure number
cus
#[1] 1889
datain[cus,1] # CUSUM signal date
#[1] 31-Aug-2005
```

```
#cumulative observed minus expected plus CUSUM, Figure 3.22
Observed<-cumsum(a)
Procedures<-1:length(Observed)
Expected<-cumsum(p)
O<-Observed/Procedures
E<-Expected/Procedures
n<-Procedures
L2<-0
for (i in 1:length(n)){
Z<-.02275;P<-E[i];N<-n[i]
X<-0
if (1-pbeta(P,X+1,N-X)>=Z){X<-0}else{
X<-P*N
A<-1
bl<-F
while (bl==F){
X<-X-A
K<-1-pbeta(P,X+1,N-X)
if (K<=Z){bl<-T}
}
A<-.01
bl<-F
while (bl==F){
X<-X+A
K<-1-pbeta(P,X+1,N-X)
if (K>=Z){bl<-T}
}
}
L2[i]<-X/n[i]
}
U2<-0
for (i in 1:length(n)){
Z<-.02275;P<-E[i];N<-n[i]
X<-N
if (pbeta(P,X,N-X+1)>=Z){X<-N}else{
X<-N*P
A<-1
bl<-F
while (bl==F){
X<-X+A
K<-pbeta(P,X,N-X+1)
if (K<Z){bl<-T}
}
A<-.01
bl<-F
while (bl==F){
X<-X-A
K<-pbeta(P,X,N-X+1)
if (K>=Z){bl<-T}
}
}
U2[i]<-X/n[i]
}
On<-O*n
En<-E*n
Un<-U2*n
```

```
Ln<-L2*n
On<-On-En
Un<-Un-En
Ln<-Ln-En
ma<-max(c(On,Un))
mi<-min(c(On,Ln))
c2<-rep(0,length(d))
for (i in 1:length(d)){if (i%%50==0){c2[i]<-ma/20}}
tv<-"Cumulative O - E."
m<-months(d)
y<-substr(years(d),3,4)
Dates<-paste(m,y,sep="")
P<-paste("Cumulative O - E plus RA Bernoulli CUSUM"," from ",Dates[1]," to ",
Dates[length(Dates)],".",sep="")
th1<-"Observed Blue, 95% Limits Red, Arrows CUSUM Signals,"
th2<-" Tick Marks Every 50 Units.";th<-paste(th1,th2,sep="")
par(xaxs="i")
plot(On,col="blue",lwd=2,type="l",ylim=c(mi,ma),main=P,ylab=tv,xlab="",
axes=F)
box()
par(cex=.7)
axis(side=1,tick=F,labels=Dates,at=Procedures)
axis(side=c(2,3,4))
par(cex=1)
lines(Un,col="red",lwd=2)
lines(Ln,col="red",lwd=2)
lines(c2,type="l",col="green4",lwd=2)
mtext(text=th,side=1,line=2)
arrows(1889,mi,1889,On[1889],lwd=3,col="black")
```

The Steiner CUSUM was employed for comparison. It signaled at row 1857 on 26 August 2005 (row 1889 was on 31 August). The two charts appear similar.

3.20.2   The EWMA

A suitable weight (w) must be selected for the EWMA. For individual observations, Cook [A,B] and colleagues recommend a value between 0.005 and 0.02, depending on the average of the predicted outcome probabilities (the smaller the mean of the predicted AEs, the lower the value of w), and the level of smoothing required. For the data used in the example below (average expected rate .01), w = .005 has been selected. The function bewmacusum() can be used to perform this analysis.

$$\text{EWMA(observed)} = w \times O_i + (1-W) \times (O_{i-1})$$

$$\text{EWMA(predicted)} = w \times \pi_i + (1-W) \times (\pi_{i-1}),$$ where π_i is the ith predicted outcome probability.

When the average of the predicted outcome probabilities is sufficiently large, a control limit (CL) can be obtained for EWMA(predicted). For the ith observation $CL_i = \text{EWMA(predicted)}_i \pm Z \times w \times \sqrt{(\sum_i[(1-w)^{(2\times i)} \times (\pi_i \times (1-\pi_i)])}$, where for a two standard deviation limit $Z=2$ and π_i is the ith predicted value. For very low rate AEs a possible approach that will require formal evaluation is shown in the Appendix.

The methods described above are illustrated with complex SSI data. These data are in the file ssicomplx2005.csv. Figure 3.23 demonstrates the method.

EWMA plus RA Bernoulli CUSUM Complex SSIs from Jan-05 to Dec-05.

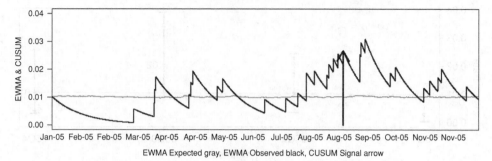

EWMA Expected gray, EWMA Observed black, CUSUM Signal arrow

Figure 3.23   EWMA with Bernoulli CUSUM, low rate data.

```
#EWMA plus RA Bernoulli CUSUM, Figure 3.23
library(chron)
ew<-.005
av<-mean(p)
O<-a[1]*ew+av*(1-ew)
for (i in 2:length(p)){O[i]<-O[i-1]*(1-ew)+a[i]*ew}
E<-p[1]*ew+av*(1-ew)
for (i in 2:length(p)){E[i]<-E[i-1]*(1-ew)+p[i]*ew}
m<-months(d)
y<-substr(years(d),3,4)
Dates<-paste(m,y,sep="")
P<-paste("EWMA plus RA Bernoulli CUSUM Complex SSIs"," from ",Dates[1],"
to ",Dates[length(Dates)],".",sep="")
plot(E,type="l",ylim=c(0,.04),axes=F,lwd=2,col="red",main=P,
xlab="EWMA Expected red, EWMA Observed blue, CUSUM Signal arrow",
ylab="EWMA & CUSUM")
box()
lines(O,lwd=2,col="blue")
arrows(1889,0,1889,O[1889],lwd=3,col="black")
axis(side=c(2,3,4))
axis(side=1,labels=Dates,at=1:length(d),tick=F)
```

3.20.3   Quarterly rates

Inspection of the EWMA plus CUSUM charts shows that, with these low-rate data, the smoothing of the observed data EWMA is quite variable in spite of the use of a small EWMA weight. We describe an alternative approach for obtaining an estimate of the ongoing rate that employs quarterly data. When average expected rates are low, quarterly rates may appeal to clinicians. In this chart, supported ranges or confidence intervals are presented (Figure 3.24). When these exclude the expected rate, it is possible that the process has become unpredictable and an M&M audit should be performed. However, multiple confidence intervals should be treated with caution (they are better thought of as indicating the precision of the quarterly rate). In addition, they may fail to show runs of AEs that are demonstrated by a CUSUM analysis.

```
# chart of quarterly rates
# can also use binqtrsra, output qtrs
```

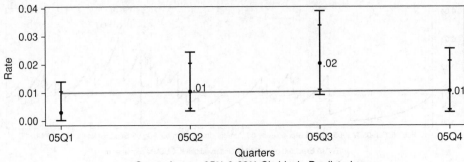

Figure 3.24   Plot of quarterly rates with confidence intervals.

```
#converting data to months
library(chron)
d<-datain[,1]
a<-datain[,2]
b<-datain[,3]
d<-chron(as.character(d),format="dd-mmm-yyyy",out.format="dd-mmm-yyyy")
o<-order(d)
d<-d[o]
a<-a[o]
b<-b[o]
y<-years(d)
m<-months(d)
dates<-paste(m,y)
aes<-tapply(a,dates,sum)
totals<-tapply(a,dates,length)
expecteds<-tapply(b,dates,sum)
month<-names(aes)
month<-paste("1",month)
month<-chron(as.character(month),format="dd mmm yyyy",out.format=
"dd-mmm-yyyy")
o<-order(month)
Month<-month[o]
aes<-as.numeric(aes)
totals<-as.numeric(totals)
expecteds<-as.numeric(expecteds)
AEs<-aes[o]
Totals<-totals[o]
Expecteds<-expecteds[o]
Table<-data.frame(Month,AEs,Totals,Expecteds)
dataout<-Table

#converting to quarters
d<-chron(as.character(dataout[,1]),format="dd-mmm-yyyy",out.format=
"dd-mmm-yyyy")
f<-dataout[,2]
n<-dataout[,3]
e<-dataout[,4]
Y<-years(d)
```

```
m<-as.numeric(months(d))
Q<-rep(0,length(m))
Q[m>=1&m<=3]<-1
Q[m>=4&m<=6]<-2
Q[m>=7&m<=9]<-3
Q[m>=10&m<=12]<-4
Tablea<-as.data.frame(xtabs(f~Q+Y))
Tableb<-as.data.frame(xtabs(n~Q+Y))
Tablec<-as.data.frame(xtabs(e~Q+Y))
Qtrs<-paste(Tablea[,2],"Q",Tablea[,1],sep="")
Table1<-data.frame(Qtrs,Tablea[,3],Tableb[,3],Tablec[,3])
names(Table1)<-c("Qtrs","AEs","Denoms","Exp")
Table1<-Table1[Table1[,3]!=0,]
LL<-length(Table1[,1])
Rate<-Table1[,2]/Table1[,3]
Expected<-Table1[,4]/Table1[,3]
s1<-Table1[1,1]
s2<-Table1[length(Table1[,1]),1]
my<-substr(Table1[,1],3,6)

#calculating precision and making chart, Figure 3.24
library(exactci)
M<-0
L<-0
U<-0
L0<-0
U0<-0
for (i in 1:LL){M<-binom.exact(Table1[i,2],Table1[i,3])$conf.int;U[i]<-M[2];
L[i]<-M[1]}
for (i in 1:LL){M<-binom.exact(Table1[i,2],Table1[i,3],
conf.level=.99)$conf.int;U0[i]<-M[2];L0[i]<-M[1]}
mx<-max(U0)
ma<-paste("Complex SSIs from ",s1," to ",s2,".",sep="")
par(xaxs="r"); par(yaxs="r")
plot(Rate,ylim=c(0,mx),col="blue",lwd=2,pch=19,axes=F,main=ma,ylab="Rate",
xlab="Quarterly rate, 95% & 99% CIs blue, Predicted red")
box()
axis(side=1,labels=as.character(my),at=1:LL)
axis(side=c(2,3,4))
lines(Expected,lwd=2,col="red")
arrows(1:LL,L0,1:LL,U0,angle=90,code=3,col="blue",length=.1,lwd=2)
points(L,lwd=2,pch="-",col="blue",cex=1.75)
points(U,lwd=2,pch="-",col="blue",cex=1.75)
mtext("Quarters",side=1,line=2)
text(Rate,labels=substr(as.character(round(Rate,2)),2,4),pos=4,offset=.3,
cex=.8,lwd=3)
```

When the expected outcome probabilities are higher, for example, CCU or ICU mortality, monthly rather than quarterly rates may be useful for clinicians.

3.21   Intervals between uncommon binary adverse events

When events are uncommon, control chart methods that monitor the intervals between events have been used to detect changes in AE rates. Intervals have the disadvantage that their distributions are severely skewed with very long right tails. A geometric distribution will often provide an approximate fit. The intervals can be placed in run charts. A run of increasing intervals following a process change provides evidence of improvement (Alemi and colleagues) while a run of short intervals may indicate a problem. Intervals can be made approximately normally distributed by transforming them using, for example, the power of 0.28. As Montgomery describes Nelson's observation, this produces approximately normally distributed data due to the transformation of the geometrically distributed data to a Weibull distribution that is approximated by the normal distribution. Other approaches are described, for example, by Benneyan. We find little use for these charts with the hospital data we analyse but describe an approach for completeness. They are undoubtedly useful for monitoring other selected uncommon event data. The data file allssicomplx.csv contains complex SSI data from a group of hospitals and includes probabilities of SSIs occurring using NNIS risk stratification. The mean rate was 1%. We use the interval information in this file to analyse the 2006 subset of the data in allssicomplx06.csv. The mean rate for the latter was 0.98%. First, we perform the analysis without using risk-adjustment.

```
g.d() # allssicomplx.csv

library(chron)
o<-order(datain[,1])
datain<-datain[o,]
m<-mean(datain[,2])
m
#[1] 0.01083109
k<-1;d1<-0;d0<-0
l<-length(datain[,1])
for (i in 1:length(datain[,1])){if (datain[i,2]==0){d1[k]<-
d1[k]+1}else{d1[k]<-d1[k]+1;d0[k]<-datain[i,1];k<-k+1;d0[k]<-0;d1[k]<-0}}
d0[k]<-datain[l,1]
d1[length(d1)]
# 184
# we leave the last interval that has no AE at the end as it is quite long
d0<-chron(d0,out.format="dd-mmm-yyyy")
me<-qgeom(.5,.01083109)
me
#
#[1] 63

dd<-d1^.28
hist(dd,main="Transformed intervals",xlab="Intervals^.28") # figure 3.25

qqnorm(dd)
qqline(dd) # Figure 3.26
shapiro.test(dd)$p.value # distribution approximately normal
#[1] 0.1520169
mean(dd)
#[1] 3.197747
sd(dd)
#[1] 0.9814481

# extracting the 2006 data
datain1<-datain[datain[,1]>"31-Dec-2005",]
s.d(datain1)
```

```
Use clipboard (c) or a data file (f) f
Enter a file name d:/allssicomplx06
```

```
g.d() # allssicomplx06.csv

library(chron)
o<-order(datain[,1])
datain<-datain[o,]
k<-1;d1<-0;d0<-0
l<-length(datain[,1])
for (i in 1:length(datain[,1])){if (datain[i,2]==0){d1[k]<-
d1[k]+1}else{d1[k]<-d1[k]+1;d0[k]<-datain[i,1];k<-k+1;d0[k]<-0;d1[k]<-0}}
d0[k]<-datain[l,1]
d1[length(d1)]
#[1] 184
# last interval has no AE at the end left as it is quite long
d0<-chron(d0,out.format="dd-mmm-yyyy")
plot(d1,type="b",axes=F,col="blue",lwd=2,pch=19,
main="Intervals between complex SSIs",
xlab="Dates of SSIs",ylab="Intervals")
box()
axis(side=1,labels=d0,at=1:k)
abline(h=68,col="red",lwd=2)
axis(side=c(2,3,4))

dd<-d1^.28
iewmachart(data.frame(d0,dd)) # Figure 3.28
```

```
Chart heading.
Enter a heading for the chart Transformed intervals
Y axis heading.
Enter a heading for the Y axis Intervals^.28
The mean value is 3.26357.
Do you want to change the mean value (Y/N) y
Enter new value for the mean 3.197747
The standard deviation is 1.01966.
Do you want to change it (Y/N) y
Enter new value for the standard deviation 0.9814481
EWMA weight.
Enter weight between 0.2 & 0.8 .2
EWMA control limit.
Enter limit between 2 & 3 2.5
```

We now re-do the analysis using the probabilities of the SSIs using NNIS stratification. The histogram, normal probability plot and intervals run chart are similar to Figures 3.25 to 3.27 and are not shown. The Shewhart/EWMA chart with risk adjustment for 2006 (Figure 3.29) is also similar.

```
g.d()# allssicomplx.csv

o<-order(datain[,1])
datain<-datain[o,]
k<-1;d1<-0;d0<-0
l<-length(datain[,1])
```

Transformed intervals

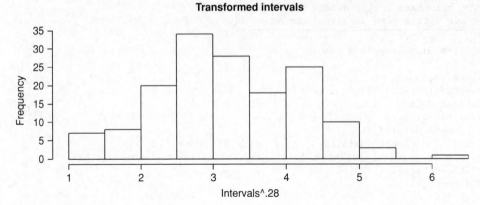

Figure 3.25   Histogram of transformed intervals between uncommon binary AEs.

```
for (i in 1:length(datain[,1]))
{if (datain[i,2]==0){d1[k]<-d1[k]+datain[i,3]}else
{d1[k]<-d1[k]+datain[i,3];d0[k]<-datain[i,1];k<-k+1;d0[k]<-0;d1[k]<-0}}
d0[k]<-datain[l,1]
d1[length(d1)]
#[1] 1.899277
# we leave the last interval that has no AE at the end as it is quite long
d0<-chron(d0,out.format="dd-mmm-yyyy")
me<-median(d1)
me
#[1] 0.6550475
dd<-d1^.28
hist(dd,main="Risk transformed intervals",xlab="Risk intervals^.28")

qqnorm(dd)
qqline(dd)
shapiro.test(dd)$p.value # distribution approximately normal
#[1] 0.2781828
```

Normal Q-Q Plot

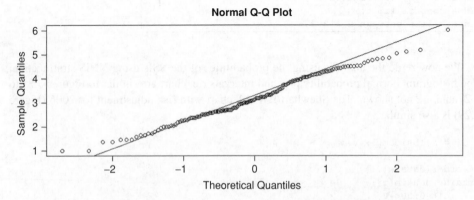

Figure 3.26   Q-Q plot of transformed intervals between uncommon binary AEs.

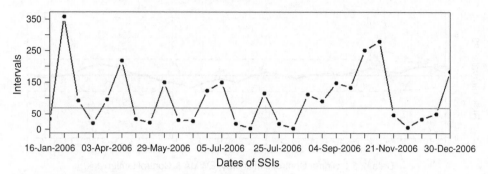

Figure 3.27 Run chart of intervals between uncommon binary AEs.

```
mean(dd)
#[1] 0.8996094
sd(dd)
#[1] 0.2785765

g.d() # allssicomplx06.csv

# run chart
library(chron)
o<-order(datain[,1])
datain<-datain[o,]
k<-1;d1<-0;d0<-0
l<-length(datain[,1])
for (i in 1:length(datain[,1]))
{if (datain[i,2]==0){d1[k]<-d1[k]+datain[i,3]}else
{d1[k]<-d1[k]+datain[i,3];d0[k]<-datain[i,1];k<-k+1;d0[k]<-0;d1[k]<-0}}
d0[k]<-datain[l,1]
d1[length(d1)]
#[1]1.899277
# last interval has no AE at the end left as it is quite long
```

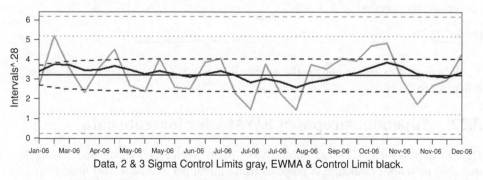

Figure 3.28 Shewhart/EWMA i chart of transformed intervals.

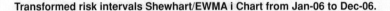

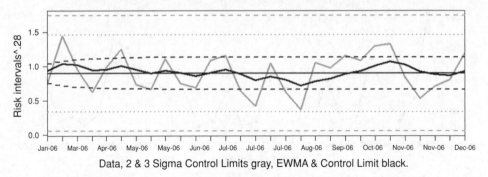

Data, 2 & 3 Sigma Control Limits gray, EWMA & Control Limit black.

Figure 3.29   Shewhart/EWMA i chart of transformed risk intervals.

```
d0<-chron(d0,out.format="dd-mmm-yyyy")
plot(d1,type="b",axes=F,col="blue",lwd=2,pch=19,
main="Risk intervals between complex SSIs",
xlab="Dates of SSIs",ylab="Risk intervals")
box()
axis(side=1,labels=d0,at=1:k)
abline(h=.655,col="red",lwd=2)
axis(side=c(2,3,4))

dd<-d1^.28
iewmachart(data.frame(d0,dd)) # Figure 3.29
```

```
Chart heading.
Enter a heading for the chart Transformed risk intervals
Y axis heading.
Enter a heading for the Y axis Risk intervals^.28
The mean value is 0.90772.
Do you want to change the mean value (Y/N) y
Enter new value for the mean .89960940
The standard deviation is 0.28329.
Do you want to change it (Y/N) y
Enter new value for the standard deviation 0.2785765
EWMA weight.
Enter weight between 0.2 & 0.8 .2
EWMA control limit.
Enter limit between 2 & 3 2.5
```

With these data, employing the risk stratification values as intervals makes no noticeable difference to the charts.

3.22   Appendix, proposed EWMA for low rate data

Obtaining limits for single observation EWMA charts when events are uncommon (e.g. less than 5%) presents a challenge. A proposal requiring further evaluation that makes repeated use of the rbinom() function with counting of the randomly generated EWMA values at each

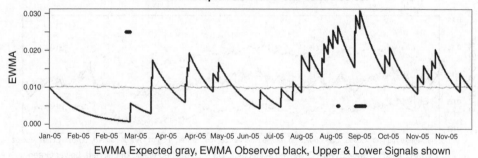

EWMA Complex SSIs from Jan-05 to Dec-05.

EWMA Expected gray, EWMA Observed black, Upper & Lower Signals shown

Figure 3.30 Proposed EWMA chart of uncommon AEs with lower and upper signals obtained by repeated random sampling from expected values.

data point is shown below. If this method proves to be useful, it may permit the detection of declining rates that may indicate under-reporting.

```
g.d.( ) # ssicomplx2005.csv

# 1% level Figure 3.30
library(chron)
ew<-.005 # EWMA weight
av<-.01 # Average rate
o<-order(datain[,1])
datain<-datain[o,]
a<-datain[,2] # AEs (0,1)
p<-datain[,3] # Predicted
d<-datain[,1] # Dates
O<-a[1]*ew+av*(1-ew)
for (i in 2:length(p)){O[i]<-O[i-1]*(1-ew)+a[i]*ew}
E<-p[1]*ew+av*(1-ew)
for (i in 2:length(p)){E[i]<-E[i-1]*(1-ew)+p[i]*ew}
m<-months(d)
y<-substr(years(d),3,4)
Dates<-paste(m,y,sep="")
P<-paste("EWMA Complex SSIs"," from ",Dates[1]," to ",Dates[length(Dates)],
".",sep="")
th1<-"EWMA Expected red, EWMA Observed blue,"
th2<-" Upper Signal Red, Lower Green";th0<-paste(th1,th2,sep="")
plot(E,type="l",ylim=c(0,.03),axes=F,lwd=1,col="red",main=P,
xlab=th0,ylab="EWMA")
box()
lines(O,lwd=3,col="blue")
axis(side=c(2,3,4))
axis(side=1,labels=Dates,at=1:length(d),tick=F)
#
l<-length(datain[,3])
ll<-length(O)
su<-rep(0,ll)
sl<-rep(0,ll)
ku<-rep(0,ll)
kl<-rep(0,ll)
```

EWMA AAA Mortality from Dec-98 to Jan-02.

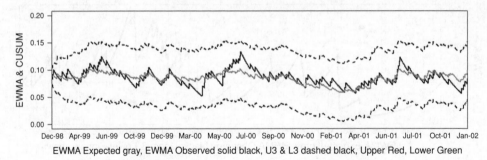

EWMA Expected gray, EWMA Observed solid black, U3 & L3 dashed black, Upper Red, Lower Green

Figure 3.31   EWMA chart (Cook and colleagues).

```
s<-0
j<-0
for (i in 1:1000){
j<-rbinom(1,1,datain[,3]);s[1]<-j[1]*ew+av*(1-ew);for (v in 2:length(j))
{s[v]<-s[v-1]*(1-ew)+j[v]*ew};
for (y in 1:length(s)){su[y]<-as.numeric(s[y]>=O[y]);ku[y]<-
ku[y]+su[y];su[y]<-0;sl[y]<-as.numeric(s[y]<=O[y]);kl[y]<-
kl[y]+sl[y];sl[y]<-0}
}
kuu<-rep(-1,length(O))
kuu[which(ku<=5)]<-.025
points(kuu,col="red",pch=19)
kll<-rep(-1,length(O))
kll[which(kl<=5)]<-.023
points(kll,col="green4",pch=19)
```

As this involves repeated generation of EWMA lines from the expected values using random sampling, there can be some variation when it is repeated. Although a little time-consuming with a large data set, it may be worth running it two or three times to get a stable result.

Cook[A,B] and colleagues EWMA for individual observations is illustrated with the abdominal aortic aneurysm(AAA) mortality data that had a rate of 8.5% (Beiles and Morton). These are composite data and display no signal. Nevertheless the rate is probably sufficiently high to illustrate the EWMA. The formulas are in sections 3.12 and 3.20.2 of this chapter.

```
g.d() # aaamort.csv

# Figure 3.31
library(chron)
o<-order(datain[,1])
datain<-datain[o,]
W<-.01
L<-3
Dates<-datain[,1]
D<-datain[,3]
mo<-months(Dates)
yr<-substr(years(Dates),3,4)
Dates<-paste(mo,yr,sep="")
```

```
M<-mean(D)
V<-D*(1-D)
E<-M*(1-W)+D[1]*W
for (i in 2:length(D)){E[i]<-E[i-1]*(1-W)+D[i]*W}
O<-datain[,2]
MO<-mean(O)
ME<-MO*(1-W)+O[1]*W
for (i in 2:length(O)){ME[i]<-ME[i-1]*(1-W)+O[i]*W}
X<-0
X<-(X^2*(1-W)^2+V[1]*W^2)
UP<-E[1]+L*X^.5
LO<-E[1]-L*X^.5
for(i in 2:length(E)){X[i]<-X[i-1]+V[i]*W^2*(1-W)^(2*(i-1));UP[i]<-E[i]+
L*X[i]^.5;LO[i]<-E[i]-L*X[i]^.5}
P<-paste("EWMA AAA Mortality"," from ",Dates[1]," to ",Dates[length(Dates)],
".",sep="")
th1<-"EWMA Expected gray, EWMA Observed solid black,"
th2<-" U3 & L3 dashed black";th0<-paste(th1,th2,sep="")
plot(ME,type="l",ylim=c(0,.2),axes=F,lwd=2,main=P,
xlab=th0,ylab="EWMA & CUSUM")
box()
lines(E,lwd=2,col="gray60")
lines(UP,lty=2,lwd=2)
lines(LO,lty=2,lwd=2)
axis(side=c(2,3,4))
axis(side=1,labels=Dates,at=1:length(E),tick=F)
```

4

Introduction to analysis of count and rate data

4.1 Introduction

We deal with count and rate data in this chapter. These data occur frequently in QI and IM work. For example, most hospital-acquired infections, excluding SSIs, can be analysed as monthly counts of events. Other examples include such adverse occurrences as patient falls, medication errors, readmissions, pressure ulcers and needlestick injuries.

These data may be grouped, for example the number of patient falls in a month or year in a single hospital, aggregated, for example, for a group of hospitals or analysed sequentially, for example, in a control chart; this chapter deals with the first of these. Its contents are summarised as follows. Aggregated data are dealt with in Chapter 5 and sequential data in Chapter 6.

```
1. Estimation and testing of a single count or rate,
2. Estimation for a series of counts or rates,
3. Comparison of two counts or rates,
4. Evaluation of more than two counts or rates,
5. The analysis of stratified data,
6. Data that display clustering and increased variability.
```

When analysing hospital-acquired infection data, its prevalence, that is, the number of patients that are carrying and potentially spreading the organism, commonly called the colonisation pressure or multiple antibiotic resistant organism (MRO) burden, is very important. We defer analysis of these often highly correlated data to Chapter 7. Other important factors

Statistical Methods for Hospital Monitoring with R, First Edition. Anthony Morton, Kerrie Mengersen, Michael Whitby and George Playford.
© 2013 John Wiley & Sons, Ltd. Published 2013 by John Wiley & Sons, Ltd.

in MRO transmission include bed occupancy, hygiene measures, particularly hand hygiene and environmental services (cleaning, particularly of high touch surfaces), antibiotic usage, prevalence in the community surrounding the hospital, the characteristics of the organism, the adequacy of the hospital's screening and isolation facilities, the services the hospital provides and discharge planning. Recent work on complex systems and networks has emphasised the importance of the complex contact patterns involving patients, nurses, and medical and other staff in the transmission of hospital-acquired organisms (Ueno and Masuda, Temime and colleagues).

First, we begin with methods for single samples, followed by methods for two independent samples. Next we describe methods for stratified data. Following this, we discuss the common problem of breakdown of independence and the likely ensuing increase in variation. In discussing medication errors, we briefly introduce power law distributions.

4.2   Rate and count data

During a three-month surveillance period there were 12 unplanned readmissions for 32,190 occupied bed-days in a small teaching hospital and during the same months in the succeeding year there were 28 similar unplanned readmissions for 37,440 occupied bed-days.

The number of readmissions was greater in the second period but the hospital's bed occupancy was also higher. Also the numbers of readmissions could have been greater in the second period because the surveillance may have been more effective. However, for the present purpose, we shall use these data as if ascertainment were similar in the two periods. The rates for the two periods were respectively 0.37 ($12 \times 1000/32190$) and 0.75 ($28 \times 1000/37440$) per 1000 occupied bed-days.

Certain patients are much more prone to requiring readmission than others and some may need repeated admissions. This may lead to increased variability and may cause the methods of this section that are based on the Poisson distribution to give misleading results. It is therefore advisable whenever possible to check that the mean and variance of these and similar count data are alike before using the methods of this section.

During an 11-month period of relatively constant bed occupancy, the following monthly counts of unplanned readmissions were observed: 4, 5, 5, 2, 9, 6, 4, 6, 3, 7 & 7. The mean of these counts is 5.3 and the variance is 4. Although one would hope to base these calculations on more data, for example 20 to 24 monthly counts, there is no evidence of excessive variation; perhaps the majority of the repeated admissions were not unplanned. This is very important because many adverse events (AEs) are not fully independent, for example becoming a carrier of an MRO requires transmission from another source. When the variance of a series of observations exceeds their mean, a not uncommon occurrence with AE count data, their analysis becomes more challenging as the use of conventional methods based on the Poisson distribution can mislead. We mostly employ the negative binomial distribution instead of the Poisson distribution with these data.

4.3   Single count or rate

The reader is referred to the beginning of Chapter 1 for a discussion of sample and population values. The ideas apply equally to counts and rates.

If X is the number of events and N is the person-time of exposure, then the observed rate is R=X/N. (Note that in Chapter 1, we used the notation $\hat{p}$ for R.) A measure of the precision of the rate, its confidence interval (CI), is also required. In likelihood terms, this tells us the range of possible values of the rate that are supported by the data.

4.3.1   Confidence interval

To obtain an accurate confidence interval (CI), we employ the inverse gamma function. For the lower 95% limit qgamma(0.025,X,1)/N and for the upper value qgamma(0.975,X+1,1)/N are employed in R (if there is only a count, N=1). We may obtain identical results using the R function poisson.exact() in the exactci library. Occupied bed-days is a frequently used denominator and rates are often expressed as per 1000 or 10,000 bed-days.

In Chapter 1 we described mid-P intervals. These are thought to be superior with count data as the exact intervals are considered to be conservative due to the discrete nature of the Poisson distribution. Calculation for small counts is difficult and, unlike proportion data, there appears currently to be no R library with a CI function for their calculation. For small counts we employ tables (Cohen and Yang) and for larger counts we use the method of Kulkarni and colleagues. Cohen and Yang also describe an accurate mid-P approximation, $((X+.5)^{.5} \pm Z/2)^2$, where for a 95% limit Z=1.96.

```
# Cohen and Yang mid-P approximation
x<-12
N<-32190
midp.lower95<-((x+.5)^.5-1.96/2)^2
midp.lower95*1000/N
#[1]  0.2028814
midp.upper95<-((x+.5)^.5+1.96/2)^2
midp.upper95*1000/N
#[1]  0.633428
#
midp.lower99<-((x+.5)^.5-2.575829/2)^2
midp.lower99*1000/N
#[1]  0.1569367
midp.upper99<-((x+.5)^.5+2.575829/2)^2
midp.upper99*1000/N
#[1]  0.7227603

# tables (Cohen and Yang)
# 95%
#[1]  0.2019261
#[1]  0.6337372
# 99%
#[1]  0.1615409
#[1]  0.7331469

# Kulkarni and colleagues
# 95%
#[1]  0.2000325
#[1]  0.6354976
# 99%
#[1]  0.1573399
#[1]  0.7344832
```

4.3.2   Significance test

It is often desirable to compare the observed rate with a reference rate. For example, the unplanned readmission rate for a surveillance period may be compared with a rate, obtained for a large group of hospitals, which is regarded as a reference rate.

To illustrate the method, suppose that the reference rate was 0.45 per 1000 occupied bed-days and it is to be compared with the rate of 28 readmissions in 37,440 occupied bed-days that occurred in the second surveillance period. For these data, the expected count is $E=.45 \times 37440/1000 = 16.848$.

We employ the gamma distribution function in R. When the expected count E is greater than X, employ $2 \times (1-\text{pgamma}(E,X+1,1))$ and when X is greater than E, use $2 \times \text{pgamma}(E,X,1)$ to obtain two tailed p-values. With these data the two tailed P-value is 0.0158. For these calculations, it is convenient to use poisson.exact() from the exactci library. Note that R has a function poisson.test() that can give a slightly different result because it deals with the two tails of the Poisson distribution separately instead of employing the more conventional method of doubling the one tailed P-value and this distribution has a longer right than left tail when samples are small.

The exact P-value can be considered to be too conservative due to the discrete nature of the Poisson distribution and a mid-P value may be preferred. This employs half the probability of the observed outcome plus the probability of all possible outcomes with a lesser probability and, for these data, it is 0.012. An approximation described by Vollset can be used to obtain the mid-P P-value. This involves taking the P-value for the observed and expected counts and then, if the observed count is greater than the expected adding one to it, otherwise if the observed count is smaller than the expected count subtracting one from it (provided it is not zero) and again obtaining the P-value for this new result. The mid-P value is then approximately the average of these. The value of the Z-score, the standard normal deviate, can be obtained using the qnorm function and $\text{abs}(\text{qnorm}(0.0158/2))=2.41$ or $-0.862+(0.743-2.404 \times \log(P))^{.5}=2.41$ (Bland and Altman).

```
abs(qnorm(0.0158/2))
#[1] 2.413503
-0.862+(0.743-2.404*log(0.0158))^.5
#[1] 2.411252
#
cat(paste("1/",as.character(round(1/exp(-2.41^2/2),0)),sep=""),"\n")
#1/18
```

In addition, the likelihood ratio is calculated using, for a Z-score of Z= 2.41, cat(paste("1/",as.character(round(1/exp(-Z^2/2),0)),sep=""),"\n") = 1/18. This means that the support from the data for the expected rate of 0.45 per 1000 is small. These calculations are in the function rate().

```
#using the rate() function
rate()
```

```
Enter numerator 28
Is there a denominator (y/n) y
Enter the denominator 37440
Is a reference rate available? y
Enter reference rate .00045
```

```
Rate = 0.00075, lower 95% limit = 5e-04, upper limit = 0.00108
Mid-P 95% limits are 0.00051 and 0.00107.
P = 0.016, LR = 1/18.
Mid-p value = 0.012, LR = 1/23.
```

Byar's approximation (Rothman and Boice) is a useful alternative for the significance test. Z-score$=\sqrt{(9\times OB)}\times(1-1/(9\times OB)-(E/OB)^{1/3})$, where OB=X if X>E or OB=X+1 if X<E. Funnel plots are described in Chapter 5 and corrections for overdispersion that require Z-scores may be needed. When there is marked overdispersion, a Z-score obtained with the gamma distribution as described above and then the qnorm() function can report infinity. When this occurs Byar's approximation can be used. This approximation can also be used to obtain confidence limits. Where N=37440. L95=X$\times(1-1/(9\times X)-1.96/(3\times\sqrt{X}))^3$/N=0.000496836   and   U95=(X+1)$\times(1-1/(9\times(X+1))+1.96/(3\times\sqrt{(X+1)}))^3$/N= 0.001080918 with P-value=0.0158702, similar to the results employing rate(). Byar's method employs a chi-squared approximation; the chi-squared and gamma distributions are closely related.

```
# Byar's CI
X<-28
L95<-X*(1-1/(9*X)-1.96/(3*X^.5))^3/37440
U95<-(X+1)*(1-1/(9*(X+1))+1.96/(3*(X+1)^.5))^3/37440
L95;U95
#
#[1] 0.000496836
#[1] 0.001080918
#
# Byar's P-value
E<-16.848
OB<-X # as X>E, if X<E, OB=X+1
Z.score=(9*OB)^.5*(1-1/(9*OB)-(E/OB)^(1/3))
P.value<-exp(-0.717*Z.score-0.416*Z.score^2)
Z.score;P.value
#
#[1] 2.409696
#[1] 0.0158702
```

Byar's formula can also be used to obtain approximate mid-P intervals but it works less well with very small counts.

```
X<-28
L95<-(X+.5)*(1-1/(9*(X+.5))-1.96/(9*(X+.5))^.5)^3/37440
U95<-(X+.5)*(1-1/(9*(X+.5))+1.96/(9*(X+.5))^.5)^3/37440
L95
#[1] 0.0005077
U95
#[1] 0.001065


X<-12
L95<-(X+.5)*(1-1/(9*(X+.5))-1.96/(9*(X+.5))^.5)^3/32190
U95<-(X+.5)*(1-1/(9*(X+.5))+1.96/(9*(X+.5))^.5)^3/32190
L95
#[1] 0.0002036
U95
#[1] 0.0006314
```

The function rate() can also be accessed via IMenu(). Enter IMenu() at the R prompt, then 2 and 1.

4.4   Confidence limits for columns of counts and rates

Scientists in IM and QI departments are required to present periodic reports that involve summarising rows of counts or rates. Calculating confidence limits for each of the individual counts or rates is time-consuming and prone to error. The required confidence limits can be obtained for multiple counts or rates (e.g. rate per 1000 occupied bed-days) using the qgamma() function. If the latter are required, multiply the counts by 1000 and divide by the bed-days denominator. Data are in the file bacttable.csv. The second and third columns are employed. The function multiplecounts() calculates the required confidence intervals.

```
g.d() # bacttable.csv
```

```
Loading data.
Data from clipboard (C) or file (F) c
Do data column(s) have heading(s) (Y/N) y
Is column 1 a date column (Y/N) n
```

```
#using the multiplecounts() function
multiplecounts(datain[,2])
```

```
      s      sl95     sl997     su95    su997
1    60   45.7863   39.5891   77.232    86.80
2   205  177.8964  165.0988  235.066   251.21
3    96   77.7603   69.5057  117.232   128.84
4   190  163.9430  151.6824  219.022   234.63
5   136  114.1045  103.9776  160.873   174.35
6    69   53.6861   46.9273   87.324    97.45
7    94   75.9616   67.8100  115.032   126.54
8    12    6.2006    4.2451   20.962    26.32
9    42   30.2699   25.3374   56.772    65.08
10   32   21.8880   17.7762   45.174    52.67
11   48   35.3914   30.0121   63.641    72.39
12   18   10.6679    7.9545   28.448    34.56
13   14    7.6539    5.4298   23.490    29.11
14    3    0.6187    0.2197    8.767    12.55
15   27   17.7932   14.1388   39.284    46.32
16   15    8.3954    6.0434   24.740    30.49
17   13    6.9220    4.8298   22.230    27.73
18    5    1.6235    0.8113   11.668    15.89
19    5    1.6235    0.8113   11.668    15.89
20    8    3.4538    2.1032   15.763    20.52
21    6    2.2019    1.2000   13.059    17.47
The data are in ss
```

```
# The data are in ss; use s.d(ss) with clipboard to export
# to get rates per 1000 bed-days
ss*1000/datain[,3]
```

```
          s        sl95     sl997      su95     su997
1    0.14465  0.110384  0.095443  0.18619  0.20925
2    0.15477  0.134310  0.124648  0.17747  0.18966
3    0.12706  0.102919  0.091994  0.15516  0.17053
4    0.18903  0.163109  0.150911  0.21791  0.23343
5    0.21647  0.181617  0.165499  0.25606  0.27751
6    0.14735  0.114651  0.100217  0.18649  0.20810
7    0.09429  0.076199  0.068022  0.11539  0.12694
8    0.02880  0.014881  0.010188  0.05031  0.06317
9    0.07922  0.057095  0.047791  0.10708  0.12275
10   0.11248  0.076933  0.062481  0.15878  0.18512
11   0.11851  0.087382  0.074100  0.15713  0.17874
12   0.04920  0.029158  0.021741  0.07775  0.09445
13   0.07809  0.042693  0.030287  0.13102  0.16240
14   0.02932  0.006047  0.002147  0.08569  0.12262
15   0.08894  0.058609  0.046572  0.12940  0.15259
16   0.11084  0.062035  0.044656  0.18281  0.22531
17   0.05875  0.031281  0.021826  0.10046  0.12529
18   0.06460  0.020977  0.010483  0.15077  0.20527
19   0.06675  0.021673  0.010831  0.15577  0.21208
20   0.09988  0.043122  0.026259  0.19681  0.25624
21   0.03412  0.012522  0.006824  0.07427  0.09936
```

The function multiplecounts can be accessed via IMenu().

```
IMenu(datain[,2])
```

```
Introductory Menu

1. Proportiom data,
2. Count and rate data.
2
1. Single count or rate,
2. Confidence intervals for a series of counts or rates,
3. Two counts or rates,
4. More than two counts or rates,
5. Weighted average of rates.
2
       s       sl95      sl997      su95     su997
1    60   45.7863   39.5891    77.232    86.80
2   205  177.8964  165.0988   235.066   251.21
3    96   77.7603   69.5057   117.232   128.84
4   190  163.9430  151.6824   219.022   234.63
5   136  114.1045  103.9776   160.873   174.35
6    69   53.6861   46.9273    87.324    97.45
7    94   75.9616   67.8100   115.032   126.54
8    12    6.2006    4.2451    20.962    26.32
9    42   30.2699   25.3374    56.772    65.08
10   32   21.8880   17.7762    45.174    52.67
11   48   35.3914   30.0121    63.641    72.39
12   18   10.6679    7.9545    28.448    34.56
13   14    7.6539    5.4298    23.490    29.11
14    3    0.6187    0.2197     8.767    12.55
15   27   17.7932   14.1388    39.284    46.32
16   15    8.3954    6.0434    24.740    30.49
```

```
17 13   6.9220   4.8298   22.230  27.73
18  5   1.6235   0.8113   11.668  15.89
19  5   1.6235   0.8113   11.668  15.89
20  8   3.4538   2.1032   15.763  20.52
21  6   2.2019   1.2000   13.059  17.47
The data are in ss
```

4.5   Two independent rates

The need to compare two independent rates can arise in IM and QI studies. Usually this is accomplished by using the rate ratio as an estimator of the magnitude of the difference between the two rates. In Chapter 1 we described the number needed to treat (NNT). Although we are now dealing with count rather than proportion data, we believe that the same approach is worth following. The inverse of the rate difference can be thought of as the person-time or bed-days needed to treat to prevent one complication.

We restate our concerns about comparing data from institutions that may differ in the services they provide when risk adjustment or stratification is, with count data AEs, in the early stages of development. Comparisons of hospitals may be made after seeing the data and the hospitals being compared may be among a number of related institutions. Funnel plots and other methods used for the display of data from a number of institutions do so relative to an average value. Post-hoc comparisons should always be treated with caution. Adjustments for multiple comparisons, using for example, the Benjamini-Hochberg procedure, may not have been made. Random variation within predictable limits that is related to regression to the mean can result in institutions varying their ranking from year to year with no change in their systems. In a judgemental environment AEs may be hidden and therefore they may be unavailable for learning. Apart from the potential bias and the statistical difficulties involved, we query the usefulness of making comparisons when the foremost question to be answered about an institution is whether or not it has instituted a sound program of compliance with evidence-based systems and bundles together with a system for sequential monitoring of its AE data.

As illustration, during one year there were $X1=88$ cases of intravenous device-related bacteraemia in $N1=274187$ occupied bed-days (OBDs) (rate $= 2.991295$ per 10000 OBDs). In the ensuing 6 months, following a system change, there were $X2=26$ cases in $N2=147836$ OBDs (rate $= 1.758706$ per 10000 OBDs). The difference was 1.450783, equivalent to a decrease of one intravenous device-related bacteraemia in approximately 5700 OBDs (i.e. approximately three cases prevented each month). However, even if this estimator is not used, it has been our experience that staff working in IM and QI departments tend to have a better intuitive understanding of the magnitude of difference estimators than they do of ratio estimators. For these reasons we prefer the rate difference to the rate ratio when dealing with count data, although we employ both estimators and their confidence intervals.

4.5.1   Confidence interval

Newcombe's method for confidence intervals for differences between proportions can easily be adapted for count and rate data difference CI calculation. First, one must obtain the confidence limits for each rate, for example by using the methods described above for a single rate. Then the formulas are $D_U = D + \sqrt{\{(R_2 - L_2)^2 + (U_1 - R_1)^2\}}$ and $D_L = D - \sqrt{\{(R_1 - L_1)^2 + (U_2 - R_2)^2\}}$ where L_1, L_2 and U_1, U_2 are the lower and upper confidence limits for the two rates (R_1=X1/N1 and R_2=X2/N2) and D, D_L and D_U are the rate difference and its lower and upper confidence limits respectively. When employing these limits, it is preferable to use mid-P values for the two rates. The method is in the function tworates(). Data may be entered from the keyboard using tworates() or from a data.frame e.g. d<-data.frame(28,37440,12,32190) then tworates(d). If counts are available without denominators use d<-data.frame(Count1,1,Count2,1) to enter data from a data.frame or enter the two counts from the keyboard.

For the rate ratio a score method described by Graham and colleagues is implemented in tworates(). Let $A=2\times X_1\times X_2$, $B=Z^2\times(X_1+X_2)$, $C=\sqrt{\{Z^2\times(X_1+X_2)[4\times X_1\times X_2+Z^2\times(X_1+X_2)]\}}$ and $D=2\times X_2^2$. Then $L=(N_1/N_2)\times(A+B-C)/D$ and $U=(N_1/N_2)\times(A+B+C)/D$, where X1 and X2 are the two counts, N1 and N2 the two denominators and L and U are the confidence limits. For comparison we show the results using poisson.exact() from the R exactci library in section 4.5.2. These are conservative due to the discrete nature of the Poisson distribution.

```
#using tworates() function
tworates() # Newcombe difference intervals, Graham ratio intervals
```

```
Are denominators available? y
Enter first numerator 28
Enter first denominator 37440
Enter second numerator 12
Enter second denominator 32190
Rate ratio = 2.006.
Lower 95% limit = 1.033, upper limit = 3.897.
Difference between rates = 0.00038.
Lower 95% limit = 2e-05, upper limit = 0.00074,
p-value = 0.039, LR = 1/8
```

4.5.2   Hypothesis test

A conservative significance test method is to regard the $X_1/(X_1+X_2)$ as a proportion with expected value $N_1/(N_1+N_2)$ where X_1 and X_2 are the two counts and N_1 and N_2 are the corresponding denominators (Rosner). For the above data the resulting P-value is 0.055. This result can be obtained by using the exactci library and entering at the R prompt poisson.exact(c(28,12),c(37440,32190))$p.value. This is suggestive, but not significant, at a level of 0.05. The rate ratio CI may be obtained by omitting the $p.value; it is 0.98 to 4.33 and provides the same inference about a suggestive, but not significant difference since it (just) contains one. Due to the conservative nature of this method, we decided to employ mid-P values with a result of 0.039 which is significant at the 5% level (poisson.exact(c(29,11),c(37440,32190))$p.value is 0.024 and (.055+.024)/2=0.0395). An alternative approach, when apparent indecision or discordance exists between the P-value and the confidence interval, is to adopt Lin's method of obtaining an approximate P-value from a confidence interval and vice-versa. This is described by Altman and Bland and is illustrated in Chapter 1 section 1.4.3.

Here we illustrate Lin's method with the log rate ratio values. The logs of the ratio CIs may be more likely to display necessary symmetry about the log of the rate ratio than the corresponding difference and its CIs. In other situations, published work may display either a P-value or CI and we may wish to obtain an approximate value for the missing estimate. Therefore we illustrate all combinations.

```
#P-value from rate ratio CI
R<-2.006
L<-1.033
U<-3.897
SE<-abs((log(U)-log(L))/(2*1.96))
Z<-abs(log(R)/SE)
Z
#
#[1] 2.055282
p.value<-exp(-0.717*Z-0.416*Z^2)
p.value
#[1] 0.03952203
```

The function IMenu() can be used to access tworates().

```
d<-data.frame(28,37440,12,32190)
IMenu(d)
```

```
Introductory Menu

1. Proportiom data,
2. Count and rate data.
2
1. Single count or rate,
2. Confidence intervals for a series of counts or rates,
3. Two counts or rates,
4. More than two counts or rates,
5. Weighted average of rates.
3
Rate ratio = 2.006.
Lower 95% limit = 1.033, upper limit = 3.897.
Difference between rates = 0.00038.
Lower 95% limit = 2e-05, upper limit = 0.00074,
p-value = 0.039, LR = 1/8.
```

4.5.3   Bayesian approach

The literature on Bayesian approaches for assessing two independent rates is growing. Although currently beyond the scope of these notes, the reader is referred to the books by Woodworth and Spiegelhalter[F]. Bayesian methods may be destined to assume increasing importance in IM and QI work in hospitals.

4.6   Chi-squared and trend tests for count and rate data

We illustrate the chi-squared and trend tests for comparing rates using the following bacteraemia data from five large hospitals. These tests are included in the manyrates() function. Since these are a sample from a group of hospitals, they could often be considered exchangeable and suitable for analysis using random effects methods. Analysis of count and rate data among groups of hospitals is dealt with in Chapter 5.

The formula for the chi-squared test is $\sum\{(O_i-E_i)^2/E_i\}$, where O_i is the observed count i and E_i is the corresponding expected value. The degrees of freedom are one less than the number of counts. It is a large sample test and will give incorrect results when there are small Es, for example, Es of one or less or many less than 5. It will often be possible to amalgamate counts with very small expected values or in some cases such as counts of bacteraemias to remove and subject them to separate audit.

However, there may have been reason to suspect that AE rates could for example be related to hospital size and so a trend test may be indicated to see if the number of bacteraemias is related to the size of the hospital; hospitals would then not be exchangeable and standard methods would be required. Also, if a trend is present, any departure from trend can also be assessed. The χ_1 trend test involves allotting scores (S) for each level. Then $\chi_1=(\sum(S\times(O-E)))^2/(\sum(E\times S^2)-(\sum(E\times S))^2/\sum(O))$, and $\sum E=\sum O$. An alternative formula that uses the counts (O) and denominators (N) is $\chi_1=((\sum(O\times S)-\mu\times\sum(O))^2)/(R\times(\sum(N\times S^2)-\sum(N)\times\mu^2))$, $R=\sum O/\sum N$ and $\mu=\sum(N\times S)/\sum N$. The calculations are in the manyrates() function.

```
#using manyrates() function
Count<-c(60,136,96,190,205)
OBD<-c(414792,628268,755547,1005113,1324524)
level1<-data.frame(Count,OBD)
o<-order(level1[,1])
level1<-level1[o,]
level1
```

	Count	OBD
1	60	414792
3	96	755547
2	136	628268
4	190	1005113
5	205	1324524

```
manyrates(level1)
```

```
#The R editor appears so data entered from the keyboard can
be checked. Click on close button after checking
```

	O	D	E	Z
1	60	414792	69.02744	-1.028142
2	136	628268	104.55296	2.908734
3	96	755547	125.73404	-2.703900
4	190	1005113	167.26546	1.695697
5	205	1324524	220.42011	-1.005261

```
Global chi-squared = 21.84 P-value = 2e-04
Is a trend test required y
Trend test chi-squared = 1.232 P-value = 0.267
Departure from trend test chi-squared = 20.608 P-value = 1e-04
```

There is no evidence of a trend. The second hospital had more AEs than expected and the third less. These differences are likely to reflect the differing services provided by these hospitals. Risk-adjustment of bacteraemia rates using the services the hospitals provide is described by Tong and colleagues and we provide an illustration at the end of Chapter 5. Risk adjustment for count and rate AE data is currently undergoing development.

The function manyrates() can also be accessed via IMenu().

```
IMenu(level1)
```

```
Introductory Menu

1. Proportiom data,
2. Count and rate data.
2
1. Single count or rate,
2. Confidence intervals for a series of counts or rates,
3. Two counts or rates,
4. More than two counts or rates,
5. Weighted average of rates.
4
       O        D        E        Z
1    60   414792    69.03  -1.028
2    96   755547   125.73  -2.704
3   136   628268   104.55   2.909
4   190  1005113   167.27   1.696
5   205  1324524   220.42  -1.005

Global chi-squared = 21.84 Pvalue = 2e-04
Is a trend test required y
Trend test chi-squared = 1.232 Pvalue = 0.267
Departure from trend test chi-squared = 20.61 Pvalue = 1e-04
```

Had these hospitals been regarded as exchangeable, a random effects analysis may have been indicated. This is now illustrated. Although this is a very small number of hospitals, the analysis shows how regarding the hospitals as a random sample of hospitals may change inferences. The common stratifying agents in IM and QI work are years and hospitals. The former will usually be a fixed agent and the latter may sometimes be regarded as a random agent.

```
library(hglm)
library(exactci)
Hosp<-1:5
P<-0
Z<-0
E<-OBD*sum(Count)/sum(OBD)
for (i in 1:5){P[i]<-poisson.exact(Count[i],E[i])$p.value}
Z<--0.862+(0.743-2.404*log(P))^.5
for (i in 1:5){if (E[i]>Count[i]){Z[i]<--Z[i]}}
Z<-round(Z,2)
Exp<-round(E,0)
h<-
hglm(fixed=Count~1,random=~1|as.character(Hosp),offset=log(
E),family=poisson(link=log),fix.disp=1)
Zrnd<-round(as.numeric(h$ranef)/as.numeric(h$SeRe),2)
data.frame(Count,Exp,Z,Zrnd)
```

	Count	Exp	Z	Zrnd
1	60	69	−1.04	−0.71
2	136	105	2.91	1.96
3	96	126	−2.70	−1.70
4	190	167	1.69	1.08
5	205	220	−1.01	−0.48

4.7   Stratified count and rate data

The stratifying agent with IM and QI data is frequently years. When these count and rate data are stratified, it may be to obtain a summary rate for a single hospital using for example yearly data or to compare summary rates of yearly data from two hospitals. In each case it will often be desirable to give more weight to the most recent data; therefore standard fixed effects methods are required. When making comparisons involving these data, it is important to look for overdispersion and group by stratum interaction as P-values may otherwise be too small or summary measures inappropriate.

4.7.1   Obtaining a summary rate

A summary rate can be obtained using the function stratifiedratesn(). Data entry can be manual via the R editor or as a data.frame. Since manual entry can be tedious and error prone, the latter method may be preferred. We illustrate with yearly bacteraemia data from a single hospital.

```
#using stratifiedratesn() function (n is for Newcombe)
# Newcombe's method described in Chapter 1, section 1.4.1
#data may be entered from the keyboard using stratifiedratesn()
#or as a data.frame e.g. from a data file
Saureus<-c(23,35,31,42,43,31)
OBD<-c(188514,214805,218009,229590,234446,239160)
W<-1:6
stratifiedratesn(data.frame(Saureus,OBD,W))
#
#The R editor appears so entered data can be checked
#Click on close button after checking
#geometrically increasing weights, may be changed in the Data Editor
#weights can be changed from 1 to 6
```

```
Weighted average = 0.00016.
Lower 95% limit = 0.00014, upper limit = 0.00018.
```

The function stratifiedratesn() can also be accessed via IMenu().

```
d<-data.frame(Saureus,OBD,W)
IMenu(d)
```

```
Introductory Menu

1. Proportiom data,
2. Count and rate data.
2
```

```
1. Single count or rate,
2. Confidence intervals for a series of counts or rates,
3. Two counts or rates,
4. More than two counts or rates,
5. Weighted average of rates.
5
Weighted average = 0.00016.
Lower 95% limit = 0.00014, upper limit = 0.00018.
```

We look for heterogeneity among the yearly bacteraemias. There is no evidence that the within stratum rates differ sufficiently to invalidate the summary rate. When the data are aggregated, the rate is little changed although the weighting is no longer available.

```
# test for homogeneity
manyrates(data.frame(Saureus,OBD))
```

```
        O       D        E            Z
1      23   188514   29.17680   -1.0560239
2      35   214805   33.24592    0.2449758
3      31   218009   33.74182   -0.3612039
4      42   229590   35.53424    1.0018858
5      43   234446   36.28581    1.0310935
6      31   239160   37.01541   -0.9023473
Global chi-squared = 5.019 P.value = 0.4135
```

```
#aggregated rate
sum(Saureus)
#[1]  205
sum(OBD)
#[1]  1324524

rate()
```

```
Enter numerator 205
Is there a denominator (y/n) y
Enter the denominator 1324524
Is a reference rate available? n
Rate = 0.00015, lower 95% limit = 0.00013, upper limit = 0.00018
Mid-P 95% limits are 0.00014 and 0.00017.
```

4.7.2   Stratified count and rate data, two sets of rates

Adverse event (Caesarean section SSI's) data for two hospitals, a specialised obstetric hospital (Group1) and a medium sized general hospital (Group2), were stratified by Elective and Emergency and by NNIS risk index giving six strata each with sparse numerators. It is usual to expect the Emergency strata to have higher SSI rates than the corresponding Elective strata. The NNIS risk-index is described in Chapter 3.

Although these are proportion data rather than counts or rates, each proportion is small so the methods of this section should be suitable for their analysis (Armitage and colleagues). The rates are for in-hospital SSIs only and therefore appear artificially low. We wish to calculate summary rates for these data, in this case the stratifying agent being the patients' risk strata and to compare them.

```
# stratified count data
Group1<-c(2,1420,3,575,1,21,5,1850,3,905,0,64)
Group2<-c(5,708,2,206,0,6,4,1023,3,334,0,10)
ssi1<-data.frame(Group1,Group2)
row.names(ssi1)<-
c("Stratum1Failures","Stratum1Procedures","Stratum2Failures",
"Stratum2Procedures","Stratum3Failures","Stratum3Procedures",
"Stratum4Failures","Stratum4Procedures","Stratum5Failures",
"Stratum5Procedures","Stratum6Failures","Stratum6Procedures")
ssi1
```

	Group1	Group2	
Stratum1Failures	2	5	(elective/risk-index0)
Stratum1Procedures	1420	708	
Stratum2Failures	3	2	(elective/risk-index1)
Stratum2Procedures	575	206	
Stratum3Failures	1	0	(elective/risk-index2)
Stratum3Procedures	21	6	
Stratum4Failures	5	4	(emergency/risk-index0)
Stratum4Procedures	1850	1023	
Stratum5Failures	3	3	(emergency/risk-index1)
Stratum5Procedures	905	334	
Stratum6Failures	0	0	(emergency/risk-index2)
Stratum6Procedures	64	10	

The stratifying variable here is type of patient requiring surgery, a fixed agent. These data are too sparse to test for homogeneity but there is none obvious on visual inspection. However, if it were present it would be necessary to examine the data within the individual strata.

4.7.3   Indirect standardisation

In indirect standardisation the observed count of the outcomes is compared to an expected count obtained by calculating the number that would have occurred if some reference rate were applied to the observed group denominators.

For a group of hospitals the expected in-hospital SSI rate for elective/risk-index0 operations was 0.336%, elective/risk-index1 operations 0.876%, elective/risk-index2 operations 2.41%, emergency/risk-index0 operations 0.705%, emergency/risk-index1 operations 1.377% and for emergency/risk-index2 operations it is 3.597%.

Applying these rates to the Hospital 1 (Group 1) data, the expected number (E) of SSIs would have been $E = 0.00336 \times 1420 + 0.00876 \times 575 + 0.0241 \times 21 + 0.00705 \times 1850 + 0.01377 \times 905 + 0.03597 = 38.11798$. The observed number was O=14. The Group 2 values were $E = 0.00336 \times 708 + 0.00876 \times 206 + 0.0241 \times 6 + 0.00705 \times 1023 + 0.01377 \times 334 + 0.03597 \times 10 = 16.49766$ and O=14. Although indirectly standardised rates can be subject to bias and methods for their analysis should be used with caution, the methods for a single rate may now be applied. The mid-P 95% confidence interval for the 14 observed count is 7.97 to 22.93. For the first hospital the standardised morbidity ratio (SMR) was 14/38.12=0.37 with a

95% CI from 7.97/38.12=0.21 to 22.93/38.12=0.60. When the observed 14 SSIs is compared with the expected 38.12, the P-value is less than 0.0001. For the second hospital the SMR was 14/16.5=0.85 with a 95% CI from 7.97/16.5=0.48 to 22.93/16.5=1.39, P-value=0.56). The ratio of the SMRs was 0.43 with a 95% CI of 0.2 to 0.92. The approximate Z-score and P-value for the latter comparison are 2.19 and 0.028 respectively.

```
# using indirect standardisation
S1<-sum(Group1[c(1,3,5,7,9,11)])
S2<-sum(Group2[c(1,3,5,7,9,11)])
StratRt<-c(0.336, 0.876, 2.41, 0.705, 1.377,3.597)
Exp1<-sum(Group1[c(2,4,6,8,10,12)]*StratRt/100)
Exp2<- sum(Group2[c(2,4,6,8,10,12)]*StratRt/100)
S1;S2;Exp1;Exp2
```

```
S1 14 (first hospital observed SSIs)
S2 14 (second hospital observed SSIs)
Exp1 38.12073 (first hospital expected SSIs)
Exp2 16.49907 (second hospital expected SSIs)
```

```
#mid-P CI for count of 14 using tables (Cohen and Yang)
x1<-14
xl<-
c(0,0.051,0.336,0.764,1.271,1.832,2.432,3.062,3.716,4.39,5.08,5.785,6.502,
7.231,7.969,8.717,9.472,10.234,11.004,11.779,12.56)
xu<-
c(2.996,4.931,6.607,8.164,9.648,11.082,12.479,13.847,15.191,16.516,17.824,
19.119,20.4,21.671,22.932,24.184,25.429,26.666,27.896,29.12,30.339)
L<-xl[x1+1];U<-xu[x1+1]
L;U
```

```
L 7.97  (lower CL for 14)
U 22.93 (upper CL for 14)
```

```
library(exactci)
#mid-P P-values
#Group 1
(poisson.exact(14,38.11798)$p.value+poisson.exact(13,38.11798)$p.value)/2
#[1] 9.16328e-06
#
#Group 2
(poisson.exact(14,16.49766)$p.value+poisson.exact(13,16.49766)$p.value)/2
#[1] 0.5586621
```

```
#comparison of group SMRs (see two sets of rates below)
#CIs
R1<-14/38.11798 # Group 1 SMR
R1L<-7.97/38.11798 # lower CI
R1U<-22.93/38.11798 # upper CI
R2<-14/16.49766 # Group 2 SMR
R2L<-7.97/16.49766 # lower CI
R2U<-22.93/16.49766 # upper CI
RR<-R1/R2 # Ratio
# Newcombe-Zou-Donner method for CI of ratio
RL<-exp((log(R1)-log(R2))-((log(R1)-log(R1L))^2+(log(R2U)-log(R2))^2)^.5)
```

```
RU<-exp((log(R1)-log(R2))+((log(R2)-log(R2L))^2+(log(R1U)-log(R1))^2)^.5)
RR;RL;RU
```

```
Ratio of SMRs 0.4328052
Lower CL      0.2046718
Upper CL      0.9152231
```

```
#Z-scores & P-values (Bland and Altman)
R<-RR
L<-RL
U<-RU
SE<-abs((log(U)-log(L))/(2*1.96))
Z<-abs(log(R)/SE)
P.value<-exp(-0.717*Z-0.416*Z^2)
Z;P.value
```

```
Approximate Z-score 2.191855
Approximate P-value 0.02815253
```

We can employ the binomial method used for the analysis of two independent sample proportion data without stratification. O_1 is binomial with denominator O_1+O_2 and expected value $E_1/(E_1+E_2)$. For the SSI data described above $O_1=14$, $E_1=38.12$, $O_2=14$ and $E_2=16.5$, $E_1/(E_1+E_2)=0.698$ and the P-value$=0.044$. This is conservative and the mid-P value is 0.03.

```
# using proportion()
proportion()
```

```
Enter numerator 14
Enter denominator 28
Is a reference proportion available? y
Enter reference proportion .698
Proportion = 0.5, lower 95% limit = 0.306, upper limit = 0.694
Mid-P lower 95% limit = 0.32, upper limit = 0.68.
P = 0.044, LR = 1/8.
Mid-P P = 0.03, LR = 1/10.
```

The following formula may also be used: $Z=2 \cdot (\sqrt{(O_1/E_1)}-\sqrt{(O_2/E_2)})/\sqrt{(1/E_1+1/E_2)}$.

```
z<-2*((14/38.12)^.5-(14/16.5)^.5)/(1/38.12+1/16.5)^.5
z
#[1] -2.138636
2*pnorm(z)
#[1] 0.03246517
#
```

4.7.4   Direct standardisation

Direct standardisation requires knowledge of suitable standardising weights for each stratum. For example, it is known that, for a large group of hospitals, the proportions in stratum 1 to 6 respectively were 0.32170857, 0.11022284, 0.0032055, 0.416444599, 0.143050245 and 0.005368246. (The weights should sum to one.)

Some hospitals may treat more patients in one of the higher risk groups than others and this will bias comparisons. However, this problem can be overcome if the data for each hospital are weighted using the same set of standardising weights.

The directly standardised rate is $R=\sum W_i(X_i/N_i)$, where the W_i are the weights for the strata and X_i and N_i are the numerator and denominator for stratum i. For the Hospital 1 data, the value of R with these data is $R=0.32170857\times2/1420+0.11022284\times3/575+0.0032055\times1/21+0.416444599\times5/1850+0.143050245\times3/905+0.005368246\times0/64=0.002780555$ and for Hospital 2, $R=0.32170857\times5/708+0.11022284\times2/206+0.0032055\times0/6+0.416444599\times4/1023+0.143050245\times3/334+0.005368246\times0/10=0.006255287$.

A suitable confidence interval estimate can be obtained for each institution using Newcombe's square-and-add method. The formula for Newcombe's method is described for stratified proportion data in Chapter 1. For Hospital 1 (Group1) the rate was .00278 and its mid-P confidence interval was 0.00179 to 0.00502. For the Hospital 2 (Group2) data, the rate was 0.00626 with the mid-p 95% confidence interval from 0.00402 to 0.01164.

```
x1<-Group1[c(1,3,5,7,9,11)]
n1<-Group1[c(2,4,6,8,10,12)]
w<-c(0.32170857,0.11022284,0.0032055,0.416444599,0.143050245,0.005368246)
stratifiedratesn(data.frame(x1,n1,w))
#
x11<-Group2[c(1,3,5,7,9,11)]
n11<-Group2[c(2,4,6,8,10,12)]
stratifiedratesn(data.frame(x11,n11,w))
```

```
Group 1
Weighted average = 0.00278.
Lower 95% limit = 0.00179, upper limit = 0.00502.
Group 2
Weighted average = 0.00626.
Lower 95% limit = 0.00402, upper limit = 0.01164.
```

We can compare two sets of directly standardised rates using the Newcombe-Zou-Donner procedures provided the weights and number of strata for the two samples are the same. Although this does not provide a P-value the Altman and Bland method can be used to obtain an approximate P-value if samples are sufficiently large for the difference or the log(ratio) confidence intervals to be symmetric. An alternative is to use the Mantel-Haenszel method but it is a large sample approach that employs weights that may not be optimal with yearly data, the most recent of which may be required to have the largest weight. The function stratified2ratesn() performs this analysis. First, we employ the Caesarean section SSI data.

```
x1<-Group1[c(1,3,5,7,9,11)]
n1<-Group1[c(2,4,6,8,10,12)]
x2<-Group2[c(1,3,5,7,9,11)]
n2<-Group2[c(2,4,6,8,10,12)]
w<-c(0.32170857,0.11022284,0.0032055,0.416444599,0.143050245,0.005368246)
stratified2ratesn(data.frame(x1,n1,x2,n2,w))
```

```
Newcombe's method using mid-P Poisson 95% confidence limits
Weighted average in first group 0.002780555
First group confidence limits 0.001790455 to 0.005024027
```

```
Weighted average in second group 0.006255287
Second group confidence limits 0.004015604 to 0.01164421

Weighted difference -0.003474732
Difference confidence limits -0.00895386 to -0.0003046615
Ratio 0.4445127
Ratio confidence limits 0.207573 to 0.9309332
Approximate Z-score 2.117835
Approximate P-value 0.03389995
```

We now use bacteraemia data from two hospitals over six years to further illustrate the analysis.

```
#using stratified2ratesn() & two hospitals 6 years bacteraemia data
#data are not adjusted for differing services the hospitals provided
#used only to demonstrate analysis
bact1 <- c(16,26,24,35,14,21)
denom1 <- c(77212,97257,104877,108771,117737,122414)
bact2 <- c(11,18,23,15,16,13)
denom2 <- c(118992,135263,124805,127658,123388,125441)
w<-1:6
twohosps<-data.frame(bact1,denom1,bact2,denom2,w)

stratified2ratesn(twohosps) #uses weights 1 to 6
```

```
Newcombe's method using mid-P Poisson 95% confidence limits
Weighted average in first group 0.0002066359
First group confidence limits 0.0001750354 to 0.0002496137
Weighted average in second group 0.000126268
Second group confidence limits 0.000103192 to 0.0001598039

Weighted difference 8.036791e-05
Difference confidence limits 3.42892e-05 to 0.000129149
Ratio 1.636487
Ratio confidence limits 1.226801 to 2.157647
Approximate Z-score 3.419724
Approximate P-value 0.0006642443
```

It is important to determine whether the data within the strata are homogeneous as the presence of substantial heterogeneity would suggest that, while within years comparisons might be justified, a stratified analysis may not. There appears to be some heterogeneity among the strata.

```
R<-0 # Rate ratios
for (i in 1:6){R[i]<-
twohosps[i,1]*twohosps[i,4]/(twohosps[i,2]*twohosps[i,3])}
R
#[1] 2.2416111 2.0089031 1.2417528 2.7384934 0.9169972 1.6553291
P<-0 # P-values for comparing the two groups
for (i in 1:6){P[i]<-
poisson.exact(c(twohosps[i,1],twohosps[i,3]),
c(twohosps[i,2],twohosps[i,4]))$p.value}
P
#[1] 0.057511580 0.031292678 0.549090002 0.001040365 0.958031366 0.202946938
```

```
Z<-0 # Z-scores
for (i in 1:6){if (R[i]<1){Z[i]<-qnorm(P[i]/2)}else{Z[i]<--qnorm(P[i]/2)}}
Z
#[1]  1.89940246  2.15333095  0.59912429  3.27937708 -0.05262416  1.2732004
TwoHosps<-data.frame(twohosps[,-5],R,P,Z)
names(TwoHosps)<-c("Outc1","Denom1","Outc2","Denom2","RR","P","Z")
TwoHosps
```

	Outc1	Denom1	Outc2	Denom2	RR	P	Z
2001	16	77212	11	118992	2.2416111	0.057511580	1.89940246
2002	26	97257	18	135263	2.0089031	0.031292678	2.15333095
2003	24	104877	23	124805	1.2417528	0.549090002	0.59912429
2004	35	108771	15	127658	2.7384934	0.001040365	3.27937708
2005	14	117737	16	123388	0.9169972	0.958031366	−0.05262416
2006	21	122414	13	125441	1.6553291	0.202946938	1.27320040

4.8   Mantel-Haenszel, homogeneity and trend tests

4.8.1   Fixed effects analysis, stratification by years

A Mantel-Haenszel analysis described by Rosner was performed on the bacteraemia data using epi.2by2() in the epiR library. The rate ratio was 1.71 ($\chi^2_1=16.35$). The Z-score was $\sqrt{16.35}=4.04$ with a P-value of 0.00005. The confidence interval was 1.32 to 2.22. Homogeneity χ^2_5 is not reported by epi.2by2() but an approximate value can be calculated from the output of epi.2by2() as shown below. Homogeneity χ^2_5 was 7.19, P=0.21. In addition, the conventional large sample method using the logarithm of the rate ratio and inverse variance weights is included and the results are in fairly close agreement. The Mantel-Haenszel analysis yields similar results to the Newcombe analysis although the methods employ different weights.

```
# Mantel-Haenszel analysis using epiR
library(epiR)
dat <- data.frame(strata = rep(c(as.character(1:6)), each = 2),
exp = rep(c("+","-"), times = 6), dis = rep(c("+","-"), times = 6))
dat$exp <- factor(dat$exp, levels = c("+", "-"))
dat$dis <- factor(dat$dis, levels = c("+", "-"))
dat <- table(dat$exp, dat$dis, dat$strata,dnn =
c("Exposure", "Disease", "Strata"))
dat[1,1,] <- c(16,26,24,35,14,21)
dat[1,2,] <- c(77212,97257,104877,108771,117737,122414)
dat[2,1,] <- c(11,18,23,15,16,13)
dat[2,2,] <- c(118992,135263,124805,127658,123388,125441)
d<-epi.2by2(dat,method="cohort.time",conf.level=0.95,verbose=T)
d$IRR.strata[,1] # Stratum Rate Ratios
#[1] 2.2416111 2.0089031 1.2417528 2.7384934 0.9169972 1.6553291

M<-log(d$IRR.strata[,1])
d$IRR.mh # Summary Rate Ratio
#
#       est         se    lower    upper
#1 1.714257 0.1328408 1.321301 2.224079
#
```

```
M0<-log(d$IRR.mh[,1])
d$chisq.mh #Summary Rate Ratio test
#  test.statistic df      p.value
#1       16.32238  1 5.342913e-05

#Homogeneity test
V<-1/twohosps[,1]+1/twohosps[,3] #approximate variance of log(RR)
w<-1/V
H<-sum(w*(M-M0)^2)
DF<-length(M)-1
P0<-1-pchisq(H,DF)
H #Homogeneity χ²
#[1] 7.194043
P0 #P-value
#[1] 0.2066044

#Stratified Rate Ratio with inverse variance weights
x1<-twohosps[,1];x2<-twohosps[,3];n1<-twohosps[,2];n2<-twohosps[,4]
x1[x1==0]<-0.5;x2[x2==0]<-0.5
RR<-x1*n2/(x2*n1)
LRR<-log(RR)
VLRR<-1/x1+1/x2
VLRR0<-1/sum(1/VLRR)
LRR0<-sum((1/VLRR)*LRR)/sum(1/VLRR)
RR0<-exp(sum((1/VLRR)*LRR)/sum(1/VLRR))
#Rate Ratio and CI
RRU<-exp(LRR0+1.96*VLRR0^.5)
RRL<-exp(LRR0-1.96*VLRR0^.5)
RR0 #Rate Ratio
#[1] 1.702261
RRL #lower CI
#[1] 1.306589
RRU #upper CI
#[1] 2.217754
#
#Rate Ratio significance test
z<-abs(LRR0/VLRR0^.5)
p0<-2*(1-pnorm(z))
z #Z-score
#[1] 3.941357 (χ²=15.5236)
p0 #P-value
#[1] 8.102203e-05

#Homogeneity test
W<-1/VLRR
ch<-sum(W*(LRR0-LRR)^2)
I<-length(x1)
p<-1-pchisq(ch,(I-1))
ch
#[1] 7.191336 (Homogeneity χ² on 5 DF)
p #P-value
#[1] 0.2067949
#
#Trend test
XX<-1:length(x1)
A<-sum(W*XX*LRR);B<-sum(W*LRR);D<-sum(XX*W);E<-sum(W);F0<-sum(W*XX^2)
Lxy<-A-B*D/E
```

```
Lxx<-F0-D^2/E
ch.sq<-Lxy^2/Lxx
P<-1-pchisq(ch.sq,1)
ch.sq #Trend test χ² on 1 DF
#[1] 0.7687804
P #P-value
#[1] 0.3805946
```

With a nonsignificant homogeneity test in spite of some evidence of heterogeneity, a Poisson regression analysis may be useful. We see that there is some overdispersion present and the stratification agent is probably necessary (anova P-value=.053). When the overdispersion is controlled using quasipoisson, the P-value is much larger especially with weighting. We have emphasised the difficulties involved with making comparisons of this nature between hospitals and we have questioned its utility. When overdispersion is present, the Newcombe analysis could easily mislead. Overdispersion is common with QI and IM count and rate data. It can be seen that, apart from potential bias in the data and the questionable utility of making such comparisons, the statistical analysis even with relatively small data sets can be challenging.

```
#using Poisson regression
Hospital1<-data.frame(bact1,denom1)
names(Hospital1)<-c("Saureus","OBD")
Hospital2<-data.frame(bact2,denom2)
names(Hospital2)<-c("Saureus","OBD")
gl<-rep(1,6)
ga<-data.frame(gl,Hospital2)
gl<-rep(2,6)
gb<-data.frame(gl,Hospital1)
g12<-rbind(ga,gb)
stratum<-c(rep(1:6),rep(1:6))
g12<-data.frame(g12,stratum)
names(g12)<-c("Hosp","Saureus","OBD","Stratum")

g<-glm(Saureus~Hosp+as.factor(Stratum),family=quasipoisson,offset=log(OBD),
data=g12)
summary(g) # abbreviated
```

	Estimate Std.	Error	t value	Pr(>|t|)	
(Intercept)	−9.68240	0.34008	−28.471	1e-06	***
Hosp	0.54202	0.16198	3.346	0.0204	*
as.factor(Stratum)2	0.30475	0.29645	1.028	0.3511	
as.factor(Stratum)3	0.36201	0.29298	1.236	0.2715	
as.factor(Stratum)4	0.39307	0.28978	1.356	0.2330	
as.factor(Stratum)5	−0.15257	0.32201	−0.474	0.6556	
as.factor(Stratum)6	−0.05791	0.31297	−0.185	0.8605	

```
   (Dispersion parameter for quasipoisson family taken to be 1.470192)
     Null deviance: 34.5112 on 11 degrees of freedom
Residual deviance:  7.3181 on  5 degrees of freedom
```

```
g1<-glm(Saureus~Hosp,family=quasipoisson,offset=log(OBD),data=g12)

anova(g1,g)
```

```
Model 1: Saureus ~ Hosp
Model 2: Saureus ~ Hosp + as.factor(Stratum)
  Resid. Df Resid. Dev Df Deviance
1       10    18.2300
2        5     7.3181  5   10.912
1-pchisq(10.912,5)=0.05315295
```

```
w<-c(1:6,1:6) # Poisson regression with weights
g2<-glm(Saureus~Hosp+as.factor(Stratum),family=quasipoisson,offset=log(OBD),
data=g12,weight=w)
summary(g2)
```

```
                     Estimate Std.    Error   t value   Pr(>|t|)
(Intercept)          -9.60349  0.52719  -18.216  9.16e-06  ***
Hosp                  0.49014  0.17067    2.872   0.0349   *
as.factor(Stratum)2   0.30608  0.52529    0.583   0.5854
as.factor(Stratum)3   0.36532  0.50167    0.728   0.4992
as.factor(Stratum)4   0.39655  0.48965    0.810   0.4548
as.factor(Stratum)5  -0.14767  0.49939   -0.296   0.7793
as.factor(Stratum)6  -0.05275  0.48925   -0.108   0.9183
  (Dispersion parameter for quasipoisson family taken to be 5.700443)
     Null deviance: 116.804 on 11 degrees of freedom
Residual deviance:  28.565 on  5 degrees of freedom
```

4.8.2   Random effects analysis, stratification by hospitals

A major problem when analysing data that are stratified is dealing with excessive variability and stratum by group interaction. Spiegelhalter[B,C,D] has described two approaches for dealing with overdispersed rate data from groups of hospitals that are described in Chapters 2 and 5. One of the methods involves the random effects analysis using an approximation proposed by derSimonian and Laird. The file staphbact.csv contains *Staphylococcus aureus* data from a group of hospitals between 2001 and 2006. We select 10 of the hospitals that are exchangeable and therefore suitable for a random effects analysis. The issue of interest is whether bscteraemia rates fell in the later data (2005 and 2006). We see that there is no statistical evidence of a difference but there is considerable heterogeneity and the random effects variance is relatively large. We discuss the effect of overdispersion on count and rate data in section 4.9 of this chapter and illustrate approaches to the analysis of those data.

```
g.d() # staphbact.csv

obd<-read.table("clipboard",T) # obd.csv

# using inverse variance weights and log rate ratio
library(chron)
d<-datain[,2]
d<-chron(as.character(d),format="dd-mmm-yy",out.format="dd-mmm-yyyy")
staphbefore<-datain[d<"01-Jan-2005",]
staphafter<-datain[d>"31-Dec-2004",]
count1<-table(staphbefore[,1])
```

```
count2<-table(staphafter[,1])

d<-chron(as.character(obd[,2]),format="d-mmm-yy",out.format="dd-mmm-yyyy")
obdbefore<-obd[d<"01-Jan-2005",]
obdafter<-obd[d>"31-Dec-2004",]
denom1<-tapply(obdbefore[,3],obdbefore[,1],sum)
denom2<-tapply(obdafter[,3],obdafter[,1],sum)

staphbef<-
data.frame(row.names(count1),as.numeric(count1),as.numeric(denom1))
names(staphbef)<-c("Hosp","Bact","OBD")
staphaft<-
data.frame(row.names(count2),as.numeric(count2),as.numeric(denom2))
names(staphaft)<-c("Hosp","Bact","OBD")

o<-order(staphaft[,2],decreasing=T)
staphaft<-staphaft[o,]
staphbef<-staphbef[o,]
safter<-staphaft[1:10,]
sbefore<-staphbef[1:10,]

Hospbacts<-data.frame(safter,sbefore[,-1])
names(Hospbacts)<-c("Hosp","BactBefore","OBDBefore","BactAfter","OBDAfter")

#Stratified Rate Ratio with inverse variance weights
x1<-Hospbacts[,2];x2<-Hospbacts[,4];n1<-Hospbacts[,3];n2<-Hospbacts[,5]
x1[x1==0]<-0.5;x2[x2==0]<-0.5
RR<-x1*n2/(x2*n1)
LRR<-log(RR)
VLRR<--1/x1+1/x2
VLRR0<-1/sum(1/VLRR)
LRR0<-sum((1/VLRR)*LRR)/sum(1/VLRR)
RR0<-exp(sum((1/VLRR)*LRR)/sum(1/VLRR))
#Rate Ratio and CI
RRU<-exp(LRR0+1.96*VLRR0^.5)
RRL<-exp(LRR0-1.96*VLRR0^.5)
RR0 #Rate Ratio
#[1] 0.9703705
RRL #lower CI
#[1] 0.8487964
RRU #upper CI
#[1] 1.109358

#Rate Ratio significance test
z<-abs(LRR0/VLRR0^.5)
p0<-2*(1-pnorm(z))
z #Z-score
#[1] 0.4404022
p0 #P-value
#[[1] 0.6596458

#Homogeneity test
W<-1/VLRR
ch<-sum(W*(LRR0-LRR)^2)
I<-length(x1)
```

```
p<-1-pchisq(ch,(I-1))
ch
#[1] [1] 21.4501 (Homogeneity χ2 on 9 DF)
p #P-value
#[1] 0.0107951

# derSimonian-Laird random effects
W1<-sum(W)-(sum(W^2)/sum(W))
Q<-max(0,ch-I+1)
Q/W1 # random effects variance
#[1] 0.06748909
qw<-Q/W1
rvlor<-VLRR+qw
w2<-1/rvlor
rlor<-sum(w2*LRR)/sum(w2)
vrvlor<-1/sum(w2)
L<-exp(rlor-1.96*vrvlor^.5)
U<-exp(rlor+1.96*vrvlor^.5)
Z<-abs(rlor/vrvlor^.5)
P<-exp(-0.717*Z-0.416*Z^2)
cat("Adjusted
RR=",round(exp(rlor),2),"\nL95=",round(L,2),"\nU95=",round(U,2),
"\nZ-score=",round(Z,2),"\nP-value=",round(P,5),"\n",sep="")
```

```
Adjusted RR=0.95
L95=0.76
U95=1.18
Z-score=0.44
P-value=0.6711
```

As a check, we repeat the analysis using epi.2by2 from the epiR library. There is a warning message but the Mantel-Haenszel result appears to be reported correctly. The result is very similar to the above: no difference but considerable heterogeneity and a large random effects variance. The homogeneity test and derSimonian-Laird random effects analysis are reported for odds ratios but not rate ratios so the required approximate values have been extracted from the output of epi.2by2.

```
# Mantel-Haenszel analysis using epiR
Hospbacts<-read.table("clipboard",T) # hospbacts.csv

library(epiR)
dat <- data.frame(strata = rep(c(1:10), each = 2),exp = rep(c("+","-"),
times = 10),dis = rep(c("+","-"), times = 10))
dat$exp <- factor(dat$exp, levels = c("+", "-"))
dat$dis <- factor(dat$dis, levels = c("+", "-"))
dat <- table(dat$exp, dat$dis, dat$strata,dnn = c("Exposure", "Outcome",
"Strata"))
dat[1,1,] <- Hospbacts[,2]
dat[1,2,] <- Hospbacts[,3]
dat[2,1,] <- Hospbacts[,4]
dat[2,2,] <- Hospbacts[,5]
d<-epi.2by2(dat,method="cohort.time",conf.level=0.95,verbose=T,units=1)
# note warnings
Z<-as.numeric((d$chisq.strata[1])^.5)
```

```
RR<-d$IRR.strata[[1]]
V<-(log(RR)/Z)^2
RR0<-d$IRR.mh[[1]]
RR0 # MH RR
#[1] 0.9576858
d$chisq.mh # MH test
#  test.statistic df   p.value
#1     0.3687883  1 0.5436655


w<-1/V
I<-length(w)
H<-sum(w*(log(RR)-log(RR0))^2)
H
#
#[1] 21.86509  homogeneity test
1-pchisq(H,I-1)
#
#[1] 0.009316513


W<-sum(w)-(sum(w^2)/sum(w))
Q<-max(0,H-I+1)
qw<-Q/W # random effects variance
qw
#[1] 0.06912746


rvlor<-V+qw
w1<-1/rvlor
rlor<-sum(w1*log(RR))/sum(w1)
vrvlor<-1/sum(w1)
L<-exp(rlor-1.96*vrvlor^.5)
U<-exp(rlor+1.96*vrvlor^.5)
Z<-abs(rlor/vrvlor^.5)
P<-exp(-0.717*Z-0.416*Z^2)
cat("Adjusted
RR=",round(exp(rlor),2),"\nL95=",round(L,2),"\nU95=",round(U,2),
"\nZ-score=",round(Z,2),"\nP-value=",round(P,5),"\n",sep="")
```

```
Adjusted RR=0.95
L95=0.76
U95=1.18
Z-score=0.45
P-value=0.66816
```

4.9   Illustration of dealing with overdispersed rates

Spiegelhalter[D] has described how adding the random effects variance to the variance for each of the members of a group of overdispersed hospital rates can be used in funnel plots to adjust control limits for the excessive variability. This is an additive correction. He also describes a multiplicative correction using the square root of the mean of the squared Z-scores for each hospital's rate and Laney (Mohammed and Laney[A]) suggests adjusting control limits with the standard deviation of the Z-scores. We employ Laney's correction in Chapters 5 and 6. We illustrate the methods using the Bactafter data in Hospbacts. The methods are described in section 1.10 of Chapter 1. See also the Appendix to Professor Spiegelhalter's paper.

```
Hospbacts<-read.table("clipboard",T)

AllS<-Hospbacts[,c(1,4,5)]
o<-order(AllS[,1])
AllS<-AllS[o,]
l<-length(AllS[,1])
M<-sum(AllS[,2])/sum(AllS[,3]) # mean rate
O<-AllS[,2]
N<-AllS[,3]
R<-O/N # rate
E<-M*N # expected count
V0<-M/N # null variance
V<-R/N # non-null variance
w<-1/V
Z<-(R-M)/V0^.5 # Z-score
CH<-sum(w*(R-M)^2) # homogeneity chi-squared
W<-sum(w)-sum(w^2)/sum(w)
Q<-(CH-(1-1))/W # derSimonian-Laird variance
ZDSL<-(R-M)/(V0+Q)^.5 # Spiegelhalter's additive correction
Hosp<-AllS[,1]
data.frame(Hosp,O,N,R,E,Z,ZDSL)
```

	Hosp	O	N	R	E	Z	ZDSL
1	A	43	319325	1.347e-04	45.57	−0.3806	−0.1626
2	B	66	624624	1.057e-04	89.14	−2.4507	−0.7841
3	D	46	273292	1.683e-04	39.00	1.1208	0.5097
4	E	23	348797	6.594e-05	49.78	−3.7951	−1.5630
5	F	131	850918	1.540e-04	121.43	0.8684	0.2414
6	G	67	506718	1.322e-04	72.31	−0.6246	−0.2193
7	H	19	178551	1.064e-04	25.48	−1.2838	−0.6856
8	I	74	462423	1.600e-04	65.99	0.9860	0.3603
9	J	31	258701	1.198e-04	36.92	−0.9740	−0.4526
10	K	101	388117	2.602e-04	55.39	6.1290	2.4138

```
sd(Z) # Laney's correction

#[1] 2.668

(mean(Z^2))^.5 # Spiegelhalter's multiplicative correction

#[1] 2.532

ZL<-Z/sd(Z)
ZS<-Z/(mean(Z^2))^.5
data.frame(Hosp,Z,ZDSL,ZS,ZL)
```

	Hosp	Z	ZDSL	ZS	ZL
1	A	-0.3806	-0.1626	-0.1504	-0.1427
2	B	-2.4507	-0.7841	-0.9680	-0.9185
3	D	1.1208	0.5097	0.4427	0.4201
4	E	-3.7951	-1.5630	-1.4991	-1.4224
5	F	0.8684	0.2414	0.3430	0.3255
6	G	-0.6246	-0.2193	-0.2467	-0.2341
7	H	-1.2838	-0.6856	-0.5071	-0.4811
8	I	0.9860	0.3603	0.3895	0.3695
9	J	-0.9740	-0.4526	-0.3847	-0.3650
10	K	6.1290	2.4138	2.4210	2.2971

The hglm library can be used to obtain the random effects values. This uses Poisson regression and empirical Bayes methods to obtain these values that are likely to be superior to estimates based on the derSimonian-Laird procedure. The latter clearly overcorrects as do the Laney and Spiegelhalter multiplicative procedures. To deal with this, Spiegelhalter describes the use of winsorising. As we have only 10 hospitals, the demonstration of winsorising is somewhat artificial, however the method is illustrated with these data. We winsorise the largest and smallest Z-scores, equivalent to 20% winsorising.

```
library(hglm) # random effects analysis
H<-1:1
h<-
hglm(fixed=AllS$Bact~1,random=~1|H,offset=log(AllS$OBD),
family=poisson(link=log),fix.disp=1)
ZH<-data.frame(h$ranef/h$SeRe)
names(ZH)<-"ZH"
row.names(ZH)<-AllS[,1]
data.frame(ZH)
```

	ZH
A	-0.03749
B	-1.45120
D	1.07874
E	-2.85895
F	0.86895
G	-0.14969
H	-0.83028
I	0.97985
J	-0.53620
K	4.18118

```
# 20% winsorising
Z1<-Z
Z1[4]<-Z1[2]
Z1[10]<-Z1[3]
sd(Z1) # Laney's correction

#[1] 1.403 # sd(Z)=2.668

Z1L<-Z/sd(Z1) # Z-score with Laney's correction
```

```
data.frame(ZH,Z1L)
```

```
            ZH       Z1L
A     -0.03749   -0.2712
B     -1.45120   -1.7462
D      1.07874    0.7986
E     -2.85895   -2.7041
F      0.86895    0.6187
G     -0.14969   -0.4451
H     -0.83028   -0.9147
I      0.97985    0.7025
J     -0.53620   -0.6940
K      4.18118    4.3671
```

The winsorised Z-scores using Laney's correction now agree fairly well with the empirical Bayes estimates. Finally, the effect on control limits can be seen.

```
M+3*V0^.5 # upper 3 SD limits, no correction

#[1] 0.0002061 0.0001881 0.0002113 0.0002034 0.0001816 0.0001931 0.0002275
#[8] 0.0001954 0.0002132 0.0002002

M+3*sd(Z)*V0^.5 # Laney's correction

#[1] 0.0003119 0.0002637 0.0003256 0.0003046 0.0002464 0.0002770 0.0003690
#[8] 0.0002833 0.0003307 0.0002962

M+3*sd(Z1)*V0^.5 # Laney's correction with winsorising

#[1] 0.0002317 0.0002063 0.0002389 0.0002279 0.0001972 0.0002134 0.0002617
#[8] 0.0002167 0.0002416 0.0002234
```

4.10   The importance of count data variation

The formulas described earlier in this chapter are suitable for performing significance tests and calculating confidence intervals for approximately Poisson distributed count data. The variance of a series of counts must be approximately equal to their mean for these methods to be appropriate, and for this to occur, individual observations must be independent. Device related infections and medication errors usually occur independently provided they do not involve repeated episodes in the same patients. However, in many cases variation is increased and this is frequently referred to as overdispersion.

With some IM and QI data, independence cannot be assumed. For example, the number of readmissions, pathology tests or hospital acquired infections may be counted rather than the number of patients being readmitted, or having pathology tests or infections. It will usually be correct to count the number of patients, not events.

Nevertheless, it is sometimes necessary to count the number of events, and when this happens, methods are needed that take into account the clustering and increased variability that occurs due to some patients having repeated admissions, tests or infections. The statistical methods then become more complex and expert advice may need to be sought.

In addition, when a patient carrying a contagious organism such as MRSA is admitted to a ward, potential spread from this patient will ensure that further colonisations or infections in the ward do not occur independently. Also, many adverse outcomes such as patient falls, readmissions, pressure ulcers, needlestick injuries and bacteraemias may exhibit overdispersion because some staff and patients are more susceptible than others and they may not be distributed randomly about the hospital.

Thus some hospital areas have much higher rates than others for some adverse outcomes. When a number of different processes produce Poisson distributed count data with different mean rates and they are considered together, the resulting amalgamated data may have greater variation than would be expected for a Poisson process. For example, patients in an ICU may be more exposed to and more susceptible to colonisation by an MRO than patients in general wards.

When this mixing occurs, one of two different processes may arise. First, when the mixing is random, the result is a linear function and it is also approximately Poisson distributed. Second, if mixing is nonrandom, the result is a weighted sum of Poissons and this is not Poisson distributed.

As a result of the above breakdowns in independence, variation will often be increased and employing Poisson distribution methods will then result in low P-values and narrow confidence limits that are incorrect.

Frequently the negative binomial distribution will describe these data better than the Poisson distribution. The negative binomial distribution is also a compound Poisson distribution with the mean count having a gamma distribution. This property makes it valuable for modelling count data that have large variability. Alternatives that we have discussed include the corrections described by Spiegelhalter[B,C,D] and Laney (Mohammed[A] and Laney).

Unfortunately, there is as yet little guidance for dealing with these data in the hospital epidemiology literature. We illustrate the problem with several trivial contrived examples. It is hoped that this discussion will stimulate interest in this important problem among hospital epidemiologists, and that statisticians will begin to describe reliable simple approximate methods for analysing these and similar data. A particular problem occurs when there are a series of counts (e.g. monthly) with varying denominators (e.g. occupied bed-days). A suitable program that finds the relevant parameters by negative binomial maximum likelihood when there are varying denominators is, so far as we are aware, currently unavailable in R. Although a simple approximation appears to be satisfactory for inclusion in, for example, control charts, the availability of an accurate method that is straightforward to use would be desirable.

Suppose that a department has $F=4$ needlestick injuries in one month and its staff wish to calculate a confidence interval for this count. Using the Poisson methods already described, the 95% confidence interval is calculated to be 1.09 to 10.24. However, suppose it is known that the mean monthly count for needlestick injuries is $M=6$ and its variance is $V=12$ and not approximately 6 as would be expected for Poisson distributed data.

The negative binomial distribution has two parameters that we label S and P. S represents a fixed number of successes in a series of Bernoulli trials and P the probability of success in each trial. We label the observed value F for failures. Unlike the binomial distribution where S is a variable and $S+F=N$ is fixed, the negative binomial variable is F and S is fixed.

When data follow a negative binomial distribution, we can calculate approximately $S=M^2/(V-M)$ and $P=M/V$. For the above data, $S=6^2/(12-6)=6$, and $F=4$. We can now use the beta distribution to obtain 95% confidence limits for F. Let $A=qbeta(0.025,S,F+1)$ and $B=qbeta(0.975,S,F)$. Then the upper 95% confidence interval for F is $U=(S-A\times S)/A$

and the lower limit is L=(S-B×S)/B. The 95% confidence limits are 0.95 to 16.87. These are much wider than the corresponding Poisson limits.

It is possible to test whether an observed monthly count differs from a mean value. For example, suppose that the count for the current month is 12. Does this differ significantly from 6? Using the conventional count data method that employs the Poisson distribution, the two-tailed p-value is 0.04 so that a conventional test would suggest that a difference probably exists.

When the negative binomial distribution is employed, the P-value is 0.14. When M=6 and V=12, P=0.5. Then pval=2×(1-pbeta(P,S,F)) when F is greater than M, and, for F less than M, pval=2×pbeta(P,S,F+1). The Camp-Poulson approximation (Bartko) is a useful alternative. Q=1-P. If F>M, F=F-1, A=(-(9×S-1)×(S×Q/(P×(F+1)))^(1/3))/ S+(9×F+8)/(F+1). B=(S×Q/(P×(F+1)))^(2/3)/S+1/(F+1). Z-score=A/(3×√B). P-value= 2×(1-pnorm(Z-score)).

Suppose now that it is of interest to determine whether the counts of 4 and 12 differ. In addition, it would be desirable to be able to calculate a confidence interval for this difference. The Poisson derived interval is 0.26 to 16.73, different from zero so significant at the conventional 95% level. An interval that takes the extra variability into account can be calculated by Newcombe's method.

The difference is 8 and its 95% confidence interval is -6.79 to 35.14. Its ratio is 3 (95% interval 0.54 to 19.24). Thus it can be seen that the Poisson methods underestimate P-values and produce confidence intervals that are too narrow when the variances of count data exceed their mean values.

```
# demonstration of overdispersion effect
F0<-4;V<-12;M<-6
P<-M/V
S<-M^2/(V-M)
A<-qbeta(0.025,S,F0+1)
B<-qbeta(0.975,S,F0)
U<-(S-A*S)/A
U
#[1] 16.86776
L<-(S-B*S)/B
L
#[1] 0.9524564
#
F0<-12
A<-qbeta(0.025,S,F0+1)
B<-qbeta(0.975,S,F0)
U<-(S-A*S)/A
U
#[1] 38.96827
L<-(S-B*S)/B
L
#[1] 4.722275
#
pval<-2*(1-pbeta(P,S,F0)) # difference of 12 from mean of 6
pval
#[1] 0.1434631

#Camp-Poulson accurate F-distribution approximation
```

```
Q<-1-P
if (F0>M){F1=F0-1}else{F1<-F0}
A<-(-(9*S-1)*(S*Q/(P*(F1+1)))^(1/3))/S+(9*F1+8)/(F1+1)
B<-(S*Q/(P*(F1+1)))^(2/3)/S+1/(F1+1)
Z<-A/(3*B^.5)
Z
#[1] 1.463743
2*(1-pnorm(1.46))
#[1] 0.1442901


# difference calculations
d2<-4
d1<-12
l2<-.95
l1<-4.72
u2<-16.87
u1<-38.97
# Newcombe's method
dl<-(d1-d2)-((d1-l1)^2+(u2-d2)^2)^.5
du<-(d1-d2)+((d2-l2)^2+(u1-d1)^2)^.5
d1-d2 #difference
#[1] 8
dl #lower limit
#[1] -6.786321
du #upper limit
#[1] 35.14191

# ratio
r<-d1/d2
#
r
#[1] 3

#Zhou and Donner extension of Newcombe's method
rl<-exp((log(d1)-log(d2))-((log(d1)-log(l1))^2+(log(u2)-log(d2))^2)^.5)
ru<-exp((log(d1)-log(d2))+((log(d2)-log(l2))^2+(log(u1)-log(d1))^2)^.5)
rl #lower limit
#[1] 0.5397549
ru #Upper limit
#[1] 19.24259
#approximate P-value, Bland and Altman
SE<-abs((log(ru)-log(rl))/(2*1.96))
Z<-abs(log(r)/SE)
Z
#[1] 1.205048
p.value<-exp(-0.717*Z-0.416*Z^2)
p.value
#[1] 0.2303604
```

There is currently much misguided interest in comparing outcomes and some managers may be tempted to compare the work of two departments such as ICUs using surveillance data, for example by analysing weekly or monthly counts of MROs. Usually such comparisons would entail employing the common Poisson count data methods that may be incorrect, and may suggest that there is a difference when one may not exist.

Such departments may have markedly differing patient populations and risk adjustment may be difficult or impossible. Moreover the distributions for the two departments may differ so that the parameters S and P may not be the same for each of them. It may be difficult to obtain sufficient monthly or weekly data during periods marked only by endemic activity to obtain stable estimates of mean values and variances. In addition, the departments may be of differing sizes so that obtaining comparable denominators may be difficult. Methods have been described for dealing with negative binomial data having denominators of varying sizes (Scheaffer and Levenworth, Bissell) but, as described above, a suitable function in R to provide maximum likelihood values when denominators differ would be valuable. Moreover, it is often difficult to determine the correct denominators. The denominator employed is often occupied bed-days. There are two difficulties with this. First, more severely ill patients are usually more susceptible to developing an AE and their monthly bed-days may fluctuate less than overall monthly bed-days. This can sometimes be seen at the Christmas New Year break in Australian hospitals when considerable low-risk elective surgery may be deferred with overall occupied bed-days decreasing but road trauma and acute illness may increase so that occupied bed-days for more severely ill, and therefore more susceptible patients, are maintained. In addition, length of stay which influences occupied bed-days is also often a risk factor.

If comparisons of this nature must be made (and we are not in favour of them), it is much more likely that sensible results will be obtained if system and process surveillance is performed and the resulting data used for making comparisons. With increasing use of bundles and checklists, surveillance of compliance with these is important. For example, is hand washing performed with equal diligence by the staff of the two departments? Are there in place sensible guidelines for the use of antibiotics and are these guidelines implemented? Is there an effective program for the detection and isolation of patients carrying potentially dangerous MROs? Is cohorting by nursing staff practiced (e.g. are there permanent staff who are assigned to particular wards and, as far as possible, patients within those wards)? Are numbers of outlier patients kept to a minimum so that unnecessary patient/staff contact is minimised, especially by staff who may be less conscientious about hand hygiene and who see patients in a number of wards)? Is environmental cleaning, especially terminal cleaning of high-touch surfaces like light switches, door handles and bed rails, effective? Are current bundles and checklists for the management and prevention of hospital-acquired infections and other AEs up to date and are they being followed correctly? Is there an effective Early Warning and Rapid Response bundle in place? Are there sufficient beds and staff to permit patient isolation or cohorting? Is an effective M&M audit bundle in place?

To use negative binomial methods, it is necessary to have data that enable mean outcome rates and their variances to be calculated. For monthly counts it would seem desirable to have at least 20 available from a period known to be free of any epidemic activity. We must gain much more experience at understanding how variation occurs with count data AEs, especially colonisations and infections due to MROs. It is possible to see variances that are similar to mean values with new isolates of some MROs when isolation procedures, antibiotic use, terminal cleaning (additional cleaning of patient areas previously occupied by an MRO carrier) and hand washing and other hygiene measures are excellent and the MRO burden is low. However, if there is less than excellent IM, for example there may be insufficient numbers of isolation beds, poor hand hygiene or inadequate terminal cleaning, variability can increase even in the absence of an outbreak. This is a difficult area and much work is needed to improve understanding. Later in these notes we discuss briefly the potential role of complex system and network analysis for this purpose. Since complex systems exhibit self-organisation and emergent behaviour, small and seemingly minor problems with a number of interacting agents may have an unexpectedly large effect.

Count data hospital-acquired infections are often better analysed in control charts that display monthly occurrence rates. Good departments examine their systems and processes regularly and constantly strive to improve them, using for example the Deming cycle and QI tools described in Chapter 8. When this is done, the sequential analysis of outcome data using control charts that, when appropriate, employ approximate negative binomial control limits, provides reliable information for making decisions. An alternative is to employ a generalised additive model (GAM) chart that we describe in detail in Chapters 3, 6 and 7.

Statistical methods are frequently employed to detect substandard performance, for example using league tables and star ratings. However, to prevent substandard performance it is necessary for management to have a firm understanding of systems and evidence, and the courage, resources and authority to act when there is an environment that is known to be associated with unsatisfactory outcomes (Lilford and colleagues, Morton[C] and colleagues). Future development of the complex system methods of agent-based modelling and pattern (system) dynamics (www.science.org.au) will aid in understanding hospital systems. Data analysis, for example, using a control chart, is a valuable adjunct, especially for the detection of unexpected variation.

Consider the situation where one AE is expected. It takes at least four or five to occur in a similar time period for statistical significance to be attained. When AEs are uncommon this may take considerable time. Reliance on statistical analysis will thus result in unacceptable delay if it is possible, employing evidence and systems analysis, to determine that an environment exists in which excess AEs may be expected to occur. In addition, when an institution first analyses its systems and institutes evidence-based bundles and checklists, stable average values may not at first be available and it may be preferable to employ a simple run chart of GAM chart (AE numbers may increase initially because of improved reporting). Then, when stable baseline data make it possible to obtain reliable estimates of average values and variation, monitoring and analysis of relevant data using statistical methods such as control charts can be an invaluable adjunct to systems analysis, M&M audits and implementation of bundles and checklists based on evidence.

4.11   Complex systems, networks and variation

Hospitals have been described as complex dynamic systems (Plsek and Greenhalgh). It is also useful to think of large hospitals as networks. Variability in networks is often dominated by power law distributions. This can be seen in some length of stay and other data including the severity and numbers of medication errors. While we do not go into this problem in detail, there is an important practical implication – the probability of the occurrence of uncommon major events, often adverse in nature, can be greatly underestimated. Thus a norovirus outbreak may result in the need to close a ward unexpectedly or the advent of a previously unknown virus could wreak havoc with the functioning of a hospital system. How do we guard against an unanticipated future major event that may have an unknown cause? Syndromic surveillance programs, particularly in Accident and Emergency Departments, may provide early warning of a major problem. There are systems for dealing with epidemics, natural disasters, major traffic accidents or terrorist attacks. However, any specifically directed safety system may be of limited value in the event of an unanticipated threat of an unknown nature.

As suggested by Orrell, Network Science suggests that systems can be made more resilient by employing modularity, diversity, redundancy and capacity for controlled shutdown. The emphasis is particularly on diversity and redundancy that Network Science has learned from studying Nature. Hospital policy, on the other hand, has been dominated by efficiency and productivity. It is known that overcrowding, for example, can cause access block and increase AEs and it is probable that a significant quantity of the work of super-efficient hospitals involves dealing with AEs that have resulted from their super-efficiency. Complex systems can become increasingly efficient but at the same time they become less stable and more prone to failure. As Ehsani and colleagues have reported, AEs were found in one study to be responsible for over 18% of total inpatient hospital budgets and that it is probable that at least one third would have been potentially preventable. Further research in this area is needed. As Evans and colleagues describe, the development of epidemiologically sound and clinically relevant clinical-quality registries is needed to improve available evidence. We refer to complex systems and networks in succeeding chapters, especially Chapter 8.

5

Tables and charts for aggregated count data

In this chapter we describe count and rate data from multiple institutions and their presentation using, for example, funnel plots (Morton[A,D,E] and colleagues). The following topics are discussed.

```
1. Risk-adjustment,
2. Tabulations,
3. Confidence intervals and Z-scores,
4. Corrections for multiple testing,
5. Corrections for excessive variability (overdispersion),
6. Funnel plots,
7. Random-effects (shrinkage) analysis,
      The lmer() and hglm() libraries in R
      OpenBUGS gamma-Poisson random-effects analysis.
```

5.1 Introduction, data, limitations of aggregated count data analysis

Annual in-hospital healthcare-associated *Staphylococcus aureus* bacteraemia count data for a group of hospitals are in hasaureusbact.csv. The data in the original data table have been simplified by removing columns that are not relevant to the analysis that follows. There are six remaining columns: 1. Hospital code; 2. Infection date; 3. *Staphylococcus aureus* TRUE; 4. In-hospital 1; 5. Intravenous device-related; and 6. MRSA. It has been shown that monitoring bacteraemias due to *Staphylococcus aureus* provides a reliable means for monitoring bacteraemias in hospitals (Collignon and colleagues). Groups of bacteraemias to be monitored

Statistical Methods for Hospital Monitoring with R, First Edition. Anthony Morton, Kerrie Mengersen, Michael Whitby and George Playford.
© 2013 John Wiley & Sons, Ltd. Published 2013 by John Wiley & Sons, Ltd.

frequently include all in-hospital infections due to *Staphylococcus aureus* (including MRSA), all device-related in-hospital infections due to *Staphylococcus aureus* (including MRSA), all in-hospital bacteraemias due to MRSA, all in-hospital bacteraemias due to *Staphylococcus aureus* (including MRSA) occurring during the most recent year and all noninpatient healthcare-associated bacteraemias due to *Staphylococcus aureus* (including MRSA) such as those associated with periodic renal dialysis, haematology/oncology or outpatient intravenous nutrition. We illustrate the analysis using all in-hospital healthcare-acquired bacteraemias due to *Staphylococcus aureus*. In addition, other groups of interest include criterion 1 bacteraemias (i.e. those due to recognised pathogens as opposed to possible contaminants), and criterion 1 bacteraemias related to intravenous devices or urinary tract catheterisation. Although monitoring *Staphylococcus aureus* bacteraemias may be most important, it is as well to remember that, for example, *Escherichia coli* bacteraemia also occurs frequently.

Denominator and hospital type (level) data are also required and occupied bed-days and level data are in the files obd.csv and levels.csv. The former provides suitable denominators for the in-hospital data. Device-days denominators for device-related infections would have been preferable but were not available. There were three hospital levels: level 1 refers to tertiary referral centres; level 2 to larger general hospitals; and level 3 to smaller general hospitals. They are used to stratify the data, although as Tong and colleagues demonstrate, and we illustrate later in the chapter, better methods for stratification and risk adjustment that involve the services hospitals provide are becoming available. The data need to be aggregated as we illustrate in Table 5.1.

```
#uses the files hasaureusbact.csv, levels.csv & obd.csv
#important to check that hospital names and times correspond
g.d() #hasaureusbact, the first column is not a date column

bact<-datain
#
g.d() #levels, the first column is not a date column

level<-datain
#
g.d() #obd, the first column is not a date column

obd<-datain
#
AllInHospSaureusBact<-xtabs(bact[,3]~bact[,1])
OBD<-tapply(obd[,3],obd[,1],sum)
hasaurbact<-
data.frame(names(AllInHospSaureusBact),as.numeric(AllInHospSaureusBact),
level[,2],as.numeric(OBD))
names(hasaurbact)<-c("Hosp","AllInHospSaureusBact","Level","OBD")
o<-order(hasaurbact[,3])
hasaurbact<-hasaurbact[o,]
a<-0;a1<-0
x<-max(hasaurbact[,3])
for (i in 1:x){
a<-hasaurbact[hasaurbact[,3]==i,]
a<-a[,4]*sum(a[,2])/sum(a[,4])
a1<-c(a1,a)
}
```

```
Exp<-round(a1[-1],2)
staph<-data.frame(hasaurbact[,-3],Exp)
o<-order(staph[,1])
staph<-staph[o,]
staph # Table 5.1
```

In Chapter 2 section 2.3.3.1 we used the risk-adjusted rate when constructing a funnel plot. Unfortunately, this approach will not usually be feasible with count and rate data because of the bias in indirectly standardised rates when there are markedly differing denominators and expected counts, often accompanied by excessive variability and clustering (overdispersion). These may be due, for example, to differing hospital patient services on which data may have been unavailable for risk adjustment by regression modeling or stratification, or breakdown of independence within institutions due to transmission of hospital-acquired organisms (Morton[D] and colleagues).

Hospitals offer differing specialist services of differing size that have differing expected rates, for example, for bacteraemias. Stratification by hospital level is available with the *Staphylococcus aureus* bacteraemia data but some level 1 hospitals have oncology and haematology or other high risk departments of varying size (higher expected bacteraemia rates) and others have varying size maternity, plastic surgery or other low risk departments (lower expected bacteraemia rates). These differences make the calculation of expected rates based on hospital level of limited value although Tong and colleagues have risk-adjusted hospitals by stratifying them by the services they provide and the method is being refined (see section 5.8 of this chapter).

	Hosp	AllInHospSaureusBact	OBD	Exp
		Table 5.1		
1	A	69	468258	41.48
2	B	94	996889	88.31
3	C	12	416680	36.91
4	D	60	414792	69.03
5	E	42	530172	46.97
6	F	205	1324524	220.42
7	G	96	755547	125.73
8	H	32	284507	25.20
9	I	190	1005113	167.27
10	J	48	405020	35.88
11	K	136	628268	104.55
12	L	15	135334	9.20
13	M	13	221283	15.04
14	N	5	77394	5.26
15	O	18	365871	32.41
16	P	14	179278	15.88
17	Q	5	74908	5.09
18	R	8	80094	5.45
19	S	3	102317	9.06
20	T	27	303590	26.89
21	U	6	175836	11.95

These differences can bias indirectly standardised rates. However, it is possible to calculate confidence (precision) limits about the observed values and control (prediction) limits about the expected values and for the latter to sort the results by the size of the expected values. They can then be presented in, for example, a funnel plot. Since observed/expected ratios (SMRs) are frequently used and the SMR for each hospital is independent of the others, it seems reasonable to employ Poisson based limits. However, there is often evidence of excessive variability (overdispersion). This suggests that Poisson-based limits may, in some cases, be too narrow and should then be used for preliminary screening only, or with adjustment using the methods described by Spiegelhalter[B,C,D] or Laney (Mohammed[A] and Laney). This should be combined with careful application of the methods described by Lilford and colleagues and Mohammed[B] and colleagues (look first for data or analysis error, then for problems with risk adjustment if used, then for system errors, and finally for problems involving staff). An additional problem, described in Chapter 2, is that, especially when precision limits are used, any variation in the expected values is ignored as is any observed-expected covariation.

Methods for dealing with excessive variability (overdispersion), in, for example, funnel plots, involve calculating Z-scores from the observed and expected values for each hospital or unit. Spiegelhalter[B,C,D] describes using the square root of mean of squared Z-scores and Laney (Mohammed[A] and Laney) the standard deviation of Z-scores. There is usually little difference between them although Laney's correction is typically slightly larger. Either is used to widen prediction limits usually by increasing the standard deviation. However, since we obtain prediction limits by using, for example, the gamma distribution, the distance between the expected values and the corresponding prediction limits is widened by either of the correction factors. As Spiegelhalter[B,C,D] has described, when overdispersion is severe, winsorising may further improve the plots because either correction factor may otherwise result in limits that are too wide. Twenty per cent winsorising involves reducing the 10% highest and 10% lowest outlier values to the next highest and lowest values. When severe overdispersion is present it is possible that the basis for the analysis may be flawed and seeking to understand the reason for its occurrence is important. Concentrating on the application of the best available evidence, for example, in bundles and checklists, and analysing within-institution data sequentially is always a sensible approach. This process may be aided by the development of epidemiologically sound, clinically relevant data in clinical-quality registries as described by Evans and colleagues.

An alternative is to employ a random-effects model that provides shrinkage predictions. This has the advantage of treating the collection of units or hospitals of interest as a group having its own distribution. However, in general when stratification is by hospital level, it is important to realise the limitations of the resulting expected values (Tong and colleagues).

The methods described by Spiegelhalter and Laney and the use of winsorising are illustrated although we have not included them in the funnel plot functions of this chapter.

5.2   Confidence intervals for *Staphylococcus aureus* bacteraemia SMR data

Confidence intervals (CIs) for the observer/expected ratio (SMR) are calculated using Poisson-based limits for each hospital and are shown in Figure 5.1. In addition, CIs are calculated using Laney's correction (Figure 5.2 with 20% winsorising and Figure 5.3 with 10% winsorising). Our preference is to avoid corrections if possible but to use Laney's correction with winsorising if essential. It is unlikely that hospital scientists would be required to undertake these analyses and they may wish to seek expert advice if confronted with these decisions.

```
#Table 5.2 and Figure 5.1, multiple Poisson-based confidence intervals
Hosp<-staph[,1]
O<-staph[,2];E<-staph[,4]
oe<-staph[,2]/staph[,4]
l2<-qgamma(0.025,O,1)/E
u2<-qgamma(0.975,O+1,1)/E
l3<-qgamma(0.0015,O,1)/E
u3<-qgamma(0.9985,O+1,1)/E
Tbl<-
data.frame(Hosp,round(oe,2),round(l2,2),round(l3,2),round(u2,2),round(u3,2))
names(Tbl)<-c("Hospital","SMR","L2","L3","U2","U3")
Tbl #Table 5.2
```

	Hospital	SMR	L2	L3	U2	U3
			Table 5.2			
1	A	1.66	1.29	1.13	2.11	2.35
2	B	1.06	0.86	0.77	1.30	1.43
3	C	0.33	0.17	0.12	0.57	0.71
4	D	0.87	0.66	0.57	1.12	1.26
5	E	0.89	0.64	0.54	1.21	1.39
6	F	0.93	0.81	0.75	1.07	1.14
7	G	0.76	0.62	0.55	0.93	1.02
8	H	1.27	0.87	0.71	1.79	2.09
9	I	1.14	0.98	0.91	1.31	1.40
10	J	1.34	0.99	0.84	1.77	2.02
11	K	1.30	1.09	0.99	1.54	1.67
12	L	1.63	0.91	0.66	2.69	3.31
13	M	0.86	0.46	0.32	1.48	1.84
14	N	0.95	0.31	0.15	2.22	3.02
15	O	0.56	0.33	0.25	0.88	1.07
16	P	0.88	0.48	0.34	1.48	1.83
17	Q	0.98	0.32	0.16	2.29	3.12
18	R	1.47	0.63	0.39	2.89	3.77
19	S	0.33	0.07	0.02	0.97	1.38
20	T	1.00	0.66	0.53	1.46	1.72
21	U	0.50	0.18	0.10	1.09	1.46

```
mi<-min(c(oe,l3))
ma<-max(c(oe,u3))
n<-1:length(oe)
par(xaxs="r")
hdr0<-"In-hospital Staphylococcus aureus Bacteraemias with"
hdr1<-"\n2 and 3 SD equivalent Poisson confidence limits."
hdr<-paste(hdr0,hdr1,sep="")
plot(oe,axes=F,col="blue",pch=19,ylim=c(mi,ma),
xlab="Hospitals.",ylab="SMR.",
main=hdr)
box()
abline(h=1)
axis(side=1,labels=Hosp,at=1:length(n))
axis(side=c(2,3,4))
arrows(1:length(n),as.numeric(l2),1:length(n),as.numeric(u2),
angle=90,code=3,col="blue",lwd=2,length=.05)
```

**In-hospital Staphylococcus aureus Bacteraemias
with two and three standard deviation equivalent Poisson confidence limits.**

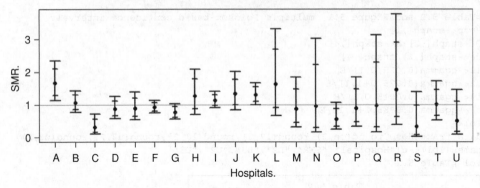

Figure 5.1   Chart for aggregated data, multiple confidence intervals (Poisson).

```
arrows(1:length(n),as.numeric(l3),1:length(n),as.numeric(u3),
angle=90,code=3,col="blue",lwd=2,length=.1)


#Z-scores for overdispersion methods (Laney & Spiegelhalter)
#using observed and expected values
library(exactci)
k<-0
O<-staph[,2];E<-staph[,4]
for (i in 1:length(O)){k[i]<-as.numeric(poisson.exact(O[i],1,E[i])$p.value)}
k<-k/2
z<-0
for (i in 1:length(O))
{if (O[i]<E[i]){z[i]<-qnorm(k[i])}else{z[i]<--qnorm(k[i])}}
#
#illustrating methods for overdispersion
length(z)
#[1] 21
sd(z)
#Laney
#[1] 2.003069 (if no overdispersion should be about one)
#Spiegelhalter
(sum(z^2)/length(z))^.5
#[1] 1.957936


#winsorising 10% (largest and smallest Z-scores)
o<-order(z)
z0<-z[o]
z0[1]<-z0[2];z0[length(z0)]<-z0[(length(z0)-1)]
sd(z0) #Laney
#[1] 1.73021
#Spiegelhalter
(sum(z0^2)/length(z0))^.5
#[1] 1.68973


#winsorising 20% (2 largest and 2 smallest Z-scores)
z0[1]<-z0[3];z0[length(z0)]<-z0[(length(z0)-2)]
```

```
z0[2]<-z0[3];z0[(length(z0)-1)]<-z0[(length(z0)-2)]
#Laney
sd(z0)
#[1] 1.56112
#Spiegelhalter
(sum(z0^2)/length(z0))^.5
#[1] 1.531405

#comparison of Z-scores obtained from Staphylococcus aureus bacteraemia data
#data using Poisson and Laney's correction
# including 10% and 20% winsorising
Zpois<-round(z,3)
ZL10<-round(Zpois/1.73,3)
ZL20<-round(Zpois/1.56,3)
Table3<-data.frame(staph[,c(1,2)],round(E,2),Zpois,ZL10,ZL20)
names(Table3)<-c("Hospital","Counts","Expecteds","Zpois","Z10Lan","Z20Lan")
Table3 #Table 5.3
```

Table 5.3

	Hospital	Counts	Expecteds	Zpois	Z10Lan	Z20Lan
1	A	69	41.48	3.855	2.228	2.471
2	B	94	88.31	0.565	0.327	0.362
3	C	12	36.91	−4.632	−2.677	−2.969
4	D	60	69.03	−1.028	−0.594	−0.659
5	E	42	46.97	−0.638	−0.369	−0.409
6	F	205	220.42	−1.005	−0.581	−0.644
7	G	96	125.73	−2.704	−1.563	−1.733
8	H	32	25.20	1.240	0.717	0.795
9	I	190	167.27	1.695	0.980	1.087
10	J	48	35.88	1.874	1.083	1.201
11	K	136	104.55	2.909	1.682	1.865
12	L	15	9.20	1.661	0.960	1.065
13	M	13	15.04	−0.360	−0.208	−0.231
14	N	5	5.26	0.000	0.000	0.000
15	O	18	32.41	−2.628	−1.519	−1.685
16	P	14	15.88	−0.309	−0.179	−0.198
17	Q	5	5.09	0.000	0.000	0.000
18	R	8	5.45	0.899	0.520	0.576
19	S	3	9.06	−2.047	−1.183	−1.312
20	T	27	26.89	0.000	0.000	0.000
21	U	6	11.95	−1.674	−0.968	−1.07

```
# Poisson based limits with Laney's correction with 20%
# winsorising (1.56), Table 5.4 and Figure 5.2
d0<-staph[,1]
d1<-staph[,2]
d2<-staph[,4]
q1<-0
z1<-0
for (i in 1:length(d0)){
X<-d1[i]
Y<-d2[i]
if (X>Y){q1[i]<-pgamma(Y,X,1)}else{q1[i]<-1-pgamma(Y,X+1,1)}
if (X>Y){z1[i]<--qnorm(q1[i])}else{z1[i]<-qnorm(q1[i])}
```

```
}
Zpois<-round(z1,3)
L<-log(d1/d2)
OE<-exp(L)
SE<-abs(L/Zpois)
U2<-exp(L+1.96*1.56*SE) #Laney's correction 1.56, see above
L2<-exp(L-1.96*1.56*SE)
U3<-exp(L+2.97*1.56*SE)
L3<-exp(L-2.97*1.56*SE)
Table4<-
data.frame(staph[,1],round(OE,2),round(L2,2),round(L3,2),round(U2,2),
round(U3,2))
names(Table4)<-c("Hospital","SMR","L2","L3","U2","U3")
Table4 #Table 5.4
```

```
                   Table 5.4
     Hospital    SMR      L2      L3      U2       U3
1        A      1.66    1.11    0.90    2.49     3.07
2        B      1.06    0.76    0.64    1.49     1.78
3        C      0.33    0.15    0.11    0.68     1.00
4        D      0.87    0.57    0.46    1.32     1.64
5        E      0.89    0.52    0.40    1.53     2.01
6        F      0.93    0.75    0.67    1.16     1.30
7        G      0.76    0.56    0.48    1.04     1.21
8        H      1.27    0.70    0.52    2.29     3.10
9        I      1.14    0.90    0.80    1.43     1.61
10       J      1.34    0.83    0.65    2.15     2.75
11       K      1.30    0.99    0.86    1.72     1.98
12       L      1.63    0.66    0.42    4.01     6.38
13       M      0.86    0.25    0.13    2.98     5.64
14       N      0.95    0.40    0.25    2.28     3.58
15       O      0.56    0.28    0.20    1.10     1.57
16       P      0.88    0.25    0.13    3.07     5.83
17       Q      0.98    0.79    0.71    1.22     1.36
18       R      1.47    0.40    0.20    5.42    10.61
19       S      0.33    0.06    0.03    1.73     4.04
20       T      1.00    0.75    0.65    1.34     1.56
21       U      0.50    0.14    0.07    1.77     3.38
```

```
mi<-min(c(OE,L3))
ma<-max(c(OE,U3))
n<-as.character(d0)
o<-order(n)
OE<-OE[o]
L2<-L2[o]
L3<-L3[o]
U2<-U2[o]
U3<-U3[o]
n<-n[o]
par(xaxs="r")
hdr0<-"In-hospital Staphylococcus aureus Bacteraemias"
hdr1<-"\nwith Poisson CIs, Laney's correction & 20% winsorising."
hdr<-paste(hdr0,hdr1,sep="")
plot(OE,axes=F,col="blue",pch=19,ylim=c(mi,ma),
xlab="Hospitals.",ylab="SMR.",
main=hdr)
```

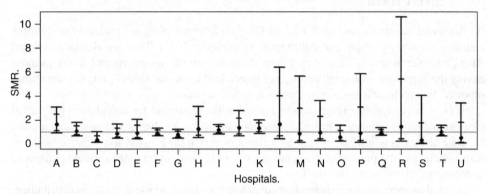

Figure 5.2   Chart for aggregated data, multiple confidence intervals Laney's correction with 20% winsorising.

```
box()
abline(h=1)
axis(side=1,labels=n,at=1:length(n))
axis(side=c(2,3,4))
arrows(1:length(n),as.numeric(L2),1:length(n),as.numeric(U2),angle=90,
code=3,col="blue",lwd=2,length=.05)
arrows(1:length(n),as.numeric(L3),1:length(n),as.numeric(U3),angle=90,
code=3,col="blue",lwd=2,length=.1)
```

Figure 5.3 code is the same as that for Figure 5.2 except that the 10% winsorising correction of 1.73 is employed instead of 1.56 for 20% winsorising.

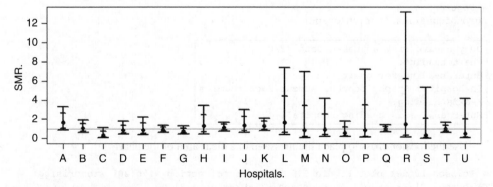

Figure 5.3   Chart for aggregated data, multiple confidence intervals (Poisson with Laney's correction with 10% winsorising).

5.3   Funnel plots for *Staphylococcus aureus* bacteraemia SMR data

As discussed earlier in section 2.3.3.1 of Chapter 2 funnel plots are preferred to multiple confidence intervals (Adap and colleagues, Spiegelhalter[B,C,D]). They are similar to control charts with the hospitals' data sorted from those having the widest control limits to those having the narrowest. Although confidence (precision) limits for funnel plots are sometimes reported, it is preferable to employ control (prediction) limits.

It is usual to employ large-sample normal approximations for calculating the funnel plot control limits. However, hospital infection data often involve small counts and a more accurate method is required that allows for the skewness of the Poisson and negative binomial distributions and the poor fit of the continuous normal distribution to the discrete count data distributions when counts are small.

A suitable approach for independent count and rate data is to use the gamma distribution, for example, the pgamma function in R. For the upper control limit U, it is necessary to find U using pgamma(E,U,1)==P where E is the expected count and P is 0.02275 for a 2 SD limit or 0.00135 for a 3 SD limit. This requires trial and error but can be automated in an R function. The SMR funnel plot centre line is one and the upper control limit vector is U/E. The lower limit L requires 1-pgamma(E,L+1,1)==P and the lower control limit vector is max(0,L/E). Figure 5.4 is a funnel plot of the *Staphylococcus aureus* data with limits based on the Poisson distribution and without Spiegelhalter's or Laney's correction. Laney's correction, if necessary with winsorising, can be employed to correct for overdispersion.

The function pgroupfunnelinstitution() can be used to produce Figure 5.4 with institutions on the horizontal axis and pgroupfunnelprocedure() Figure 5.7 with expected counts on the horizontal axis. Figure 5.5 and Figure 5.6 employ Laney's correction with 20% and 10% winsorising respectively. The functions pgroupfunnelinstitution() and pgroupfunnelprocedure() employ unadjusted Poisson based limits. Figure 5.8 is similar to Figure 5.7 but with control limits widened using Laney's correction with 20% winsorising. When a correction for overdispersion is to be employed, the Spiegelhalter or Laney methods, that appear to give similar results, can be employed although the amount of winsorising may require expert judegment.

```
#using pgroupfunnelinstitution() function (Poisson limits, no correction),
# Figure 5.4
pgroupfunnelinstitution(staph)
```

```
Do you have risk-adjusted data (Y/N) y
Chart heading.
Enter heading for chart
In-hospital Staphylococcus aureus Bacteraemias
X-axis heading.
Enter an X-axis heading Hospitals
```

Use the locator cross to place the message in a clear area of the chart.

```
# Poisson funnel plot Figure 5.5 (Laney's correction with 20% winsorising)
O<-staph[,2];E<-staph[,4];H<-staph[,1];D<-staph[,3]
TT<-E
AA<-0
```

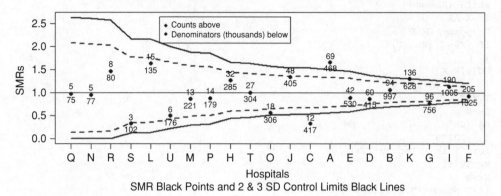

Figure 5.4   SMR funnel plot, hospitals on horizontal axis (uncorrected Poisson limits).

```
U<-0
Z<-.02275
for (i in 1:length(TT)){
M<-TT[i]
X<-M
A<-1
BL<-F
while (BL==F){
X<-X+A
K<-pgamma(M,X,1)
if (K<Z){BL<-T}
}
AA<-.001
BL<-F
while (BL==F){
X<-X-AA
K<-pgamma(M,X,1)
if (K>=Z){BL<-T}
}
U[i]<-X
}
TT<-E
AA<-0
UU<-0
Z<-.0015
for (i in 1:length(TT)){
M<-TT[i]
X<-M
A<-1
BL<-F
while (BL==F){
X<-X+A
K<-pgamma(M,X,1)
if (K<Z){BL<-T}
}
AA<-.001
```

```
BL<-F
while (BL==F){
X<-X-AA
K<-pgamma(M,X,1)
if (K>=Z){BL<-T}
}
UU[i]<-X
}
TT<-E
L<-0
AA<-0
Z<-.02275
for (i in 1:length(TT)){
M<-TT[i]
X<-0
if(1-pgamma(M,X+1,1)>=Z){X<-0}else{
A<-1
BL<-F
while (BL==F){
X<-X+A
K<-1-pgamma(M,X+1,1)
if (K>Z){BL<-T}
}
AA<-.001
BL<-F
while (BL==F){
X<-X-AA
K<-1-pgamma(M,X+1,1)
if (K<=Z){BL<-T}
}
}
L[i]<-X
}

TT<-E
LL<-0
AA<-0
Z<-.0015
for (i in 1:length(TT)){
M<-TT[i]
X<-0
if(1-pgamma(M,X+1,1)>=Z){X<-0}else{
A<-1
BL<-F
while (BL==F){
X<-X+A
K<-1-pgamma(M,X+1,1)
if (K>Z){BL<-T}
}
AA<-.001
BL<-F
while (BL==F){
X<-X-AA
K<-1-pgamma(M,X+1,1)
if (K<=Z){BL<-T}
}
```

```
}
LL[i]<-X
}
# Laney's correction with 20% winsorising
U<-E+(U-E)*1.56
UU<-E+(UU-E)*1.56
L<-E-(E-L)*1.56
LL<-E-(E-LL)*1.56
L[L<0]<-0
LL[LL<0]<-0
oe<-O/E
w<-UU-LL
o<-order(w)
O1<-O[o];E1<-E[o];H1<-H[o];D1<-D[o]
oe1<-oe[o]
L1<-L[o];L2<-L1/E1
LL1<-LL[o];LL2<-LL1/E1
U1<-U[o];U2<-U1/E1
UU1<-UU[o];UU2<-UU1/E1
hdr0<-"In-hospital Staphylococcus aureus Bacteraemias"
hdr1<-"\nwith Laney's correction & 20% Winsorising."
hdr<-paste(hdr0,hdr1,sep="")
plot(oe1,ylim=c(0,max(c(oe1,UU2))),axes=F,col="blue",pch=19,
main=hdr,xlab="SMR Blue, 2 & 3 SD Control Limits Red",ylab="SMRs")
box()
par(cex=.8)
axis(side=1,labels=H1,at=1:length(H1))
axis(side=c(2,3,4))
par(cex=1)
lines(U2,col="red",lty=2,lwd=2)
lines(L2,col="red",lty=2,lwd=2)
lines(UU2,col="red",lty=1,lwd=2)
lines(LL2,col="red",lty=1,lwd=2)
abline(h=1)
par(font=2)
text(oe1,labels=as.character(round(O1,0)),pos=3,offset=.3,cex=.8,lwd=3,
col="green4")
text(oe1,labels=as.character(round(D1/1000,0)),pos=1,offset=.3,cex=.8,
lwd=3,col="brown4")
par(font=1)
mtext("Hospitals",side=1,line=2)
legend(locator(1),legend=c("Counts Green",
"Denominators(thousands) Brown"),
pch=19,col=c("green4","brown4"),cex=.8)
```

Figure 5.6 code is the same as that for Figure 5.5 except that the 10% winsorising correction of 1.73 is employed instead of 1.56 for 20% winsorising.

```
#using pgroupfunnelprocedure() function (Poisson limits, no correction)
pgroupfunnelprocedure(staph) # Figure 5.7
```

```
Do you have risk-adjusted data (Y/N) y
Chart heading.
Enter heading for chart
In-hospital Staphylococcus aureus Bacteraemias
```

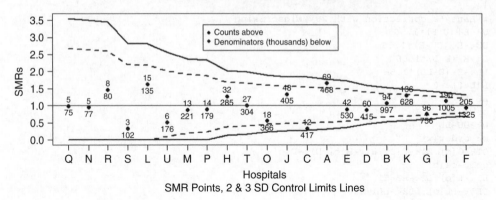

Figure 5.5   SMR funnel plot, hospitals on horizontal axis Laney's correction with 20% winsorising.

Use the locator cross to place the message in a clear area of the chart.

```
# Poisson funnel plot Figure 5.8 with Laney's correction plus
# 20% winsorising
O<-staph[,2];E<-staph[,4];H<-staph[,1];D<-staph[,3]
TT<-E
AA<-O
U<-O
Z<-.02275
for (i in 1:length(TT)){
M<-TT[i]
X<-M
A<-1
```

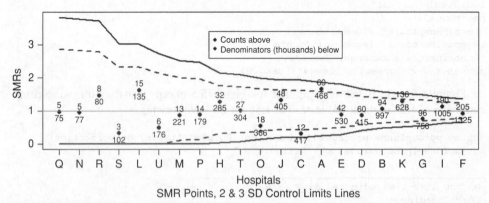

Figure 5.6   SMR funnel plot, hospitals on horizontal axis (Poisson limits with Laney's correction and 10% winsorising).

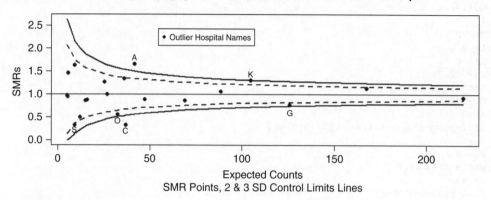

Figure 5.7 SMR funnel plot, expected counts on horizontal axis (uncorrected Poisson limits).

```
BL<-F
while (BL==F){
X<-X+A
K<-pgamma(M,X,1)
if (K<Z){BL<-T}
}
AA<-.001
BL<-F
while (BL==F){
X<-X-AA
K<-pgamma(M,X,1)
if (K>=Z){BL<-T}
}
U[i]<-X
}
TT<-E
AA<-0
UU<-0
Z<-.0015
for (i in 1:length(TT)){
M<-TT[i]
X<-M
A<-1
BL<-F
while (BL==F){
X<-X+A
K<-pgamma(M,X,1)
if (K<Z){BL<-T}
}
AA<-.001
BL<-F
while (BL==F){
X<-X-AA
K<-pgamma(M,X,1)
if (K>=Z){BL<-T}
```

```
}
UU[i]<-X
}
TT<-E
L<-0
AA<-0
Z<-.02275
for (i in 1:length(TT)){
M<-TT[i]
X<-0
if(1-pgamma(M,X+1,1)>=Z){X<-0}else{
A<-1
BL<-F
while (BL==F){
X<-X+A
K<-1-pgamma(M,X+1,1)
if (K>Z){BL<-T}
}
AA<-.001
BL<-F
while (BL==F){
X<-X-AA
K<-1-pgamma(M,X+1,1)
if (K<=Z){BL<-T}
}
}
L[i]<-X
}
L[L<0]<-0
TT<-E
LL<-0
AA<-0
Z<-.0015
for (i in 1:length(TT)){
M<-TT[i]
X<-0
if(1-pgamma(M,X+1,1)>=Z){X<-0}else{
A<-1
BL<-F
while (BL==F){
X<-X+A
K<-1-pgamma(M,X+1,1)
if (K>Z){BL<-T}
}
AA<-.001
BL<-F
while (BL==F){
X<-X-AA
K<-1-pgamma(M,X+1,1)
if (K<=Z){BL<-T}
}
}
LL[i]<-X
}
LL[LL<0]<-0
oe<-O/E
```

```
w<-E
o<-order(w)
O1<-O[o];E1<-E[o];H1<-H[o];D1<-D[o]
oe1<-oe[o]
L1<-L[o]
LL1<-LL[o]
U1<-U[o]
UU1<-UU[o]
U1<-E1+(U1-E1)*1.56 #Laney's correction with winsorising, see above
UU1<-E1+(UU1-E1)*1.56
L1<-E1-(E1-L1)*1.56
LL1<-E1-(E1-LL1)*1.56
L1[L1<0]<-0
LL1[LL1<0]<-0
plot(oe1~E1,ylim=c(0,max(c(oe1,UU1/E1))),col="blue",pch=19,
main="In-hospital Staphylococcus aureus Bacteraemias
with Laney's correction & 20% winsorising",
xlab="SMR Blue, 2 & 3 SD Control Limits Red",ylab="SMRs")
lines(U1/E1~E1,col="red",lty=2,lwd=2)
lines(L1/E1~E1,col="red",lty=2,lwd=2)
lines(UU1/E1~E1,col="red",lty=1,lwd=2)
lines(LL1/E1~E1,col="red",lty=1,lwd=2)
abline(h=1)
par(font=2)
oe2<-rep("",length(oe1))
for (i in 1:length(oe2))
{if (oe1[i]>U1[i]/E1[i]){oe2[i]<-as.character(H1[i])}}
text(oe1~E1,labels=oe2,pos=3,offset=.3,cex=.8,lwd=3,col="brown4")
oe2<-rep("",length(oe1))
for (i in 1:length(oe2))
{if (oe1[i]<L1[i]/E1[i]){oe2[i]<-as.character(H1[i])}}
text(oe1~E1,labels=oe2,pos=1,offset=.3,cex=.8,lwd=3,col="brown4")
par(font=1)
mtext("Expected Counts",side=1,line=2)
legend(locator(1),legend="Outlier Hospital Names Brown",
pch=19,col="brown4",cex=.8)
```

5.4   Tabulations and Z-scores

It may be desirable to perform further tabulations and analyses by arranging the data for example by years and searching for years during which hospitals had unusually large numbers of bacteraemias. This can be done by calculating Z-scores and subjecting data from those with values close to or above 2 to further scrutiny. In addition, data from other institutions of interest, such as those with runs of positive Z-scores, can be selected for further attention. One should also watch for persistently low counts as this may indicate under-reporting (section 3.19 of Chapter 3). We defer analysis of monthly and quarterly data from individual institutions to Chapter 6.

```
# illustration using all hospitals in 2006
# arranging by years, institutions
library(chron)
o<-order(staph[,1])
staph1<-staph[o,]
```

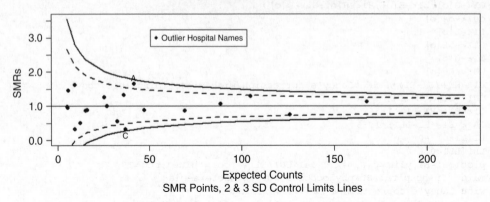

Figure 5.8 SMR funnel plot, expected counts on horizontal axis (Poisson limits with Laney's correction and 20% winsorising).

```
Hosp<-bact[,1] #from hasaureusbact.csv, see above
Date<-bact[,2]
Date<-chron(as.character(Date),format="d-mmm-yy",out.format="dd-mmm-yyyy")
Year<-years(Date)
In<-bact[,4]
Hospy<-as.data.frame(xtabs(In~Hosp+Year))
o<-order(Hospy[,1])
Hospy<-Hospy[o,]
D<-obd[,2] #from obd.csv, see above
D<-chron(as.character(D),format="d-mmm-yy",out.format="dd-mmm-yyyy")
H<-obd[,1]
O<-obd[,3]
YD<-years(D)
YOBD<-as.data.frame(xtabs(O~H+YD))
o<-order(YOBD[,1])
YOBD<-YOBD[o,]
Hosps<-data.frame(Hospy,YOBD[,3])
Exp1<-data.frame(staph1[,1],staph1[,4]/staph1[,3])
Exp2<-Exp1
for (i in 1:5){Exp2<-rbind(Exp2,Exp1)}
o<-order(Exp2[,1])
Exp2<-Exp2[o,]
Hosps1<-data.frame(Hosps,Exp2[,2]*Hosps[,4])
names(Hosps1)<-c("Hosp","Year","AE","Denom","Exp")
Hosps2<-Hosps1[Hosps1[,4]!=0,]
row.names(Hosps2)<-1:length(Hosps2[,1])
#calculating z-scores from Poisson P-values
library(exactci)
k<-0
O<-Hosps2[,3];E<-Hosps2[,5]
for (i in 1:length(O)){k[i]<-poisson.exact(O[i],E[i])$p.value/2}
z<-0
```

```
for (i in 1:length(O)){if (O[i]<E[i]){z[i]<-
qnorm(k[i])}else{z[i]<--qnorm(k[i])}}
Exp<-round(E,2)
Z<-round(z,2)
Hosps3<-data.frame(Hosps2[,-5],Exp,Z)
#selecting 2006 data for all hospitals
Hosps4<-Hosps3[Hosps3[,2]==2006,]
Hosps4
```

	Hosp	Year	AE	Denom	Exp	Z
6	A	2006	15	99938	8.85	1.79
12	B	2006	17	184379	16.33	0.08
18	C	2006	1	78350	6.94	−2.42
24	D	2006	7	69401	11.55	−1.22
30	E	2006	9	94748	8.39	0.09
36	F	2006	31	239160	39.80	−1.34
42	G	2006	13	125441	20.88	−1.69
48	H	2006	9	54548	4.83	1.57
52	I	2006	61	275760	45.89	2.08
58	J	2006	12	76556	6.78	1.70
64	K	2006	21	122414	20.37	0.07
69	L	2006	6	32847	2.23	1.93
74	M	2006	1	52483	3.57	−1.13
78	N	2006	1	27338	1.86	−0.14
83	O	2006	1	84815	7.51	−2.60
88	P	2006	2	41102	3.64	−0.54
93	Q	2006	0	18534	1.26	−0.57
98	R	2006	3	17576	1.19	1.18
107	T	2006	7	70754	6.27	0.16
112	U	2006	0	41542	2.82	−1.56

5.5   More on overdispersion, false discovery, very small expected counts

As discussed in previous chapters, overdispersion is common with count data due for example to imperfect risk-adjustment, differences in the services hospitals provide, transmission of hospital-acquired organisms or varying surveillance quality. As already referred to (Chapter 1, section 1.10 and Chapter 4, section 4.9) Spiegelhalter[B,C,D] and Laney (Mohammed[A] and Laney) have described methods to deal with this problem. The above data display overdispersion, for example, using Laney's method with the Table 5.4 data, the standard deviation (SD) of the Z-scores was 1.47. However, correcting for overdispersion does not in this case appear to be warranted, even though the expected values were derived from the hospital levels. In addition, it was largely due to several low reported rates that may indicate under-reporting. There is only one result just above 2 SD, something not unusual by chance alone with 20 institutions. We anticipate that with the further development of the methods described by Tong and colleagues we will be able to replace simple stratification by hospital level with expected values derived from regression modeling using the services the hospitals provide or stratification by revised hospital levels. In section 5.8 of this chapter we show how, by applying their modification of the hospital levels for risk adjusting MRSA bacteraemia, a large reduction in the standard deviation of the Z-scores was accomplished.

As we have indicated, we do not usually attempt to correct for overdispersion in funnel plots, although two established methods have been illustrated. However, for public reporting it may be desirable, for example Figure 5.8 may be preferred to Figure 5.7 for this purpose as in the latter nearly one third of the hospitals lie outside the two SD limits. However, what modification has been employed and the reason for its employment should also be reported. Clearly, this can be a difficult area requiring expert judgement. When there is very severe overdispersion, it may be most important to attempt to find the reason, for example insufficient numbers of hospitals for developing risk adjustment, poor or absent risk adjustment, lack of stratification of hospitals, outcomes that are not independent or varying quality of surveillance.

In addition, shrinkage (random-effects) analyses are also performed (see section 6 of this chapter). Examination of the funnel and shrinkage plots enables heterogeneity to be assessed. We believe that it should be investigated. Recently, false detection rate correction has been advocated by Jones and colleagues using the Benjamini-Hochberg procedure that is available in R (Figure 5.9). It would seem desirable if possible, when there are many institutions, to group them by the services they provide. For example hospitals with large maternity units may have few bacteraemias whereas those with oncology-haematology & renal dialysis/transplant units may expect to have more. This is discussed further in section 5.8.

Comparisons of hospitals are often advocated, although, as we have indicated, this can be subject to serious bias and to be of questionable value. When two hospitals among a group are being compared, usually after the data become available, it would seem wise to adjust P-values and Z-scores, for example, using the Benjamini-Hochberg procedure.

An additional problem with funnel plots can occur when the expected outcome count is very low, for example less than one, as the O/E ratio (SMR) can become very large. For this reason, it is wise to remove any rows where the expected count is less than one. These low values should not be ignored. A hospital with a very small chance of a particular serious infection should conduct an M&M audit, preferably involving an independent observer, whenever such an infection occurs.

```
# Benjamini-Hochberg z-score adjustment, Figure 5.9
library(exactci)
k<-0
O<-staph[,2];E<-staph[,4];hosp<-staph[,1]
for (i in 1:length(O)){k[i]<-poisson.exact(O[i],E[i])$p.value}
z<-0
for (i in 1:length(O)){if (O[i]<E[i]){z[i]<-qnorm(k[i]/2)}
else{z[i]<--qnorm(k[i]/2)}}
padj<-p.adjust(k,"BH")
q<-0
for (i in 1:length(O)){if (O[i]<E[i]){q[i]<-qnorm(padj[i]/2)}
else{q[i]<--qnorm(padj[i]/2)}}
Tabl<-data.frame(staph,round(k,4),round(z,2),round(padj,4),round(q,2))
names(Tabl)<-c("Hosp","Staph","OBD","Exp","P-value","Z-score",
"P-value(BH)","Z-score(BH)")
Tabl # Table 5.5
```

Table 5.5

	Hosp	Staph	OBD	Exp	P-value	Z-score	P-value(BH)	Z-score(BH)
1	A	69	468258	41.48	0.0001	3.86	0.0012	3.24
2	B	94	996889	88.31	0.5724	0.56	0.7512	0.32
3	C	12	416680	36.91	0.0000	−4.63	0.0001	−3.96
4	D	60	414792	69.03	0.3037	−1.03	0.5085	−0.66
5	E	42	530172	46.97	0.5233	−0.64	0.7327	−0.34
6	F	205	1324524	220.42	0.3148	−1.01	0.5085	−0.66
7	G	96	755547	125.73	0.0069	−2.70	0.0360	−2.10
8	H	32	284507	25.20	0.2151	1.24	0.4107	0.82
9	I	190	1005113	167.27	0.0900	1.70	0.2029	1.27
10	J	48	405020	35.88	0.0610	1.87	0.1829	1.33
11	K	136	628268	104.55	0.0036	2.91	0.0254	2.24
12	L	15	135334	9.20	0.0966	1.66	0.2029	1.27
13	M	13	221283	15.04	0.7188	−0.36	0.8838	−0.15
14	N	5	77394	5.26	1.0000	0.00	1.0000	0.00
15	O	18	365871	32.41	0.0086	−2.63	0.0361	−2.10
16	P	14	179278	15.88	0.7575	−0.31	0.8838	−0.15
17	Q	5	74908	5.09	1.0000	0.00	1.0000	0.00
18	R	8	80094	5.45	0.3688	0.90	0.5532	0.59
19	S	3	102317	9.06	0.0407	−2.05	0.1424	−1.47
20	T	27	303590	26.89	1.0000	0.00	1.0000	0.00
21	U	6	175836	11.95	0.0942	−1.67	0.2029	−1.27

```
o<-order(q)
q0<-q[o]
hosp0<-hosp[o]
zo<-z[o]
plot(q0,type="p",lwd=2,pch=19,col="dark blue",axes=F,
ylim=c(-5,5),xlab="Hospitals.",ylab="Benjamini & Hochberg Adjustment.",
main=" Benjamini-Hochberg Adjusted Z-scores.")
box()
axis(side=1,tick=T,labels=hosp0,at=1:length(hosp0))
axis(side=c(2,3,4))
abline(h=0)
abline(h=2,lwd=2,col="black",lty=2)
abline(h=-2,lwd=2,col="black",lty=2)
abline(h=3,lwd=2,col="black")
abline(h=-3,lwd=2,col="black")
points(zo,lwd=2,col="red")
```

5.5.1 Proposal for Benjamini-Hochberg modified funnel plot

The Benjamini-Hochberg modified P-values and Z-scores are shown in Table 5.5. We can leave the funnel plot control limits in place but bring the SMR values closer to the centre line by finding the adjusted observed values that correspond to the P-values obtained by the Benjamini-Hochberg correction (Figure 5.10).

```
# Poisson funnel plot with Benjamini-Hochberg correction
O<-staph[,2];E<-staph[,4];H<-staph[,1];D<-staph[,3]
TT<-E
AA<-O
U<-O
```

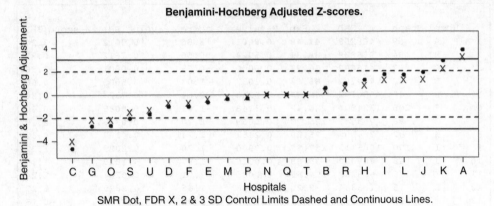

Figure 5.9   False discovery adjusted Z-scores.

```
Z<-.02275
for (i in 1:length(TT)){
M<-TT[i]
X<-M
A<-1
BL<-F
while (BL==F){
X<-X+A
K<-pgamma(M,X,1)
if (K<Z){BL<-T}
}
AA<-.001
BL<-F
while (BL==F){
X<-X-AA
K<-pgamma(M,X,1)
if (K>=Z){BL<-T}
}
U[i]<-X
}
TT<-E
AA<-0
UU<-0
Z<-.0015
for (i in 1:length(TT)){
M<-TT[i]
X<-M
A<-1
BL<-F
while (BL==F){
X<-X+A
K<-pgamma(M,X,1)
if (K<Z){BL<-T}
}
AA<-.001
BL<-F
while (BL==F){
X<-X-AA
```

```
K<-pgamma(M,X,1)
if (K>=Z){BL<-T}
}
UU[i]<-X
}
TT<-E
L<-0
AA<-0
Z<-.02275
for (i in 1:length(TT)){
M<-TT[i]
X<-0
if(1-pgamma(M,X+1,1)>=Z){X<-0}else{
A<-1
BL<-F
while (BL==F){
X<-X+A
K<-1-pgamma(M,X+1,1)
if (K>Z){BL<-T}
}
AA<-.001
BL<-F
while (BL==F){
X<-X-AA
K<-1-pgamma(M,X+1,1)
if (K<=Z){BL<-T}
}
}
L[i]<-X
}
TT<-E
LL<-0
AA<-0
Z<-.0015
for (i in 1:length(TT)){
M<-TT[i]
X<-0
if(1-pgamma(M,X+1,1)>=Z){X<-0}else{
A<-1
BL<-F
while (BL==F){
X<-X+A
K<-1-pgamma(M,X+1,1)
if (K>Z){BL<-T}
}
AA<-.001
BL<-F
while (BL==F){
X<-X-AA
K<-1-pgamma(M,X+1,1)
if (K<=Z){BL<-T}
}
}
LL[i]<-X
}
L[L<0]<-0
```

```
LL[LL<0]<-0
oe<-O/E
w<-UU-LL
o<-order(w)
O1<-O[o];E1<-E[o];H1<-H[o];D1<-D[o]
oe1<-oe[o]
L1<-L[o];L2<-L1/E1
LL1<-LL[o];LL2<-LL1/E1
U1<-U[o];U2<-U1/E1
UU1<-UU[o];UU2<-UU1/E1
hdr0<-"In-hospital Staphylococcus aureus Bacteraemias"
hdr1<-"\nwith Benjamini-Hochberg correction."
hdr<-paste(hdr0,hdr1,sep="")
plot(oe1,ylim=c(0,max(c(oe1,UU2))),axes=F,col="blue",pch=19,
xlab="SMR Blue, FDR Red, 2 & 3 SD Control Limits Red",
main=hdr,ylab="SMRs")
box()
par(cex=.8)
axis(side=1,labels=H1,at=1:length(H1))
axis(side=c(2,3,4))
par(cex=1)
lines(U2,col="red",lty=2,lwd=2)
lines(L2,col="red",lty=2,lwd=2)
lines(UU2,col="red",lty=1,lwd=2)
lines(LL2,col="red",lty=1,lwd=2)
abline(h=1)
par(font=2)
par(font=1)
mtext("Hospitals",side=1,line=2)
# Benjamini-Hochberg correction
O<-staph[,2];E<-staph[,4];H<-staph[,1];D<-staph[,3]
library(exactci)
k<-0
for (i in 1:length(O)){k[i]<-poisson.exact(O[i],E[i])$p.value/2}
padj<-p.adjust(k,"BH")
TT<-E
AA<-0
Sadj<-0
for (i in 1:length(TT)){if (O[i]>E[i]){
Z<-padj[i]
M<-TT[i]
X<-M
A<-1
BL<-F
while (BL==F){
X<-X+A
K<-pgamma(M,X,1)
if (K<Z){BL<-T}
}
AA<-.001
BL<-F
while (BL==F){
X<-X-AA
K<-pgamma(M,X,1)
if (K>=Z){BL<-T}
}
```

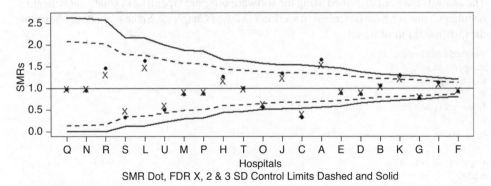

Figure 5.10 SMR funnel plot, hospitals on horizontal axis (Poisson limits and Benjamini-Hochberg false discovery adjusted SMRs).

```
Sadj[i]<-X
}else{
Z<-padj[i]
M<-TT[i]
X<-0
if(1-pgamma(M,X+1,1)>=Z){X<-0}else{
A<-1
BL<-F
while (BL==F){
X<-X+A
K<-1-pgamma(M,X+1,1)
if (K>Z){BL<-T}
}
AA<-.001
BL<-F
while (BL==F){
X<-X-AA
K<-1-pgamma(M,X+1,1)
if (K<=Z){BL<-T}
}
}
Sadj[i]<-X
}
}
for (i in 1:length(O)){if (padj[i]>.49){Sadj[i]<-E[i]}}
points(Sadj[o]/E[o],pch=19,lwd=2,col="red")
```

5.6   Bayesian shrinkage plot

Shrinkage analysis is described in Chapter 2 (section 2.3.3.5). It is assumed that the data from the hospitals of interest are, in a sense, exchangeable, and that they have their own distribution. Therefore, a large outlier may not belong to that distribution so it may be sensible to remove it for individual attention, for example, by M&M audit, and repeat the analysis with it removed. The book by Winkel and Zhang describes hierarchical model (random effects) analysis in QI.

5.6.1   Using OpenBUGS

The analysis may be performed using the software program OpenBUGS (mathstat.helsinki.fi/ openbugs/) that we have described in section 2.3.3.6 of Chapter 2. Since there are 21 hospitals, data list(n=21) must be set.

```
o<-order(staph[,1])
staph<-staph[o,]
s.d(staph[,c(2,4)])
#
#Use clipboard (c) or a data file (d) c

OpenBUGS (gammapoisson.odc).

# program window
model
{
for (i in 1:n)
{
theta[i]~dgamma(alpha,beta)
lamda[i]<-theta[i]*t[i]
x[i]~dpois(lamda[i])
}
alpha~dexp(1)
beta~dgamma(.1,.1)
}
data
list(n = 21)
inits
list(alpha = 1, beta = 1)

# data window
```

```
x[]    t[]
69     41.4808687399786
94     88.3099098303255
12     36.9118058561184
60     69.0274373317081
42     46.965551344797
205    220.420107919978
96     125.734038249677
32     25.2031946546671
190    167.265459842005
48     35.8788989340623
136    104.552956656632
15     9.2009899993332
13     15.044428377366
5      5.26180723253871
18     32.4108652212343
14     15.8814311468590
5      5.09279086460203
8      5.44537287752223
3      9.06380253379204
27     26.8936717381659
6      11.9546106486378
END
```

The above steps are described in section 2.3.3.6 of Chapter 2. There is a useful description at www.math.unm.edu/~bedrick/PIBBS/Winbugstutorial1.pdf (Woodworth). The next steps can be performed in R and the result is in Figure 5.11.

```
g.d() # data from OpenBUGS via clipboard, no headings, no date column

#data in datain
#credible intervals, use function shrink()
shrink(datain,21,40000) # for credible intervals
#Figure 5.11.
d1<-d
datain1<-staph
nn1<-datain1[,1]
P1<-datain1[,2]/datain1[,4]
mn<-0;mx<-ceiling(max(d1$u))+.1
plot(P1,col="red",pch=19,ylim=c(mn,mx),axes=F,lwd=3,
main="BUGS Shrinkage Staphylococcus aureus Bacteraemias.",
xlab="2 & 3 SD equivalent limits blue, data red.",
ylab="SMR.")
box()
points(d1$m,col="blue",lwd=3)
abline(h=1)
par(cex=.7)
axis(side=1,tick=T,nn1,at=1:length(nn1))
axis(side=c(2,3,4))
par(cex=1)
points(d1$ll,pch="-",lwd=3,col="blue",cex=1.5)
points(d1$ul,pch="-",lwd=3,col="blue",cex=1.5)
arrows(1:length(d1$m),d1$l,1:length(d1$m),d1$u,angle=90,code=3,
lwd=2,col="blue",length=.15)
mtext("Hospitals.",side=1,line=2)
```

5.6.2   Using empirical Bayes methods

An alternative approach is to use lmer() in the lme4/arm libraries or hglm() in the hglm library; see also section 2.3.3.7 of Chapter 2. These routines give broadly similar results but there

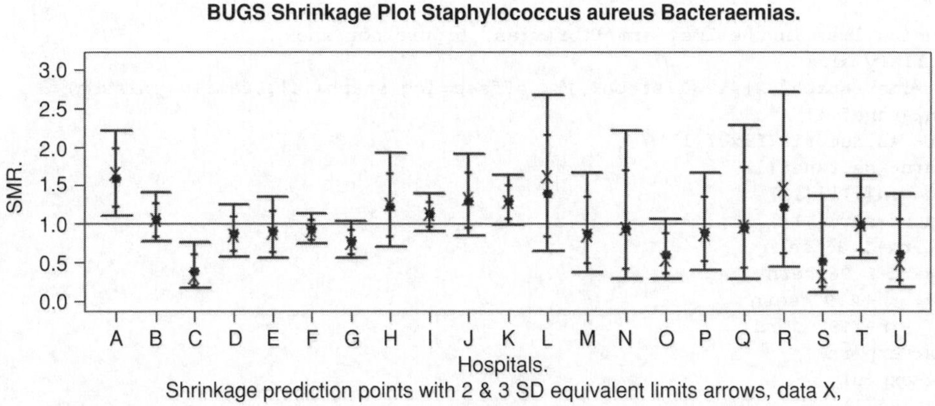

BUGS Shrinkage Plot Staphylococcus aureus Bacteraemias.

Shrinkage prediction points with 2 & 3 SD equivalent limits arrows, data X,

Figure 5.11   OpenBUGS shrinkage plot (gamma-Poisson hierarchical model).

are several clear differences (Figure 5.12). The OpenBUGS method is to be preferred since it more appropriately incorporates all of the parameter uncertainty. With these data hglm() appears to give results that are more like those of section 5.6.1 than lmer().

```
# Figure 5.12
library(hglm)
h<-hglm(fixed=staph[,2]~1,random=~1|staph[,1],offset=
log(staph[,4]),
family=poisson(link=log), fix.disp=1)
rn<-as.numeric(h$ranef)
ra<-as.numeric(h$fixef)
sern<-as.numeric(h$SeRe)
u<-rn+1.96*sern
l<-rn-1.96*sern
uu<-rn+2.97*sern
ll<-rn-2.97*sern
rn<-exp(rn)
u<-exp(u)
l<-exp(l)
uu<-exp(uu)
ll<-exp(ll)
x1<-min(ll)
x2<-max(uu)
plot(rn,axes=F,ylim=c(x1,x2),col="blue",pch=19,lwd=4,
main="HGLM Shrinkage Staphylococcus aureus Bacteraemias.",
xlab="SMR, 2 & 3 SD equivalent limits blue.",
ylab="SMR.")
box()
abline(h=1)
par(cex=.7)
axis(side=1,tick=T,staph[,1],at=1:length(staph[,1]))
axis(side=c(2,3,4))
par(cex=1)
points(l,pch="-",lwd=3,col="blue",cex=1.5)
points(u,pch="-",lwd=3,col="blue",cex=1.5)
arrows(1:length(rn),ll,1:length(rn),uu,angle=90,code=3,lwd=2,
col="blue",length=.15)
mtext("Hospitals.",side=1,line=2)


#using lmer in the lme4/arm libraries, figure not shown
library(arm)
l<-lmer(staph[,2]~1+(1|staph[,1]),offset=log(staph[,4]),family=poisson)
rn<-ranef(l)
rf<-as.numeric(fixef(l))
sern<-se.ranef(l)
rn<-rn[[1]][,1]
sern<-sern[[1]][,1]
u<-rn+1.96*sern
l<-rn-1.96*sern
uu<-rn+2.97*sern
ll<-rn-2.97*sern
rn<-exp(rn)
u<-exp(u)
l<-exp(l)
uu<-exp(uu)
```

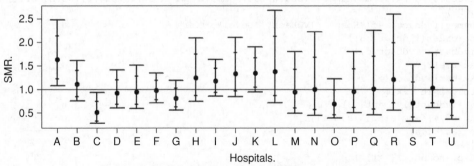

HGLM Shrinkage Plot Staphylococcus aureus Bacteraemias.

Hospitals.
Shrinkage prediction points with 2 & 3 SD equivalent limits arrows.

Figure 5.12   Empirical Bayes shrinkage plot (HGLM).

```
ll<-exp(ll)
x1<-min(ll)
x2<-max(uu)
plot(rn,axes=F,ylim=c(x1,x2),col="blue",pch=19,lwd=4,
main="LMER Shrinkage Staphylococcus aureus Bacteraemias.",
xlab="SMR, 2 & 3 SD equivalent limits blue.",
ylab="SMR.")
box()
abline(h=1)
par(cex=.7)
axis(side=1,tick=T,staph[,1],at=1:length(staph[,1]))
axis(side=c(2,3,4))
par(cex=1)
points(l,pch="-",lwd=3,col="blue",cex=1.5)
points(u,pch="-",lwd=3,col="blue",cex=1.5)
arrows(1:length(rn),ll,1:length(rn),uu,angle=90,code=3,lwd=2,
col="blue",length=.15)
mtext("Hospitals.",side=1,line=2)
```

5.7   Performing further tabulations in R

Table 5.6 is similar to Table 5.1 illustrated above but for intravenous device-related *Staphylococcus aureus* bacteraemias and Table 5.7 shows MRSA bacteraemias. In each case there is marked overdispersion, largely related to inadequate risk stratification by hospital level. However, by selecting various combinations of hospitals, years and quarters, the data can be viewed in a number of ways that may be of interest. Each of these tables may be placed in an office program for further formatting by using s.d(TableName) and the clipboard. We use the hospital level to illustrate the method for incorporating risk stratification in the analysis of these data. See section 5.8 for further discussion of risk stratification.

```
# Table 5.6, IV device-related Staphylococcus aureus bacteraemias
library(exactci)
IVDBact<-xtabs(bact[,5]~bact[,1])
```

```
OBD<-tapply(obd[,3],obd[,1],sum)
ivdbact<-data.frame(names(IVDBact),as.numeric(IVDBact),level[,2],as.numeric
(OBD))
names(ivdbact)<-c("Hosp","IVDBact","Level","OBD")
o<-order(ivdbact[,3])
ivdbact<-ivdbact[o,]
a<-0;a1<-0
x<-max(ivdbact[,3])
for (i in 1:x){
a<-ivdbact[ivdbact[,3]==i,]
a<-a[,4]*sum(a[,2])/sum(a[,4])
a1<-c(a1,a)
}
Exp<-round(a1[-1],2)
staph<-data.frame(ivdbact[,-3],Exp)
o<-order(staph[,1])
ivdstaph<-staph[o,]
k<-0
O<-ivdstaph[,2];E<-ivdstaph[,4]
for (i in 1:length(O)){k[i]<-poisson.exact(O[i],E[i])$p.value/2}
z<-0
for (i in 1:length(O)){if (O[i]<E[i]){z[i]<-qnorm(k[i])}
else{z[i]<--qnorm(k[i])}}
Exp<-round(E,2)
Z<-round(z,2)
ivdstaph<-data.frame(ivdstaph,Z)
ivdstaph
```

	Hosp	IVDBact	OBD	Exp	Z
1	A	39	468258	16.29	4.71
2	B	37	996889	34.68	0.33
3	C	6	416680	14.50	-2.31
4	D	22	414792	29.64	-1.34
5	E	11	530172	18.45	-1.70
6	F	102	1324524	94.65	0.71
7	G	29	755547	53.99	-3.62
8	H	8	284507	9.90	-0.40
9	I	92	1005113	71.82	2.25
10	J	16	405020	14.09	0.41
11	K	50	628268	44.90	0.70
12	L	3	135334	2.30	0.24
13	M	2	221283	3.76	-0.60
14	N	1	77394	1.32	0.00
15	O	9	365871	12.73	-0.90
16	P	7	179278	6.24	0.17
17	Q	2	74908	1.27	0.35
18	R	3	80094	1.36	1.01
19	S	2	102317	3.56	-0.50
20	T	6	303590	10.56	-1.29
21	U	2	175836	2.99	-0.19

Table 5.6

```
# Table 5.7, MRSA bacteraemias
library(exactci)
```

```
MRSABact<-xtabs(bact[,6]~bact[,1])
OBD<-tapply(obd[,3],obd[,1],sum)
mrsabact<-data.frame(names(MRSABact),as.numeric(MRSABact),level[,2],
as.numeric(OBD))
names(mrsabact)<-c("Hosp","MRSABact","Level","OBD")
o<-order(mrsabact[,3])
mrsabact<-mrsabact[o,]
a<-0;a1<-0
x<-max(mrsabact[,3])
for (i in 1:x){
a<-mrsabact[mrsabact[,3]==i,]
a<-a[,4]*sum(a[,2])/sum(a[,4])
a1<-c(a1,a)
}
Exp<-round(a1[-1],2)
staph<-data.frame(mrsabact[,-3],Exp)
o<-order(staph[,1])
mrsa<-staph[o,]
k<-0
O<-mrsa[,2];E<-mrsa[,4]
for (i in 1:length(O)){k[i]<-poisson.exact(O[i],E[i])$p.value/2}
z<-0
for (i in 1:length(O)){if (O[i]<E[i]){z[i]<-qnorm(k[i])}
else{z[i]<--qnorm(k[i])}}
Exp<-round(E,2)
Z<-round(z,2)
mrsa<-data.frame(mrsa,Z)
mrsa
```

	Hosp	MRSABact	OBD	Exp	Z
			Table 5.7		
1	A	24	468258	13.29	2.57
2	B	42	996889	28.29	2.35
3	C	5	416680	11.82	−2.00
4	D	4	414792	16.78	−3.52
5	E	6	530172	15.04	−2.44
6	F	54	1324524	53.58	0.01
7	G	21	755547	30.56	−1.70
8	H	6	284507	8.07	−0.51
9	I	43	1005113	40.66	0.31
10	J	13	405020	11.49	0.34
11	K	45	628268	25.42	3.45
12	L	3	135334	1.77	0.64
13	M	1	221283	2.89	−0.79
14	N	3	77394	1.01	1.39
15	O	3	365871	10.38	−2.42
16	P	2	179278	5.09	−1.19
17	Q	0	74908	0.98	−0.32
18	R	3	80094	1.05	1.34
19	S	1	102317	2.90	−0.79
20	T	13	303590	8.61	1.29
21	U	0	175836	2.30	−1.28

5.8   Adjusting hospital levels for MRSA bacteraemia

Tong and colleagues recommended that, for *Staphylococcus aureus* bacteraemias, expected counts could be estimated using a regression model with relevant hospital services as explanatory variables, for example, renal dialysis, oncology and infectious diseases. For MRSA bacteraemia they recommended, for the data in our example, modifying the hospital levels based on similar explanatory variables. We illustrate the effect of this modification on expected MRSA bacteraemia rates in Figure 5.13. The overdispersion is reduced, for example, the standard deviation of the Z-scores falls from 1.81 to 1.19 (1.16 with removal of hospitals with less than one expected bacteraemia). Table 5.8 illustrates the MRSA data using the modified hospital levels.

```
#uses data from the files hasaureusbact.csv, levels1.csv & obd.csv
#levels1.csv contains the adjusted levels for MRSA bacteraemia
g.d() #levels1, the first column is not a date column
level<-datain

library(exactci)
MRSABact<-xtabs(bact[,6]~bact[,1])
OBD<-tapply(obd[,3],obd[,1],sum)
mrsabact<-data.frame(names(MRSABact),as.numeric(MRSABact),level[,2],
as.numeric(OBD))
names(mrsabact)<-c("Hosp","MRSABact","Level","OBD")
o<-order(mrsabact[,3])
mrsabact<-mrsabact[o,]
a<-0;a1<-0
x<-max(mrsabact[,3])
for (i in 1:x){
a<-mrsabact[mrsabact[,3]==i,]
a<-a[,4]*sum(a[,2])/sum(a[,4])
a1<-c(a1,a)
}
Exp<-round(a1[-1],2)
staph<-data.frame(mrsabact[,-3],Exp)
o<-order(staph[,1])
mrsa<-staph[o,]
k<-0
O<-mrsa[,2];E<-mrsa[,4]
for (i in 1:length(O)){k[i]<-poisson.exact(O[i],E[i])$p.value/2}
z<-0
for (i in 1:length(O)){if (O[i]<E[i]){z[i]<-qnorm(k[i])}
else{z[i]<--qnorm(k[i])}}
Exp<-round(E,2)
Z<-round(z,2)
mrsa<-data.frame(mrsa,Z)
mrsa # Table 5.8 now remove hospitals with Es less than one, see section 5.5)
#
which(mrsa[,4]<1)
# [1] 14 17 18
# remove from funnel plot calculations, audit cases
#
sd(Z[-c(14,17,18)])
#
#[1] 1.161
```

```
# Poisson funnel plot Figure 5.13 (Laney's correction 1.16)
O<-mrsa[-c(14,17,18),2];E<-mrsa[-c(14,17,18),4];H<-mrsa[-c(14,17,18),1];
D<-mrsa[-c(14,17,18),3]
TT<-E
AA<-0
U<-0
Z<-.02275
for (i in 1:length(TT)){
M<-TT[i]
X<-M
A<-1
BL<-F
while (BL==F){
X<-X+A
K<-pgamma(M,X,1)
if (K<Z){BL<-T}
}
AA<-.001
BL<-F
while (BL==F){
X<-X-AA
K<-pgamma(M,X,1)
if (K>=Z){BL<-T}
}
U[i]<-X
}
TT<-E
AA<-0
UU<-0
Z<-.0015
for (i in 1:length(TT)){
M<-TT[i]
X<-M
A<-1
BL<-F
while (BL==F){
X<-X+A
K<-pgamma(M,X,1)
if (K<Z){BL<-T}
}
AA<-.001
BL<-F
while (BL==F){
X<-X-AA
K<-pgamma(M,X,1)
if (K>=Z){BL<-T}
}
UU[i]<-X
}
TT<-E
L<-0
AA<-0
Z<-.02275
for (i in 1:length(TT)){
M<-TT[i]
X<-0
```

```
if(1-pgamma(M,X+1,1)>=Z){X<-0}else{
A<-1
BL<-F
while (BL==F){
X<-X+A
K<-1-pgamma(M,X+1,1)
if (K>Z){BL<-T}
}
AA<-.001
BL<-F
while (BL==F){
X<-X-AA
K<-1-pgamma(M,X+1,1)
if (K<=Z){BL<-T}
}
}
L[i]<-X
}
TT<-E
LL<-0
AA<-0
Z<-.0015
for (i in 1:length(TT)){
M<-TT[i]
X<-0
if(1-pgamma(M,X+1,1)>=Z){X<-0}else{
A<-1
BL<-F
while (BL==F){
X<-X+A
K<-1-pgamma(M,X+1,1)
if (K>Z){BL<-T}
}
AA<-.001
BL<-F
while (BL==F){
X<-X-AA
K<-1-pgamma(M,X+1,1)
if (K<=Z){BL<-T}
}
}
LL[i]<-X
}
# Laney's correction
U<-E+(U-E)*1.16
UU<-E+(UU-E)*1.16
L<-E-(E-L)*1.16
LL<-E-(E-LL)*1.16
L[L<0]<-0
LL[LL<0]<-0
oe<-O/E
w<-UU-LL
o<-order(w)
O1<-O[o];E1<-E[o];H1<-H[o];D1<-D[o]
oe1<-oe[o]
L1<-L[o];L2<-L1/E1
LL1<-LL[o];LL2<-LL1/E1
U1<-U[o];U2<-U1/E1
```

```
UU1<-UU[o];UU2<-UU1/E1
plot(oe1,ylim=c(0,max(c(oe1,UU2))),axes=F,col="blue",pch=19,
main="In-hospital MRSA Bacteraemias with Laney's correction.",
xlab="SMR Blue, 2 & 3 SD Control Limits Red",ylab="SMRs")
box()
par(cex=.8)
axis(side=1,labels=H1,at=1:length(H1))
axis(side=c(2,3,4))
par(cex=1)
lines(U2,col="red",lty=2,lwd=2)
lines(L2,col="red",lty=2,lwd=2)
lines(UU2,col="red",lty=1,lwd=2)
lines(LL2,col="red",lty=1,lwd=2)
abline(h=1)
par(font=2)
text(oe1,labels=as.character(round(O1,0)),pos=3,offset=.3,cex=.8,lwd=3,
col="green4")
text(oe1,labels=as.character(round(D1/1000,0)),pos=1,offset=.3,cex=.8,
lwd=3,col="brown4")
par(font=1)
mtext("Hospitals",side=1,line=2)
legend(locator(1),
legend=c("Counts Green","Denominators(thousands) Brown"),
pch=19,col=c("green4","brown4"),cex=.8)
```

	Hosp	MRSABact	OBD	Exp	Z
			Table 5.8		
1	A	24	468258	22.02	0.35
2	B	42	996889	46.88	−0.63
3	C	5	416680	9.12	−1.23
4	D	4	414792	9.07	−1.62
5	E	6	530172	11.60	−1.58
6	F	54	1324524	62.29	−0.99
7	G	21	755547	16.53	0.98
8	H	6	284507	6.22	0.00
9	I	43	1005113	47.27	−0.53
10	J	13	405020	8.86	1.20
11	K	45	628268	29.55	2.59
12	L	3	135334	2.96	0.00
13	M	1	221283	2.25	−0.41
14	N	3	77394	0.79	1.68
15	O	3	365871	3.72	−0.03
16	P	2	179278	1.83	0.00
17	Q	0	74908	0.76	−0.08
18	R	3	80094	0.82	1.64
19	S	1	102317	1.04	0.00
20	T	13	303590	6.64	2.08
21	U	0	175836	1.79	−0.97

5.9   Bacteraemia risk adjustment

In order to illustrate risk adjustment for bacteraemias we have employed the R geepack function geeglm(). The model has incorporated hospital services from 23 hospitals. There were five years' data divided into 10 half-yearly periods in the file staphbact.xls.

```
g.d() # staphbact.xls Sheet2
```

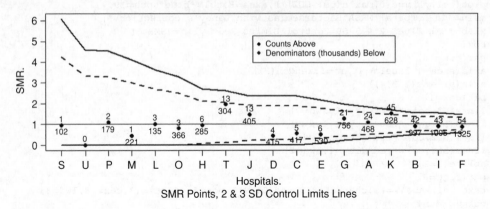

Figure 5.13 SMR funnel plot, hospitals on horizontal axis (Poisson limits with Laney's correction).

The dependent variable of interest is bacteraemias due to *Staphylococcus aureus*. The following was the best fitting model –

```
library(geepack)
g<-geeglm(inpat_staph~icu_level1+icu_level2+infectious_level1+
infectious_level2+renalrnephrology+cardiacsurgeryservices+neurosurgery+
transplantorgan, id=Hosp,data=datain,offset=log(pdays),family=poisson,
corstr="ar1")

summary(g)
```

```
Coefficients:
                                Estimate   Std.err      Wald    Pr(>|W|)
(Intercept)                      -10.287     0.288   1271.84     < 2e-16
datain$icu_level2                  1.139     0.288     15.59     7.8e-05
datain$icu_level1                  0.861     0.322      7.14      0.0075
datain$infectious_level1           0.334     0.145      5.32      0.0210
datain$infectious_level2           1.307     0.145     81.57     < 2e-16
datain$renalrnephrology            0.341     0.143      5.64      0.0175
datain$cardiacsurgeryservices      1.477     0.145    104.19     < 2e-16
datain$neurosurgery               -1.385     0.287     23.22     1.4e-06
datain$transplantorgan            -1.573     0.145    118.24     < 2e-16
Estimated Scale Parameters:
           Estimate Std.err
(Intercept)    1.27    0.182
Correlation: Structure = ar1   Link = identity
Estimated Correlation Parameters:
      Estimate Std.err
alpha    0.263  0.0518
Number of clusters:    23    Maximum cluster size: 10
```

```
# Table of observed and expected counts
library(exactci)
StaphBact<-data.frame(datain$Hosp,datain$inpat_staph,g$fitted)
```

```
Obs<-tapply(StaphBact[,2],StaphBact[,1],sum)
Emodel<-tapply(StaphBact[,3],StaphBact[,1],sum)
N<-tapply(datain$pdays,datain$Hosp,sum)
Edata<-N*sum(Obs)/sum(N)
P<-0
Z<-0
for (i in 1:length(N))
{P[i]<-poisson.exact(Obs[i],Emodel[i])$p.value}
for (i in 1:length(N)){if (Obs[i]>Emodel[i]){Z[i]<--qnorm(P[i]/2)}
else{Z[i]<-qnorm(P[i]/2)}}
PD<-0
ZD<-0
for (i in 1:length(N))
{PD[i]<-poisson.exact(Obs[i],Edata[i])$p.value}
for (i in 1:length(N)){if (Obs[i]>Edata[i]){ZD[i]<--qnorm(PD[i]/2)}
else{ZD[i]<-qnorm(PD[i]/2)}}
STAPH<-data.frame(names(Obs),Obs,Edata,ZD,Emodel,Z)
names(STAPH)<-c("Hosps","Obs","Edata","Zdata","Emodel","Zmodel")
row.names(STAPH)<-1:length(STAPH[,1])
STAPH
```

	Hosps	Obs	Edata	Zdata	Emodel	Zmodel
1	A	64	56.50	0.9341	64.24	0.00000
2	B	58	108.21	−5.2227	56.80	0.11452
3	C	37	41.69	−0.6346	33.72	0.50032
4	D	1	15.35	−4.4928	5.25	−1.84124
5	E	24	22.44	0.2562	25.35	−0.13602
6	F	65	56.23	1.0997	63.50	0.14593
7	G	159	125.69	2.8252	158.51	0.01207
8	H	82	81.54	0.0145	79.08	0.28888
9	I	47	30.22	2.7698	24.44	3.99174
10	J	204	146.57	4.4515	203.57	0.00661
11	K	28	40.57	−1.9756	32.82	−0.74097
12	L	121	73.12	5.0805	120.39	0.02561
13	M	23	22.06	0.1286	17.84	1.09706
14	N	17	31.83	−2.7460	10.88	1.62792
15	O	3	5.49	−0.8324	1.88	0.55233
16	P	11	10.96	0.0000	8.86	0.58955
17	Q	20	45.16	−4.0874	36.52	−2.86261
18	R	24	19.65	0.8778	15.90	1.81824
19	S	1	10.84	−3.5000	3.71	−1.19698
20	T	2	8.00	−2.2056	6.47	−1.70749
21	U	6	12.43	−1.7998	10.05	−1.14199
22	V	21	38.82	−3.0086	31.40	−1.84195
23	W	7	21.61	−3.4706	7.39	0.00000

```
sd(STAPH$Zmodel)
#[1] 1.43
sd(STAPH$Zdata)
#[1] 2.8
```

Unfortunately, the residuals are poorly distributed and a better model must be sought. There were a number of cells with zero entries in the data.frame. However, the general approach is illustrated and the fitted values are a considerable improvement on the expected values calculated from the data.

The data were changed to five yearly groups and four hospitals with many zero results were removed leaving 19 hospitals (a minimum for a GEE analysis) and up to five yearly periods for each hospital. The following model that resulted in approximately normally distributed residuals was developed.

```
g.d() # staphbact.xls Sheet3

g<-geeglm(inpat_staph~icu_level1+icu_level2+infectious_level2+
cardiacsurgeryservices+neurosurgery+transplantorgan,id=Hosp,data=datain,
offset=log(pdays),family=poisson,corstr="ar1")

summary(g)
```

```
Coefficients:
                                Estimate    Std.err        Wald    Pr(>|W|)
(Intercept)                     -9.98e+00   1.94e-01    2.64e+03    < 2e-16
datain$icu_level2                8.96e-01   1.94e-01    2.13e+01    3.9e-06
datain$icu_level1                6.81e-01   2.21e-01    9.45e+00     0.0021
datain$infectious_level2         9.84e-01   4.63e-06    4.51e+10    < 2e-16
datain$cardiacsurgeryservices    1.15e+00   4.69e-06    6.02e+10    < 2e-16
datain$neurosurgery             -7.82e-01   6.90e-06    1.28e+10    < 2e-16
datain$transplantorgan          -1.28e+00   6.91e-06    3.43e+10    < 2e-16
Estimated Scale Parameters:
                Estimate Std.err
(Intercept)         1.51    0.24
Correlation: Structure = ar1 Link = identity
Estimated Correlation Parameters:
        Estimate Std.err
alpha 0.299 0.156
Number of clusters:    19    Maximum cluster size: 5
```

```
# Table of observed and expected counts
library(exactci)
StaphBact<-data.frame(datain$Hosp,datain$inpat_staph,g$fitted)
Obs<-tapply(StaphBact[,2],StaphBact[,1],sum)
Emodel<-tapply(StaphBact[,3],StaphBact[,1],sum)
N<-tapply(datain$pdays,datain$Hosp,sum)
Edata<-N*sum(Obs)/sum(N)
P<-0
Z<-0
for (i in 1:length(N)){P[i]<-poisson.exact(Obs[i],Emodel[i])$p.value}
for (i in 1:length(N)){if (Obs[i]>Emodel[i]){Z[i]<--qnorm(P[i]/2)}
else{Z[i]<-qnorm(P[i]/2)}}
PD<-0
ZD<-0
for (i in 1:length(N)){PD[i]<-poisson.exact(Obs[i],Edata[i])$p.value}
for (i in 1:length(N)){if (Obs[i]>Edata[i]){ZD[i]<--qnorm(PD[i]/2)}
else{ZD[i]<-qnorm(PD[i]/2)}}
STAPH<-data.frame(names(Obs),Obs,Edata,ZD,Emodel,Z)
names(STAPH)<-c("Hosps","Obs","Edata","Zdata","Emodel","Zmodel")
row.names(STAPH)<-1:length(STAPH[,1])
STAPH
```

	Hosps	Obs	Edata	Zdata	Emodel	Zmodel
1	A	64	58.4	0.6823	51.8	1.58606
2	B	58	111.8	−5.5343	56.3	0.17743
3	C	37	43.1	−0.8432	38.3	−0.09504
4	E	24	23.2	0.0992	20.6	0.66275
5	F	65	58.1	0.8477	51.6	1.75245
6	G	159	129.9	2.4421	154.1	0.36836
7	H	82	84.2	−0.1721	81.6	0.00315
8	I	47	31.2	2.5748	27.7	3.27537
9	J	204	151.4	4.0306	204.2	0.00000
10	K	28	41.9	−2.1738	37.2	−1.46344
11	L	121	75.5	4.7734	120.4	0.02584
12	M	23	22.8	0.0000	20.2	0.52982
13	N	17	32.9	−2.9157	14.8	0.48108
14	P	11	11.3	0.0000	10.1	0.19296
15	Q	20	46.7	−4.2845	41.4	−3.57858
16	R	24	20.3	0.7274	18.0	1.26719
17	U	6	12.8	−1.9056	11.4	−1.52671
18	V	21	40.1	−3.1961	35.6	−2.52424
19	W	7	22.3	−3.6030	10.0	−0.78225

```
sd(STAPH$Zmodel)
#[1] 1.55
sd(STAPH$Zdata)
#[1] 2.78
```

This analysis, that is beyond the scope of these notes, is not meant to be definitive but rather to give readers an idea of the sort of approach described by Tong and colleagues. There is another R GEE program, gee() from the gee library that gives similar results. It is said that no statistical package does every analysis that may be required and it is possible that the above analysis may be better performed with alternative software.

We are indebted to Mrs Mohana Rajmokan MSc (Biostatistics), statistician at the Queensland Health Centre for Health Related Infection Surveillance and Prevention (CHRISP) who has continued the work of Tong and colleagues. Risk adjustment for hospital antibiotic usage has recently been described by Rajmokan and colleagues (to appear). A considerable limitation has been the relatively small number of available hospitals. Another possible limitation would be if, for example, icu_level 1 was associated with these AEs but icu_level 2 was not. This would suggest that the smaller hospitals with level 1 ICUs might be less conscientious at applying bundles for the prevention of these AEs. The object of the analysis is to make hospital rates appearing in, for example, funnel plots fairer, not to obscure important reasons for the occurrence of the AE. Work in this very important area is in its early development and it is hoped that this note, together with the work of Tong and colleagues and Rajmokan and colleagues, will stimulate interest in further developing risk adjustment for count data AEs and other relevant agents such as antibiotics.

6

Sequential count and rate data

In this chapter we describe the analysis of sequential count and rate data. Some important issues are summarised in the box.

```
 1. Tabulations,
 2. Denominators and outliers,
 3. Bar and run charts,
 4. Shewhart control charts,
 5. EWMA control charts,
 6. CUSUM charts for count data,
 7. Cumulative O-E charts for count data,
 8. Overdispersion,
 9. Autocorrelation,
10. Spline smoothing,
11. Generalised additive model (GAM) charts.
```

To aid in the selection of a suitable method, there is an appendix Control Chart Menu at the end of the introductory chapter. In addition, there is a corresponding function CCMenu() in rprogs. There is also a Supplement on the internet.

Although examining grouped and aggregated data is important, it is by analysing sequentially accumulating data that we can get timely warning of system changes or unforeseen problems. There is often some delay in acquiring these data (for example, a microbiology specimen is collected, it is processed and then the result is reported). However, for many practical purposes, analyses at the end of each month suffice provided there is a surveillance team working daily in the wards to ensure compliance with bundles and checklists (Chapter 8, section 8.4.2) and to be alert for any unusual occurrences.

Sequential analysis also has the ability to help staff resist tampering with systems in the face of changes that are predictable and often random in nature. However, a single case of an

Statistical Methods for Hospital Monitoring with R, First Edition. Anthony Morton, Kerrie Mengersen,
Michael Whitby and George Playford.
© 2013 John Wiley & Sons, Ltd. Published 2013 by John Wiley & Sons, Ltd.

unusual adverse event (AE) or unusually serious AE should be dealt with immediately using, for example, an M&M audit and systems analysis as described by Singer and by Vincent.

6.1   Grouping data

Count data hospital adverse events are often available as a column of dates that indicate when they occurred. It is usual to analyse these data by months although occasionally daily, weekly, quarterly or even yearly grouping is employed. A difficulty may occur when the data are sparse if there are periods at the beginning or end of a series that have no events. This is different from there being no events because the period of interest was not or has not yet been observed.

While it is possible to add extra weeks or months with zero occurrences in R, one must take care, especially when there are denominator data available and these must be matched with the AE data. The weeks or months need to coincide with the denominator data.

Although the above data management may involve considerable complexity, it needs only to be done once when the same adverse outcome data are being used in control charts each week, month or quarter. For example, with monthly data, one might start with two or three years of data. Then as each new month's data become available, a new chart can be produced with the most recent month added and the earliest one discarded, the required data being held in, for example, a spreadsheet from month to month.

6.2   Means and variances, predictability

An important consideration is the need to obtain, when possible, the true mean for the process (and for clustered data or excessively variable or overdispersed data, the correct variance). This may require the removal of any obvious outlier data values. Outliers should be removed carefully, since these values may be a true part of the distribution or may be a signal of a problem or changed performance. Moreover, with some data it is unrealistic to expect a meaningful average value. For example, what should the average monthly amount of an antibiotic's use be when usage will be determined by the hospital's changing microbial population? This is also often the case with multiple antibiotic resistant organism prevalence (MRO Burden). In addition, some data, such as length of stay (LOS) have markedly skewed distributions that may sometimes resemble, at least approximately, fractal (power law) distributions. Such distributions have no interpretable mean value. In these cases, conventional control charts fail and alternative methods such as spline regression (generalised additive model or GAM) charts are a useful alternative. We deal with these data particularly in Chapter 7.

When surveillance is commencing and the system of interest is yet to be brought into a predictable state, the numbers of AEs may increase substantially due to better reporting. For analysis in a control chart, predictable data must be available so that reliable patterns, expected or mean values and associated variation can be determined. Tabulation or a run or GAM chart (Morton[B] and colleagues) may be valuable when predictable data are unavailable.

Many hospital AE counts can be modelled as having a Poisson distribution. Under the Poisson distribution, the observations are independent and the standard deviation (SD) is approximately equal to the square root of the mean. Thus one way of assessing whether this distribution is indeed appropriate is to evaluate if this relationship holds. However, may AEs such as multiple antibiotic resistant organism (MRO) colonisations and infections cannot be modelled as Poisson since they are not independent and variation is frequently greater than expected under these distributions. A common alternative is to employ the negative binomial distribution to describe these data. The weighted variance approach described by Bissell can be used when there are differing denominators. Excessive variability can be dealt with using the method described by Mohammed[A] and Laney; this is straightforward to implement and in most cases it appears to provide control limits that are very similar to those produced by the negative binomial approach. See Chapter 5 (sections 1, 2 3, 5, 8) and the internet Supplement for further discussion and R code.

As already noted, in some cases it is impossible to determine a stable mean value and we then use a GAM analysis and chart to display and analyse the data. Occasionally, monthly count data display autocorrelation. Although a moving average EWMA (MAEWMA) chart, as described by Montgomery, can be used in this situation, its interpretation can be difficult and we also prefer to employ a GAM chart with these data.

For finding the variance for data that have differing denominators (e.g. monthly MRSA colonisations and occupied bed-days denominators), the weighted variance of the mean count (Bissell[A,B]) can be calculated $[V^* = \{1/(N-1)\} \times \{W_i(X_i/W_i-M)^2\}]$, where N is the number of time periods and M is the mean count $(\sum X_i/N)$. X_i is the count for time period i and W_i is the denominator for that time period (D_i) divided by the mean of the denominators $(\sum D_i/N)$. This differs from the variance of the weighted mean $M^{**} = \sum(X_i \times D_i)/\sum D_i$. The variance of the weighted mean $V^{**} = \sum(D_i \times (X_i-M)^2)/(((N-1)/N) \times \sum D_i)$. For the remainder of the chapter we use the Bissell weighted variance of the mean, for example, in the negative binomial Shewhart and EWMA control charts.

6.3   Tabulations

First we use the data in mrsabact.csv and obd0111.csv to illustrate tabulations by months and quarters, and the calculation of the weighted variance. It is important to get the correct time period. Surveillance may start before and end after adverse events (AEs) of interest occur. Inspection of the denominator data, if available, will help to identify the required time period.

```
g.d() # getting mrsabact.csv data into R in data.frame datain
```

```
Loading data.
Data from clipboard (C) or file (F) c
Do data column(s) have heading(s) (Y/N) y
Is column 1 a date column (Y/N) y
Date format.
  6-Feb-01
Date format.
Enter the required date format d-mmm-yy
```

```
head(datain)
```

	DATE
1	06-Feb-2001
2	12-Aug-2001
3	03-Dec-2001
4	14-Jan-2002
5	14-Jan-2002
6	19-Jan-2002

Using function monthlycounts() to tabulate by months
monthlycounts(datain) # monthly counts in dataout

```
The first date is 06-Feb-2001
Is an earlier date required (Y/N) y
Enter the new starting date 1-Jan-2001
The last date is 30-Dec-2011
Is a later date required (Y/N) y
Enter the new finishing date 31-Dec-2011
```

head(dataout)

	Dates	Counts
1	01-Jan-2001	0
2	01-Feb-2001	1
3	01-Mar-2001	0
4	01-Apr-2001	0
5	01-May-2001	0
6	01-Jun-2001	0

```
# using function countquarters() to tabulate by quarters
countquarters(dataout)

# data are in countqtr
s.d(countqtr) # to data file
```

```
Use clipboard (c) or a data file (f) f
Enter a file name h:/countquarters
```

```
#getting corresponding monthly denominator data obd0111.csv
g.d()

# matching the monthly counts and denominators
ae<-data.frame(dataout,datain[,2])
names(ae)<-c("Months","Counts","Denoms")
head(ae)
```

	Months	Counts	Denoms
1	01-Jan-2001	0	18279
2	01-Feb-2001	1	19604
3	01-Mar-2001	0	19527
4	01-Apr-2001	0	16504
5	01-May-2001	0	21187
6	01-Jun-2001	0	20496

```
# using function ratequarters() to tabulate by quarters
ratequarters(ae)

#data in rateqtr
s.d(rateqtr) # to data file
```

```
Use clipboard (c) or a data file (f) f
Enter a file name h:/ratequarters
```

```
#using function wtdvar() to obtain mean and weighted variance
wtdvar(ae[,2],ae[,3]) # monthly data
```

```
The mean count is 0.818.
The mean denominator is 23263.
The weighted variance (V) is 0.734.
```

```
wtdvar(rateqtr[,2],rateqtr[,3]) # quarterly data
```

```
The mean count is 2.455.
The mean denominator is 69790.
The weighted variance (V) is 3.164.
```

6.4   Denominators

The most frequently used denominator for hospital adverse outcome count data is occupied bed-days. Device related denominators include central line days and ventilator days. Occupied bed-days data are usually readily available either daily or, more frequently, aggregated by months. Central line days in intensive care and oncology-haematology units are usually monitored and the method can be employed for ventilator days. However, the diagnosis of ventilator-related pneumonia (VAP) can be imprecise and, although ICUs apply VAP bundles and checklists and carefully review cases presenting with fever, leukocytosis, purulent sputum and pulmonary infiltrates, statistical monitoring of VAP and ventilator-days does not appear to be universal.

There are several ways that central line days can be counted (www.clabsi.com.au/clabsi-surveillance). Ideally, when there is suitable computerisation, the number of days each patient has one or more central lines in place can be calculated. Alternatively, the number of patients with a central line in place each day can be counted. Bundles for the prevention of central line associated bloodstream infections and ventilator related pneumonia including advice on calculating device days and infection rates are available, for example, from the Institute of Healthcare Improvement (IHI).

There are difficulties with these denominators. First, occupied bed-days include patients having a wide spectrum of susceptibility. For example, when counting new infections with MROs during the Christmas–New Year period in Australia, overall occupied bed-days may be reduced because of suspension of some more minor routine surgery. However, these patients are usually at low risk of developing MRO colonisation or infection. At this time there may be no reduction in the number of seriously ill and injured and therefore at risk patients. This problem may be partially dealt with by counting patients and bed-days within departments such as intensive care, renal-dialysis and oncology-haematology that are less susceptible to this fluctuation. In addition, these data may be displayed using functions for plotting counts and denominators separately on the same chart; see, for example, the R routines shewcountdenom() and ewmacountdenom().

A further difficulty is that these denominators can include causes as well as denominators. For example, patients requiring long periods of mechanical ventilation or long periods of treatment requiring central lines or urinary catheters are likely to be more at risk of infection than patients requiring these devices for short periods. One department may have a large number of patients requiring short-term mechanical ventilation and another department fewer patients but requiring ventilation for longer periods. Their device-days denominators may be similar but their susceptibilities to device related infections differ. This can also apply to central line days (McLaws and Berry) and occupied bed-days. It is useful to record the number of patients with devices and the length of time the devices have been employed as well as the number of device days so that device usage can be assessed. Process surveillance of device usage should be employed to ensure compliance with current evidence-based practice incorporated in bundles and checklists. Analysis of sequential data from individual hospitals or units within them where workloads are relatively stable should minimise this problem.

The above difficulties with denominators are more likely to produce error when hospitals or departments are being compared. Since individual hospitals and units within them often have relatively stable workloads, assessing their AEs sequentially in control charts or time-series charts is less likely to mislead. Where device usage or bed occupancy does not vary greatly, charting the counts of the AE and the relevant denominator separately can be valuable. Then, if there is a change in the count for which assignable causes cannot be found, examination of the denominator data may show an unusual pattern of usage at that time and this may explain the anomalous result. If this approach is adopted, it is important to account for nonrandom changes in the denominator of interest, such as the addition or closure of beds.

However, in searching for causes, we must realise that hospitals and their component units are complex systems. It is well known that surveillance of AEs with feedback can reduce their rate of occurrence, sometimes called a Hawthorne effect (Wadsworth and colleagues). What may be happening is that subtle improvements in a number of interacting agents that contribute to the occurrence of the AE may occur with the result that the self organisation of the relevant complex system exhibits improved emergent behaviour. We may need to re-think our ideas about the Pareto effect, where most of the problems are believed to have few causes, and about root cause analysis. Instead of one or a few major root causes there may be emergent behaviour resulting from the interaction of a number of less obvious agents.

Denominator data must be employed thoughtfully. Aggregation of daily denominator data by weeks, months or quarters can be performed in R, for example, for months by using the function monthlynumbers() that we refer to in Chapter 7. When using these data in control charts, they need to coincide with the relevant AE, for example with monthly data the counts of the AE and the denominators must refer to the same months. For uncommon AEs the count for some months may be zero, especially at the beginning or end of the series. This is different from having a zero count when there is no surveillance. Once a data table is created in, for example, a spreadsheet, adding the AE counts and denominator values for each succeeding time period requires minimal extra work.

6.5 Shewhart, EWMA and GAM control charts without denominators

The Shewhart control chart is perhaps the best known and most frequently used of the control charts (Montgomery). For a standard Shewhart control chart method, count data require analysis in a C chart for counts or a U chart for rates. This chart is usually based on the Poisson distribution as the monthly counts are conventionally regarded as being independent. As we have described in section 6.2, some hospital count data AEs may not be independent and their variances may be larger than their means; in these cases the negative binomial distribution may be more appropriate than the Poisson distribution for obtaining control chart limits or Poisson based limits can be widened, for example, by the methods described by Spiegelhalter[B,C,D] or Laney (Mohammed[A] and Laney).

The mean count for a conventional Shewhart chart is $M=\sum C_i/N$, where C_i is the number of bacteraemias in month i and N is the number of months. The Poisson based upper 2 SD warning control limit can then be calculated as $U_2=M+2\times\sqrt{M}$ and the other control limits are calculated similarly. However we prefer to calculate exact control limits using the gamma distribution as hospital adverse event samples are often too small for the large sample normal approximation to be accurate. For the U_2 limit, this involves starting with X equal to M rounded upwards and increasing it progressively until, in R notation, pgamma(M,X,1)=0.02275. X is increased continually by one until pgamma(M,X,1)<0.02275. It is then decreased continually by .001 until pgamma(M,X,1)>=0.02275. For example, if M=5, pgamma(M,X,1)<0.02275 when X=11. Then when X=10.411, pgamma(M,X,1)=0.02275. Similar calculations are performed for the other control limits except for the lower limits it is convenient to start at zero and reverse the process using 1-pgamma(M,X+1,1) as X is frequently zero. For the negative binomial counterpart, the upper control limit calculations are similar to the Poisson based calculations except that 1-pbeta(P,R,X) replaces pgamma(M,X,1), where P=M/V, and $R=M^2/(V-M)$ with V the variance. For the lower limit calculations it is again convenient to start at zero and reverse the process using pbeta(P,R,X+1).

We note here two issues in developing these conventional charts. First, there must be sufficient data to make the charts practicable. When the AE is uncommon, for example for monthly data when there may be less than two AEs on average expected each month, it may be preferable to employ a count data CUSUM and cumulative observed minus expected (O-E) chart similar to those described in Chapter 3. There must be sufficient data that are stable, predictable and do not display a trend (e.g. they are in statistical control), so that reliable control limits can be calculated. Otherwise, as discussed in section 6.2, a table, run chart or GAM chart may be a useful alternative to a control chart.

Second, the distributional assumptions on which the chart is based must be valid. Bacteraemias, medication errors and device related infections are usually independent and the mean and variance are often similar so that the conventional Poisson based methods for count data are appropriate. However, many count data AEs such as patient falls, MRO infections and colonisations, needle-stick injuries, pressure ulcers and sometimes bacteraemias tend to cluster and display increased variability. Carriers of MROs are likely to spread the organism to others so these events may not be independent. Patients may have very differing susceptibility to AEs like patient falls, bacteraemias and pressure ulcers and, for staff needle-stick injuries, and these people are often not distributed randomly in the hospital; this too can cause clustering and increased variability. See section 6.2 for further discussion of the problem and possible solutions. If excessive variability is ignored, control limits in control charts will be too narrow, thus predisposing to the occurrence of excessive false positive signals.

We now illustrate some of the suggested approaches to dealing with excessively variable counts. Figure 6.1 is a barchart and Figure 6.2 a negative binomial Shewhart C chart for weekly bacteraemias occurring in 1996. These data are in the file bactdata.csv with conversion to weekly data in the data.frame dataout. Because weeks and years do not necessarily coincide, the first week begins on the last Sunday before the start of the data collection period and ends on the last Saturday after it concludes. The name of the first data period for the chart is then changed to the date that data collection began. Figure 6.3 is a Poisson chart illustrating the

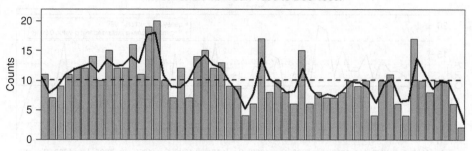

Hospital-acquired bacteraemias by weeks
bar chart from Jan-1996 to Dec-1996.

Data gray, median dashed, smooth continuous.

Figure 6.1 Bar chart.

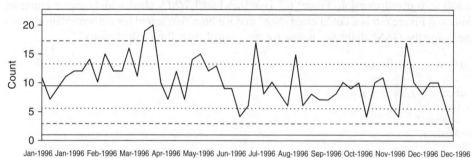

Weekly bacteraemia data
Shewhart chart from Jan-1996 to Dec-1996.

Data black, shewhart limits 1 SD dots, 2 SD dashes, 3 SD continuous.

Figure 6.2 Count data Shewhart chart (negative binomial).

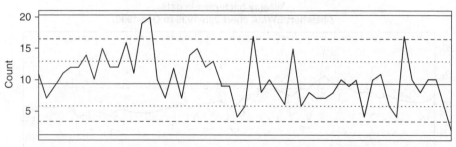

Weekly bacteraemia data (Poisson)
Shewhart chart from Jan-1996 to Dec-1996.

Data black, shewhart limits 1 SD dots, 2 SD dashes, 3 SD continuous.

Figure 6.3 Count data Shewhart chart (Poisson).

Weekly bacteraemia data (Poisson limits & Laney's correction)
shewhart chart from Jan-1996 to Dec-1996.

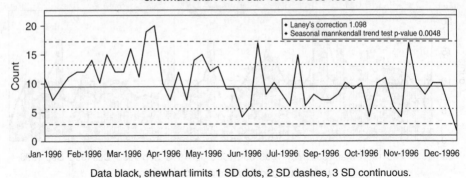

Data black, shewhart limits 1 SD dots, 2 SD dashes, 3 SD continuous.

Figure 6.4 Count data Shewhart chart (Poisson with Laney's correction).

effect of underestimating the variance, Figure 6.4 is a Poisson chart with Laney's correction to deal with overdispersion, Figure 6.5 is a Shewhart/EWMA chart with negative binomial limits and Figure 6.6 is a GAM chart. Note that we have first tested for autocorrelation when employing the GAM chart. See below for the control chart limit calculations.

```
g.d() # bactdata.csv

# arranging data by weeks
d<-datain[,1]
o<-order(d)
d<-d[o]
d[1]
#
#[1] 02-Jan-1996

weekdays(d[1])
#[1] Tue
```

Weekly bacteraemia data
Shewhart/EWMA chart Jan-1996 to Dec-1996.

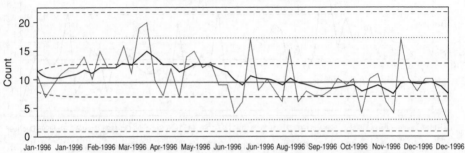

Data & 2, 3 SD shewhart limits gray, EWMA line continuous, EWMA limits dashes.

Figure 6.5 Count data Shewhart/EWMA chart (negative binomial).

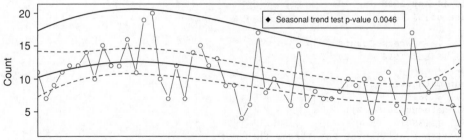

Data gray, fitted GAM thick continuous, 95% CI dashed, control limit black.

Figure 6.6   GAM chart count data, 3 degrees of freedom.

```
weekdays(d[length(d)])
#[1] Tue
fst<-d[1]-2 #last Sunday before data collection period
lst<-d[length(d)]+4 #first Saturday after data collection period
s<-seq.dates(from=fst,to=lst,by="weeks")
k<-NA
for (i in 1:(length(s)-1)){k[i]<-sum(d>=s[i]&d<s[i+1])}
k[length(s)]<-sum(d>=s[length(s)])
s[1]<-d[1]-1 # start of data collection period 01-Jan-1996
dataout<-data.frame(s,k)
names(dataout)<-c("Weeks","Counts")

# using function barnodenom()
barnodenom(dataout)
```

```
Chart heading.
Enter heading for chart Hospital-acquired Bacteraemias by weeks
```

```
# the data appear quite variable
mean(dataout[,2])
#
#[1] 10.11321
var(dataout[,2])
#
#[1] 14.98694
#variance is 48% greater than the mean

locator() # use to define run of more stable data, end with right-click
#
#$x
#[1] 16.04191 50.50187
#$y
#[1] 10.29226 10.19258
# more stable data between 16th and 51st values
#
dataout[16,]
```

```
#
#          Weeks Counts
#16 14-Apr-1996       10
dataout[51,]
#
#          Weeks Counts
#51 15-Dec-1996       10
#
mean(dataout[16:51,2])
#[1] 9.361111
var(dataout[16:51,2])
#[1] 11.38016
# variance still over 20% larger than mean

# search for an overall trend
library(Kendall)
d<-dataout[,2]
s<-SeasonalMannKendall(ts(d))
s
#tau = -0.277, 2-sided pvalue =0.0046315
#time-series Mann-Kendall test suggests a marked overall downward trend

d<-d[16:51] # look for trend in more stable data
s<-SeasonalMannKendall(ts(d))

#tau = -0.0617, 2-sided pvalue =0.61063
# no trend in more stable data, ? a change point not a trend (Chapter 7)

# control chart now OK to use as stable mean and variance
# available from the latter section of the data series

# using function countshew(), Figure 6.2
countshew(dataout) # note change in mean and variance
```

```
The mean count is 10.113.
Do you want to change the mean value (Y/N) y
Enter new value for the mean 9.36
The variance is 14.987 (SD 3.871 ).
Do you want to change the variance (Y/N) y
Enter new value for the variance 11.38
Chart heading.
Enter heading for chart Weekly Bacteraemia Data
```

```
which(dataout[,2]>9.36) # counts above mean value
#[1]  1  4  5  6  7  8  9 10 11 12 13 14 15 16 18 20 21 22 23
28 30 33 39 41 43 44 47 48 50 51
```

There is a run of 13 consecutive data values above the mean (weeks 4 to 16) including a run-sum of 7. Run-sum charts are described in section 3.11 of Chapter 3. These data are therefore unpredictable.

It was noted that the variance of these data exceeded the mean by about 48% when all the data were included and, when the more stable data between the 16th and 51st observations were used, the variance was still about 20% greater than the mean. Figure 6.2 control limits were therefore calculated using the approximate method for the negative binomial. For comparison we have included Figure 6.3 where the control limits were obtained from the Poisson distribution and Figure 6.4 where they were obtained using the Poisson distribution but including Laney's correction. This involves calculating the expected weekly counts and using them to obtain Z-scores (standard normal deviates). Since these are expected to have a mean of zero and a standard deviation of one, the Poisson control limits can be corrected by widening them using the standard deviation of the Z-scores. Figure 6.2 shows contiguous weeks in late March and early April 1996 having counts above the two sigma equivalent line. Figure 6.3 shows, incorrectly, two additional occasions when the upper two sigma equivalent warning limits would have been exceeded. Although Laney's correction was quite modest at just under 10% with these data, Figure 6.4 also correctly classified these two data points, although it may also be incorrect (see below and the internet Supplement).

In addition, with Figure 6.4 we have included the result of the seasonal MannKendall trend test described above that indicates the presence of a significant overall downward trend. However, as we describe in section 6.5.1 of this chapter, there is in this case a possible change point. The R code for Figure 6.3 and 6.4 is in the internet code file, with that for the latter shown below. For Figure 6.3, use countshew() as above, and enter 9.36 for both the mean and the variance. Figure 6.6 is a GAM chart. Further examples are included later in this chapter.

```
# using function countshew(), Figure 6.3
countshew(dataout)
```

```
The mean count is 10.113.
Do you want to change the mean value (Y/N) y
Enter new value for the mean 9.36
The variance is 14.987 (SD 3.871 ).
Do you want to change the variance (Y/N) y
Enter new value for the variance 9.36
Chart heading.
Enter heading for chart
Weekly Bacteraemia Data (Poisson)
```

```
#Shewhart chart Poisson limits & Laney's correction, Figure 6.4
dz<-dataout[,1]
dz<-chron(as.character(dz),format="dd-mmm-yyyy",out.format="dd-mmm-yyyy")
d1<-dataout[,2]
o<-order(dz)
dz<-dz[o];d1<-d1[o]
s1<-paste(months(min(dz)),years(min(dz)))
s2<-paste(months(max(dz)),years(max(dz)))
da1<-paste(months(dz),years(dz))
lda1<-1:length(da1)
#m<-mean(d1)
m<-9.36
#v<-var(d1)
v<-m # variance overridden so Poisson limits calculated
AA<-0
BE<-T
if (v<m*1.05){mstar<-m
vstar<-mstar
BE<-F
```

```
}else{
mstar<-m
vstar<-v}
#lower Poisson control limits
if (BE==F){
L1<-0;L2<-0;L3<-0
for (I in 1:3){
if (I==1){Z<-.15866}
if (I==2){Z<-.02275}
if (I==3){Z<-.00135}
LO<-0
for (i in 1:length(mstar)){
M<-mstar[i]
X<-0
if(1-pgamma(M,X+1,1)>=Z){X<-0}else{
A<-1
BL<-F
while (BL==F){
X<-X+A
K<-1-pgamma(M,X+1,1)
if (K>Z){BL<-T}
}
AA<-.001
BL<-F
while (BL==F){
X<-X-AA
K<-1-pgamma(M,X+1,1)
if (K<=Z){BL<-T}
}
}
LO[i]<-X
}
if (I==1){L1<-LO}
if (I==2){L2<-LO}
if (I==3){L3<-LO}
}
#lower negative binomial control limits
}else{
L1<-0;L2<-0;L3<-0
for (I in 1:3){
if (I==1){Z<-.15866}
if (I==2){Z<-.02275}
if (I==3){Z<-.00135}
LO<-0
for (i in 1:length(mstar)){
M<-mstar[i];V<-vstar[i]
P<-M/V
R<-M^2/(V-M)
X<-0
if(pbeta(P,R,X+1)>=Z){X<-0}else{
A<-1
BL<-F
while (BL==F){
X<-X+A
K<-pbeta(P,R,X+1)
if (K>Z){BL<-T}
```

```
}
AA<-.001
BL<-F
while (BL==F){
X<-X-AA
K<-pbeta(P,R,X+1)
if (K<=Z){BL<-T}
}
}
LO[i]<-X
}
if (I==1){L1<-LO}
if (I==2){L2<-LO}
if (I==3){L3<-LO}
}
}
#upper Poisson control limits
if (BE==F){
U1<-0;U2<-0;U3<-0
for (I in 1:3){
if (I==1){Z<-.15866}
if (I==2){Z<-.02275}
if (I==3){Z<-.00135}
UO<-0
for (i in 1:length(mstar)){
M<-mstar[i]
X<-ceiling(M)
A<-1
BL<-F
while (BL==F){
X<-X+A
K<-pgamma(M,X,1)
if (K<Z){BL<-T}
}
AA<-.001
BL<-F
while (BL==F){
X<-X-AA
K<-pgamma(M,X,1)
if (K>=Z){BL<-T}
}
UO[i]<-X
}
if (I==1){U1<-UO}
if (I==2){U2<-UO}
if (I==3){U3<-UO}
}
#upper negative binomial control limits
}else{
U1<-0;U2<-0;U3<-0
for (I in 1:3){
if (I==1){Z<-.15866}
if (I==2){Z<-.02275}
if (I==3){Z<-.00135}
UO<-0
for (i in 1:length(mstar)){
```

```
M<-mstar[i];V<-vstar[i]
P<-M/V
R<-M^2/(V-M)
X<-ceiling(M)
A<-1
BL<-F
while (BL==F){
X<-X+A
K<-1-pbeta(P,R,X)
if (K<Z){BL<-T}
}
AA<-.001
BL<-F
while (BL==F){
X<-X-AA
K<-1-pbeta(P,R,X)
if (K>=Z){BL<-T}
}
UO[i]<-X
}
if (I==1){U1<-UO}
if (I==2){U2<-UO}
if (I==3){U3<-UO}
}
}
#end of control limit calculations
#Laney's correction
library(exactci)
k<-0
O<-d1;E<-rep(sum(d1)/length(d1),length(d1))
for (i in 1:length(O)){k[i]<-
poisson.exact(O[i],E[i])$p.value/2}
z<-0
for (i in 1:length(O)){if (O[i]<E[i]){z[i]<-
qnorm(k[i])}else{z[i]<--qnorm(k[i])}}
Ln<-sd(z)
U1<-m+(U1-m)*Ln
U2<-m+(U2-m)*Ln
U3<-m+(U3-m)*Ln
L1<-m-(m-L1)*Ln
L2<-m-(m-L2)*Ln
L3<-m-(m-L3)*Ln
#Trend Test
library(Kendall)
s<-SeasonalMannKendall(ts(O))
q<-d1
q1<-rep(m,length(q))
u0<-rep(U1,length(q))
l0<-rep(L1,length(q))
u1<-rep(U2,length(q))
l1<-rep(L2,length(q))
u2<-rep(U3,length(q))
l2<-rep(L3,length(q))
ma0<-"Weekly Bacteraemia Data (Poisson Limits & Laney's correction)"
ma1<-paste("\nShewhart Chart from ",s1," to ",s2,".",sep="")
ma<-paste(ma0,ma1,sep="")
```

```
qr<-paste("Data Blue, Shewhart Limits 1 SD Orange, 2 SD Brown, 3 SD Red.")
uk<-max(c(u2,q));lk<-max(c(0,min(l2)))
par(lab=c(length(da1),5,7))
par(xaxs="i")
plot(q,type="l",lwd=2,col="blue",axes=F,ylim=c(lk,uk),xlab=qr,
ylab="Count",main=ma)
lines(u0,type="l",lwd=2,col="darkorange")
if (min(L1)>0){lines(l0,type="l",lwd=2,col="darkorange")}
lines(u1,type="l",lwd=2,col="brown")
if (min(L2)>0){lines(l1,type="l",lwd=2,col="brown")}
lines(u2,type="l",lwd=2,col="red")
if (min(L3)>0){lines(l2,type="l",lwd=2,col="red")}
box()
par(cex=.8)
axis(side=1,tick=F,labels=da1,at=lda1)
axis(side=c(2,3,4))
par(cex=1)
abline(h=q1,lwd=2,col="black")
msg1<-paste("Laney's Correction ",round(Ln,3),sep="")
msg2<-paste("Seasonal MannKendall Trend Test p-value ",
round(as.numeric(s$sl),4),sep="")
legend(locator(1),legend=c(msg1,msg2),pch=19,
col=c("green4","brown4"),cex=.6)
#The Seasonal MannKendall Trend Test result can be stamped in a vacant
#area of the chart as the locator() function turns the cursor into a
#cross. Place the cursor as required and press the left mouse button.
```

The use of the Laney Z-score correction may involve hospital scientists in making difficult judgements. This is well illustrated by Figure 6.4. Laney's correction was 1.096. However, the mean value of 9.36 was obtained from the predictable data between week 16 and week 51 while, for Laney's correction, the data for the entire year was employed. When Laney's correction is calculated using the predictable data its value is 0.96 so, on this basis, no correction should be made to the Poisson-based chart (Figure 6.3). Thus Figure 6.3 under-estimates the control limits and Figure 6.4 probably includes an incorrect adjustment. Although informal comparisons with monthly data suggest that Laney's correction usually works well, in this case the negative binomial chart (Figure 6.2) is clearly less likely to mislead. An alternative that we prefer and increasingly employ with these and similar data is to use a GAM chart.

```
library(exactci)
q<-dataout[16:51,2]
P<-0
O<-q;E<-rep(sum(q)/length(q),length(q))
for (i in 1:length(O)){P[i]<-poisson.exact(O[i],E[i])$p.value}
Z<--0.862+(0.743-2.404*log(P))^.5
for (i in 1:length(O)){if (O[i]<E[i]){Z[i]<--Z[i]}}
sd(Z) # Laney
#[1] 0.9645443
```

6.5.1   Shewhart/EWMA charts

EWMA (exponentially weighted moving average) charts are generally superior to Shewhart charts for displaying smaller persistent changes in the mean count or rate (Montgomery, Morton[A] and colleagues). When used with large sample normal approximations, the EWMA chart is much less sensitive than the Shewhart chart to the requirement for the data to be approximately normally distributed.

```
#using function countewma() for Figure 6.5
countewma(dataout)
```

```
The mean count is 10.113.
Do you want to change the mean value (Y/N) y
Enter new value for the mean 9.36
The variance is 14.987 (SD 3.871 ).
Do you want to change the variance (Y/N) y
Enter new value for the variance 11.38
Chart heading.
Enter heading for chart Weekly Bacteraemia Data
EWMA weight.
Enter weight between 0.2 & 0.8 .2
EWMA control limit.
Enter limit between 2 & 3 2.5
```

To construct an EWMA chart a weight W has to be selected. This controls the degree of smoothing in the estimated values. Although different weights can give slightly better performance for false negative and false positive errors in different situations, or equivalently better run lengths when the process is in control and when it is out of control, W=0.2 is a suitable general purpose weight for these count data. When very variable or trended data are being analysed, a larger weight such as 0.4 or 0.5 may work better. Use of spline smooth or loess smooth methods and particularly the spline GAM chart approach will often be more valuable in the latter situation. This will be so especially when the data display autocorrelation.

The EWMA chart begins at zero time. We employ loess smoothing using the R function lowess() to determine a suitable starting value. At the first time that data become available, this value is multiplied by 1-W=0.8 and the first data value is multiplied by the weight W=0.2 and the results are added. Thus the EWMA at the first data period is EWMA=$0.2 \times Y_1 + 0.8 \times E$, where E is the starting value and Y_1 is the observed value. Thereafter each new value is multiplied by W=0.2 and added to 1-W=0.8 times the previous EWMA value to give the current EWMA value.

Calculation of the standard deviation for the EWMA chart is complicated for approximately the first six time periods when W=0.2 but thereafter it is straightforward: $SD_E = SD_S \times \sqrt{[W/(2-W)]}$, where SD_E is the EWMA standard deviation, SD_S is the Shewhart chart standard deviation calculated in the usual way for the large sample normal approximation, and W is the weight. Using a weight of 0.2 the formula becomes $SD_E = SD_S/3$. For small samples where control limits based on, for example, the gamma distribution may be preferred, the EWMA control limits will then be 1/3 of the distance from the centreline to the corresponding Shewhart control limit. If the complete formula is required it is $SD_E = SD_S \times \sqrt{[\{w/(2-w)\} \times \{1-(1-w)^{2 \times t}\}]}$, where t is the relevant time period. However, since this chart is useful for examining longer term changes in the process mean, the first few time periods are unlikely to be of great interest. After about six time periods, the two formulas give similar results when W=0.2 but it takes longer to reach this equivalence when W is smaller.

The first few time periods have narrower EWMA control limits because the expected value employed in the calculation of the starting value is considered not to be a variable. An easy way to incorporate this difference in the control chart when W=0.2 is to use the simple formula $SD_E=k\times SD_S/3$ and for the first six time periods k is 0.6, 0.77, 0.86, 0.91, 0.94 and 0.97 respectively; thereafter, $k\approx1$.

When calculating the upper EWMA control limit after the Shewhart limits have been determined using the pgamma() function described in section 6.5 above, the variance V is approximately equal to $((U-M)/E)^2$, where U in the upper Shewhart value for the control limit selected for the EWMA, E=2.5 for, for example, 2.5 standard deviations, and M is the mean. The EWMA control limit can then be determined by the recursive formula $U_{Ei}=M+E\times X_i$ where $X_i=(X_{(i-1)}^2\times(1-W)^2+V\times W^2)^{.5}$, where for the first limit $X_0=0$. To demonstrate the calculations, let M=10 and V=10. The calculations for the first three periods are shown. When denominators differ, these formulas require modification as described in Chapter 3.

```
# calculating the EWMA limits
M<-10
V<-10
X<-0
W<-.2
E<-2.5
# general formula
U<-M+E*V^.5*(W/(2-W))^.5 # (W/(2-W))^.5 = 1/3 when W = .2
U
#[1] 12.63523
# for the first value when W = .2
U<-M+.6*E*V^.5*(W/(2-W))^.5
U
#[1] 11.58114
# for the second value when W = .2
U<-M+.77*E*V^.5*(W/(2-W))^.5
U
#[1] 12.02913
# for the third value when w = .2
U<-M+.86*E*V^.5*(W/(2-W))^.5
U
#[1] 12.2663


# generally for the first value, standard formula
U<-M+E*V^.5*((W/(2-W))*(1-(1-W)^(2*1)))^.5
U
#[1] 11.58114
# for the second value
U<-M+E*V^.5*((W/(2-W))*(1-(1-W)^(2*2)))^.5
U
#[1] 12.02485
# for the third value
U<-M+E*V^.5*((W/(2-W))*(1-(1-W)^(2*3)))^.5
U
#[1] 12.26363


# for the first value, recursive formula
X<-0
X<-(X^2*(1-W)^2+V*W^2)^.5
```

```
U<-M+E*X
U
#[1]  11.58114
# for the second value
X<-(X^2*(1-W)^2+V*W^2)^.5
U<-M+E*X
U
#[1]12.02485
# for the third value
X<-(X^2*(1-W)^2+V*W^2)^.5
U<-M+E*X
U
#[1]  12.26363
```

It is incorrect to include multiple control limits in EWMA charts because of the correlation between successive values, so a single control limit is employed: for example 2.5 has an ARL of approximately 100 when W=0.2 and this will often be suitable with monthly count data.

As discussed in section 6.2, under the Poisson distribution the standard deviation (SD) is approximately equal to the square root of the mean. For count data that can be described using this distribution, the upper 2 SD Shewhart control limit is then $U_2=M+2\times\sqrt{M}$ and the other control limits are calculated accordingly. One and 3 SD limits are frequently included so that run-sum tests described below can be implemented.

There are two considerations when using the square root of the mean to calculate the control limit. First, the sizes of the sequential samples should be adequate for this large sample normal approximation to be used, and this requires a minimum mean value of 5. As already described in section 6.5, we employ gamma distribution exact limits in practice because counts of hospital adverse outcomes are often too small for the large sample normal approximation shown above to be accurate. Poisson based limits derived from the gamma distribution are preferred especially when counts are low but we employ them in all cases. Secondly, as described in section 6.2, the adverse events should be independent and the variance or square of the standard deviation, calculated during a period when the underlying processes are known to be predictable (i.e. it is in statistical control), should be approximately equal to the mean. In the current example, the weekly mean count was 10.11 and the variance was 14.99, nearly 50% greater. For the more stable period (weeks 16 to 51) they were 9.36 and 11.38 with the variance still exceeding the mean so using approximate negative binomial control limits would be preferable.

It can be seen in the figures that the weekly count is lower and less variable for most of the second part of the year. At about the time of this change, the processes for the care of intravenous lines and for performing blood cultures were reviewed. In addition, in the first half of the year, compliance with antibiotic guidelines and general hygiene measures such as hand washing had been improved because of the need to control concurrent *ESBL-Klebsiella pneumoniae* colonisations.

The changes in the control chart indicate that there was both a special cause problem (consecutive high weekly counts in February to April) and common cause change (subsequent change in the mean) during this period, and this is likely to account for the increased variation. In addition, there were more than seven consecutive values above the mean between February and April. We have determined the mean and variance during the most stable period between 14 April and 15 December. An alternative approach, that we would prefer with these data, is to use a GAM analysis. Figure 6.6 is the resulting chart.

Ideally when using a conventional control chart the data should be independent and they should display a run of nontrended data that are predictable (in statistical control) so that reliable control limit values can be obtained. The weekly bacteraemia data show a fall in the bacteraemia counts in the second part of the year. Figure 6.6 illustrates the alternative approach that employs nonparametric spline smoothing via a generalised additive model (GAM). The dashed lines are 95% confidence limits about the GAM spline-smoothed nonparametric trend line. The upper black line is equivalent to a Poisson two sigma control limit above the GAM smoothed line. Although requiring rigorous evaluation, this is motivated by the Poisson outbreak detection (POD) method proposed by Pelecanos and colleagues. It may help detect time periods when the data values are not typical of the time-series. Figure 6.6 suggests that there was a nonlinear trend in the weekly bacteraemia rate. The two high values in the first and second weeks of April do not appear to be outliers in relation to the predicted process mean at that time (they do not exceed the two sigma control limit above the GAM smoothed line). In the Shewhart charts (Figures 6.2 to 6.5) these appeared to be outliers. The high value in the final week of October appears to be an outlier in relation to the estimated mean at that time in the GAM chart; it does not appear to be an outlier in the Shewhart charts. The GAM chart may be superior to the Shewhart chart in the presence of such trends that make it difficult to determine the centre-line and control limits for the latter.

```
#using function countgamauto(), looking for autocorrelation (a2)
countgamauto(dataout) # chart not shown
```

```
Chart heading.
Enter heading for chart Weekly Bacteraemia Data
Change degrees of freedom (Y/N) n
```

Use the locator cross to position the seasonal trend test result.

```
Abbreviated summary:
              Estimate Std. Error t value Pr(>|t|)
(Intercept)   2.298095    0.249083   9.226 4.03e-12 ***
a2           -0.002077    0.015247  -0.136    0.892
a2 shows no evidence of autocorrelation
(Dispersion parameter for quasipoisson family taken to be 1.308088)
    Null deviance: 78.409  on 51  degrees of freedom
Residual deviance: 61.950  on 47  degrees of freedom
  (2 observations deleted due to missingness)
```

```
#using function countgam()
countgam(dataout) # Figure 6.6
```

```
Chart heading.
Enter heading for chart Weekly Bacteraemia Data
Change degrees of freedom (Y/N) n
```

Use the locator cross to position the seasonal trend test result.

```
Abbreviated summary
                    Estimate Std. Error t value Pr(>|t|)
(Intercept)          2.3103      0.1765  13.086   <2e-16 ***
(Dispersion parameter for quasipoisson family taken to be 1.261503)
    Null deviance: 78.486  on 52  degrees of freedom
Residual deviance: 62.085  on 49  degrees of freedom
The model is in mmg.
Type summary(mmg)/predict(mmg,se=T) to see.
tau = -0.277, 2-sided pvalue =0.0046315
```

Changes in default degrees of freedom (DF) are seldom necessary with routine data. However, increasing the DF may provide a better fit, particularly with large data sets. Figure 6.7 may be slightly better visually than Figure 6.6. It may also support a change-point rather than a trend.

```
#testing with 5 DF
id<-1:length(dataout[,1])
mg<-glm(dataout[,2]~bs(id),family=quasipoisson)
mg1<-glm(dataout[,2]~bs(id,df=5),family=quasipoisson)
a<-anova(mg,mg1)
a
```

```
Model 1: dataout[,2] ~ bs(id)
Model 2: dataout[,2] ~ bs(id, df = 5)
  Resid. Df Resid. Dev Df Deviance
1        49     62.085
2        47     55.136  2   6.9484
```

```
1-pchisq(a$Deviance[[2]],2)
#[1] 0.03098701
#the model with 5 degrees of freedom has a slightly better fit
countgam(dataout) # repeat using 5 DF for Figure 6.7
```

```
Chart heading.
Enter heading for chart Weekly Bacteraemia Data (5DF)
Change degrees of freedom (Y/N) y
Enter degrees of freedom 5
```

Use the locator cross to position the seasonal trend test result.

```
The model is in mmg.
Type summary(mmg)/predict(mmg,se=T) to see.
tau = -0.277, 2-sided pvalue =0.0046315
Abbreviated summary
                    Estimate Std. Error t value Pr(>|t|)
(Intercept)          2.1581      0.2389   9.033 7.67e-12 ***
(Dispersion parameter for quasipoisson family taken to be 1.175266)
    Null deviance: 78.486  on 52  degrees of freedom
Residual deviance: 55.136  on 47  degrees of freedom
```

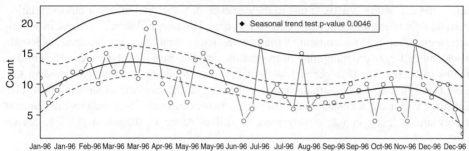

Data gray, fitted GAM thick continuous, 95% CI dashed, control limit black.

Figure 6.7   GAM chart count data, 5 degrees of freedom.

The GAM predicted log mean at the start of the series was 2.31 (log standard error se=0.18); at the peak in mid-March (week 13) it was 2.53 (se=0.080); at its lowest point in November (week 46) it was 2.05 (se=0.094) and at the end of the series it was 2.13 (se=0.20). Using exponentiation, the four predicted values were 10.1, 12.6, 7.8 and 8.5 respectively. The z-score for the difference between the highest and lowest values was 3.9 (p-value=0.0001). This was adjusted using the Benjamini-Hochberg procedure for 53 observations to 0.005 (z=2.7). This suggests that a real difference existed in spite of these comparisons being suggested by the data and therefore to be viewed with great caution. The approximate significance of the GAM smooth terms was: P-value=1-pchisq(78.49-55.14,52-47)=0.00029 indicating substantial changes. A seasonal Mann-Kendall test suggests a substantial overall downward trend in the data values. However, since there is no evidence of autocorrelation and seasonal effects are unusual with these data, a Wilcoxon test can be used to look for a change-point (Pettitt, Siegel and Castellan).

```
library(Kendall)
#overall trend
SeasonalMannKendall(ts(dataout[,2]))
#tau = -0.277, 2-sided pvalue =0.0046315
#
#change point at 16
wilcox.test(dataout[1:15,2],dataout[16:52,2])$p.value
#[1] 0.001592226
#
#no evidence of trend during the second part of the year
SeasonalMannKendall(ts(dataout[16:53,2]))
#tau = -0.149, 2-sided pvalue =0.20442
```

Both the SeasonalMannKendall test and the Wilcoxon test applied to the data for the whole year are highly significant. However, when the SeasonalMannKendall test is applied to the data for the second part of the year, there is no evidence of a trend. Figures 6.1 and 6.2 suggest a stable process during the second part of the year. A change point is therefore more probable. As Montgomery emphasises, the key is to know the process. For example, was a change in the care of central lines implemented before the putative changepoint in response to an elevated bacteraemia rate? If so, how rapid and effective was its implementation? Another issue is the use of the Wilcoxon test in the presence of a seasonal effect or autocorrelation. Seasonal effects are unlikely with bacteraemia data. If autocorrelation is present in weekly bacteraemia data, it is uncommon to see it when bacteraemia data are grouped by months so selecting a larger grouping may overcome the problem provided there are sufficient data for this to be feasible (Runger and Willemain). An alternative is to apply a median test. There is a difficulty when there are many values tied at the median. As shown below, their placement can make a considerable difference. However, even when the ties are removed or they are assigned conservatively there is still evidence to suggest a possible change point.

```
d<-dataout[,2]
m<-median(d)
m
#[1] 10
w<-which(d==m) # ties at median
w
#
#[1]  8 16 30 39 41 43 48 50 51
k<-ifelse(d>m,1,0) # ties not included with larger values
k1<-ifelse(d>=m,1,0) # ties included with larger values (conservative)
s<-rep(1,length(d))
s[1:15]<-0
fisher.test(table(k,s))$p.value
#[1] 0.0003405125
fisher.test(table(k1,s))$p.value
#[1] 0.006369436
d1<-d[d!=m]
s1<-s[d!=m]
k2<-ifelse(d1>m,1,0)
fisher.test(table(k2,s1))$p.value # ties removed
#[1] 0.0009047252
```

6.6   Shewhart, EWMA and GAM control charts with denominators

In routine surveillance practice, it will usually be more stable and still adequately informative to use monthly rather than weekly data. The data in the file bactsall.csv are for 1999 and the first 10 months of 2000. The denominator data are in bactdenom.csv. Figure 6.8 is a barplot that shows the monthly counts and Figure 6.9 and Figure 6.10 are Shewhart and EWMA charts with the bacteraemia counts and the denominators shown separately. Figure 6.11 and Figure 6.12 show rates of bacteraemias per 1000 occupied bed-days in Shewhart and Shewhart/EWMA charts. The mean rate for the Shewhart chart is $M=\sum C_i/\sum N_i$, where C_i is the number of bacteraemias in month i and N_i is the number of occupied bed-days for that month. The U_2 control limit can then be calculated as $U2=M+2\times\sqrt{(M/N_i)}$. These are then multiplied by 1000 for rates per 1000 occupied bed-days. The other control limits are calculated similarly. However we prefer to calculate exact control limits using the gamma

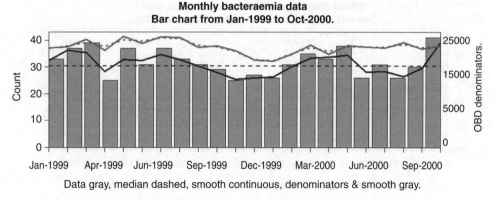

Figure 6.8   Bar chart with superimposition.

distribution as hospital adverse event samples are often too small for the large sample normal approximation to be accurate. Figure 6.13 is a GAM chart.

To implement the gamma distribution control limit approach for rates, the expected count for data period i is $E_i=N_i\times M$. To obtain the 2 SD upper limit, X_i begins at round(E_i) and is increased successively by one until pgamma($E_i,X_i,1$)<.02275. It is then decreased successively by .001 until pgamma($E_i,X_i,1$)>=.02275. The required upper 2 SD value for period i is then X_i/N_i. Similar calculations are performed for the other control limits except for the lower limits it is convenient to start at zero and reverse the process using 1-pgamma($E_i,X_i+1,1$) as the lower limit is frequently zero.

First, we obtain the data in bactsall.csv and group them by months, for example, using monthlycounts(). Next, we get the corresponding denominator data in bactdenom.csv and unite the data and denominators in a data.frame. The two files must come from matching time periods. However, it is necessary to be careful as with sparse data there may be no AEs in some time periods, for example, because there are no data in the first or last time period due to no AEs occurring. This is not the same as there being no surveillance during those periods.

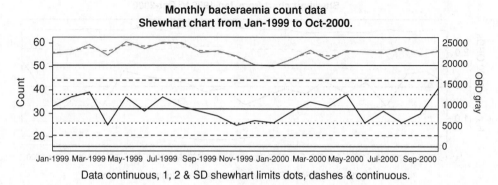

Figure 6.9   Shewhart chart, denominator data separate.

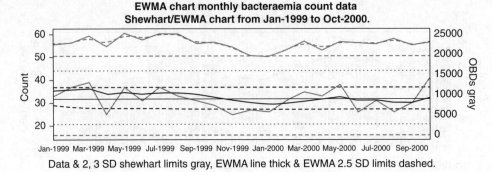

Figure 6.10   Shewhart/EWMA chart, denominator data separate.

Inspection of the denominator data reveals that the period of observation was from January 1999 to October 2000.

```
g.d() # bactsall.csv

# preparing data by months
library(chron)
d<-datain[,1]
o<-order(d)
d<-d[o]
fst<-chron("01/01/1999")
lst<-chron("10/31/2000")
s<-seq.dates(from=fst,to=lst,by="months")
k<-NA
for (i in 1:(length(s)-1)){k[i]<-sum(d>=s[i]&d<s[i+1])}
k[length(s)]<-sum(d>=s[length(s)])
s<-chron(s,format="m/d/y",out.format="dd-mmm-yyyy")
dataout<-data.frame(s,k)
names(dataout)<-c("Months","Counts")
head(dataout)
```

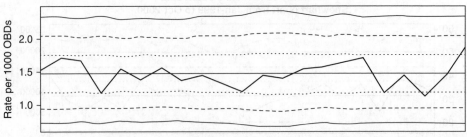

Figure 6.11   Shewhart rate chart.

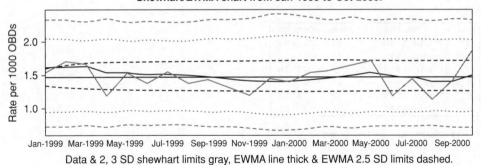

Figure 6.12   Shewhart/EWMA rate chart.

	Months	Counts
1	01-Jan-1999	33
2	01-Feb-1999	37
3	01-Mar-1999	39
4	01-Apr-1999	25
5	01-May-1999	37
6	01-Jun-1999	31

```
# using the function monthlycounts()
monthlycounts(datain)
```

```
The first date is 01-Jan-1999
Is an earlier date required (Y/N) n
The last date is 31-Oct-2000
Is a later date required (Y/N) n
data are now in dataout (see above)
```

```
g.d() # getting denominator data bactdenom.csv
```

```
# amalgamating data
ae<-data.frame(dataout,datain[,2])
```

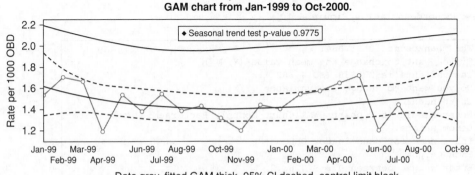

Figure 6.13   GAM chart, rate data using quasipoisson.

```
names(ae)<-c("Months","Counts","Denoms")
head(ae)
```

```
        Months   Counts   Denoms
1     01-Jan-1999     33    21482
2     01-Feb-1999     37    21722
3     01-Mar-1999     39    23415
4     01-Apr-1999     25    21025
5     01-May-1999     37    24112
6     01-Jun-1999     31    22521
```

```
# bar chart using bardenom(),
bardenom(ae) # Figure 6.8
```

```
Chart heading.
Enter heading for chart Monthly Bacteraemia Data
Denominators.
Enter denominator name OBD
```

Shewhart and Shewhart/EWMA charts are now shown, first with the counts and denominators separately and then as rates. In addition, a GAM chart analysis is performed.

```
#for displaying counts and denominators separately
#use shewcountdenom() and ewmacountdenom()
shewcountdenom(ae) # variance not greater than mean, Poisson limits
used, Figure 6.9
```

```
The mean count is 31.864.
Do you want to change the mean value (Y/N) n
The variance (V) is 23.838.
Do you want to change V (Y/N) n
Denominators.
Enter name for denominator OBD
Chart heading.
Enter heading for chart
Monthly Bacteraemia Count Data
```

```
ewmacountdenom(ae) # Figure 6.10
```

```
The mean count is 31.864.
Do you want to change the mean value (Y/N) n
The variance is 23.838 (SD 4.882 ).
Do you want to change the variance (Y/N) n
Chart heading.
Enter heading for chart EWMA Chart Monthly Bacteraemia Count Data
Denominators.
Enter name for denominator OBD
EWMA weight.
Enter weight between 0.2 & 0.8 .2
EWMA control limit.
Enter limit between 2 & 3 2.5
```

With the functions rateshew(), rateewma() and rateshewqtr() and rateewmaqtr() that display rates, it is possible to change the mean, denominator and variance, for example, if predictable data are available elsewhere. When this is so and there is also overdispersion, it is recommended that these functions be avoided as the resulting negative binomial limits may be unsatisfactory. Instead Poisson limits with Laney's correction (see overdispersed() and rateewmao() in section 6.6.1), shewcountdenom() or ewmacountdenom() could be used. Our usual preference in this situation is to use rategam() or rategamqtr().

```
#using function rateshew(), Figure 6.11
rateshew(ae) #Shewhart chart of rates
```

```
The mean count is 31.864.
Do you want to change the mean value (Y/N) n
The mean denominator is 21708.
Do you want to change the mean denominator value (Y/N) n
The weighted variance (V) is 17.112.
Do you want to change V (Y/N) n
Denominators.
Enter name for denominator OBDs
Denominators.
Per thousand (1000), hundred (100), ten (10), unit (1) OBDs 1000
Chart heading.
Enter heading for chart Monthly Bacteraemia Data
```

```
#using function rateewma(), Figure 6.12
rateewma(ae)
```

```
The mean count is 31.864.
Do you want to change the mean value (Y/N) n
The mean denominator is 21708.
Do you want to change the mean denominator value (Y/N) n
The weighted variance (V) is 17.112.
Do you want to change V (Y/N) n
Denominators.
Enter name for denominator OBDs
Denominators.
Per thousand (1000), hundred (100), ten (10), unit (1) OBDs 1000
EWMA weight.
Enter weight between 0.2 & 0.8 .2
EWMA control limit.
Enter limit between 2 & 3 2.5
Chart heading.
Enter heading for chart Monthly Bacteraemia Data
```

When denominators differ so that Shewhart control limits are not straight lines, the EWMA control limits are calculated as described in section 3.12 of Chapter 3. The Shewhart limits corresponding to the EWMA limits are obtained with the pgamma() function search (sections 6.5 and 6.6 of this chapter). They are then modified. The first upper EWMA limit will be $CL+(Us_1-CL)\times W$, the second $CL+(Us_2-CL)\times \sqrt{(W^2+W^2\times(1-W)^2)}$, the third $CL+(Us_3-CL)\times \sqrt{(W^2+W^2\times(1-W)^2+W^2\times(1-W)^4)}$, and so on, where the Us values constitute the Shewhart values corresponding to the required EWMA limit, CL is the centre line and W the

EWMA weight. This approach results in slightly unsmooth EWMA limits but appears to be satisfactory with monthly hospital AE attribute data.

For a GAM chart analysis, we first exclude autocorrelation. The analysis is similar to that described above (Figure 6.6) except that an offset, the logarithm of the denominator, is included or, as here, the rate is modeled with the denominator as a weight.

```
#using rategamauto()GAM chart function for autocorrelated data
rategamauto(ae) # autocorrelation a2 not significant
```

```
Chart heading.
Enter heading for chart Monthly bacteraemia data
Denominators.
Enter name for denominator OBD
Denominators.
Per ten thousand (10000), thousand (1000), hundred (100), ten (10),
unit (1) OBD 1000
Change degrees of freedom (Y/N) n
```

```
Abbreviated output (figure not shown)
                    Estimate Std. Error t value Pr(>|t|)
(Intercept)        -6.140937   0.305732 -20.086 8.96e-13 ***
a2                 -0.006285   0.007330  -0.857   0.404
(Dispersion parameter for quasipoisson family taken to be 0.5965643)
    Null deviance: 11.2491  on 20  degrees of freedom
Residual deviance:  9.6425  on 16  degrees of freedom
(2 observations deleted due to missingness)
```

```
#using rategam(), Figure 6.13
rategam(ae) # GAM chart function for non-autocorrelated data
```

```
Chart heading.
Enter a heading for the chart Monthly Bacteraemia Data
Denominators.
Enter name for denominator OBD
Denominators.
Per ten thousand (10000), thousand (1000), hundred (100), ten (10),
unit (1) OBD 1000
Change degrees of freedom (Y/N) n
```

```
Abbreviated summary
                 Estimate Std. Error t value Pr(>|t|)
(Intercept)      -6.42933    0.09278 -69.294   <2e-16 ***
(Dispersion parameter for quasipoisson family taken to be 0.558965)
    Null deviance: 11.320  on 21  degrees of freedom
Residual deviance: 10.252  on 18  degrees of freedom
```

These charts show data that are predictable. However, there is some underdispersion that may warrant a re-checking of the accuracy of the data. We have drawn attention to the risk of under-reporting when there is perceived to be an unjustly judgemental environment and data showing such small variation may raise suspicion, although it was known not to be the case with these data. Moreover, the function employs quasipoisson because overdispersion

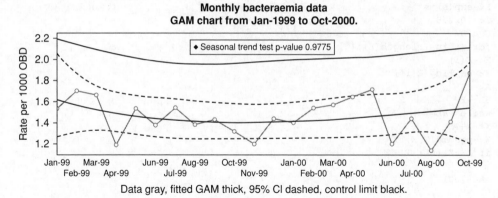

Figure 6.14   GAM chart, rate data (Poisson GLM).

is so common with these data; repeating the analysis with poisson (Figure 6.14) might be preferable although it makes little difference to the chart but could cause difficulty for a hospital scientist. There is no evidence of a trend. In the GAM chart, the change in the deviance (1.068 with 3 DF) suggests that these data displayed very little variation. Note also that there are warnings. When the outcome variable is entered into the glm as a rate with the denominator as a weight, the AIC calculation fails but the chart seems otherwise satisfactory.

```
#GAM chart using poisson, Figure 6.14
library(chron)
library(splines)
library(Kendall)
da<-ae[,1]
d2<-ae[,2]
d3<-ae[,3]
da<-chron(as.character(da),format="day-month-year",out.format=
"day-mon-year")
o<-order(da)
da<-da[o]
d2<-d2[o]
d3<-d3[o]
s1<-paste(months(min(da)),years(min(da)))
s2<-paste(months(max(da)),years(max(da)))
k<-format.Date(da,"%b%y")
eh<-"Monthly Bacteraemia Data"
ma<-paste(eh,"\nGAM Chart from ",s1," to ",s2,".",sep="")
den<-"OBD"
dn<-1000
yl<-paste("Rate per",as.character(dn),den)
df1<-3
a<-d2
s<-d3
id<-1:length(da)
mg<-glm(a/s~bs(id,df=df1),family=poisson,weight=s)
mgp<-predict(mg,se=T)
b<-mgp$fit;e<-mgp$se.fit
```

```
E<-exp(b)*s
Z<-.02275
UP<-0
for (i in 1:length(E)){
M<-E[i]
X<-ceiling(E[i])
A<-1
BL<-F
while (BL==F){
X<-X+A
K<-pgamma(M,X,1)
if (K<Z){BL<-T}
}
AA<-.001
BL<-F
while (BL==F){
X<-X-AA
K<-pgamma(M,X,1)
if (K>=Z){BL<-T}
}
UP[i]<-X
}
v1<-exp(b)*dn;v2<-exp(b+1.96*e)*dn;v3<-exp(b-1.96*e)*dn
aa<-a*dn/s
uu<-UP*dn/s
x1<-min(c(aa,v3));x2<-max(c(aa,v2,uu))
par(lab=c(length(datain[,1]),5,7))
par(xaxs="i")
plot(aa,axes=F,ylim=c(x1,x2),type="b",main=ma,ylab=yl,xlab="Data blue,
Fitted GAM red, 95% CI brown, Control limit black.",col="blue",lwd=2)
box()
par(cex=.7)
axis(side=1,tick=F,labels=k,at=id)
axis(side=c(2,3,4))
par(cex=1)
lines(v1,lwd=2,col="red")
lines(v2,lwd=2,lty=1,col="brown")
lines(v3,lwd=2,lty=1,col="brown")
lines(smooth.spline(uu,spar=.5),lwd=2)
mmg<<-mg
s<-SeasonalMannKendall(ts(aa))
print(s)
ss<-0
if(s$sl<.001){ss<-"<0.001"}else{ss<-
as.character(round(s$sl,4))}
msg2<-paste("Seasonal Trend Test p-value ",ss,sep="")
legend(locator(1),legend=msg2,pch=19,col="brown4",cex=.8)
summary(mg)
```

```
Abbreviated summary
              Estimate Std. Error z value Pr(>|z|)
(Intercept)    -6.4293     0.1241 -51.807   <2e-16 ***
(Dispersion parameter for poisson family taken to be 1)
    Null deviance: 11.320  on 21  degrees of freedom
Residual deviance: 10.252  on 18  degrees of freedom
```

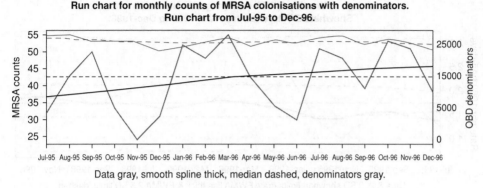

Run chart for monthly counts of MRSA colonisations with denominators.
Run chart from Jul-95 to Dec-96.

Data gray, smooth spline thick, median dashed, denominators gray.

Figure 6.15   Run chart.

6.6.1   Overdispersed data

Monthly MRSA new isolates in the hospital between July 1995 and December 1996 are in the file monthlymrsa.csv. The mean count was 42 and its variance 91 (weighted variance 86). It is clear that the variance is far larger than the mean. The differences in occupied bed-days are relatively small and could not account for this large variation. Figure 6.15 is a run chart of these data. It does not suggest any special pattern that could indicate special cause variation or a process difficulty increasing common cause variation that could be the cause of the difference between the mean and the variance. Figure 6.16 is a correlogram; there is no suggestion of autocorrelation. Figure 6.17 is a negative binomial Shewhart/EWMA rate chart, Figure 6.18 a Poisson Shewhart/EWMA rate chart, Figure 6.19 a Poisson Shewhart/EWMA rate chart with Laney's correction and Figure 6.20 is a GAM chart.

For negative binomial data, use of maximum likelihood is to be preferred but is difficult to implement in a control chart when there are differing denominators. So far as we are aware there is at this time no suitable R library in which negative binomial maximum likelihood calculations are available for data with differing denominators. A linear approximation due to Bissell appears to converge quickly and reliably to a solution but we employ

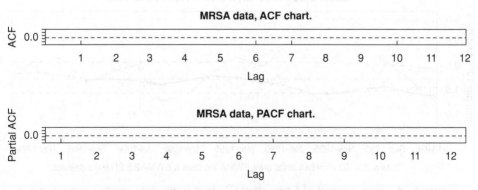

MRSA data, ACF chart.

MRSA data, PACF chart.

Figure 6.16   ACF/PACF chart.

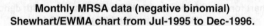

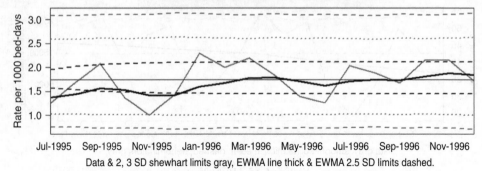

Monthly MRSA data (negative binomial)
Shewhart/EWMA chart from Jul-1995 to Dec-1996.

Data & 2, 3 SD shewhart limits gray, EWMA line thick & EWMA 2.5 SD limits dashed.

Figure 6.17   Shewhart/EWMA rate chart (negative binomial).

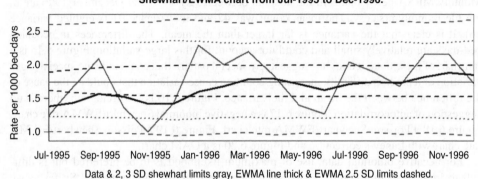

Monthly MRSA data (Poisson)
Shewhart/EWMA chart from Jul-1995 to Dec-1996.

Data & 2, 3 SD shewhart limits gray, EWMA line thick & EWMA 2.5 SD limits dashed.

Figure 6.18   Shewhart/EWMA rate chart (Poisson limits are too narrow).

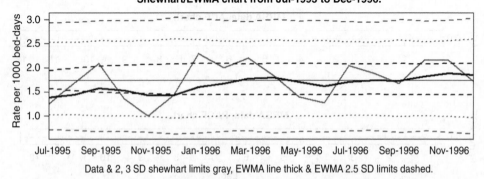

Monthly MRSA data (Laney)
Shewhart/EWMA chart from Jul-1995 to Dec-1996.

Data & 2, 3 SD shewhart limits gray, EWMA line thick & EWMA 2.5 SD limits dashed.

Figure 6.19   Shewhart/EWMA rate chart (Poisson limits with Laney's correction).

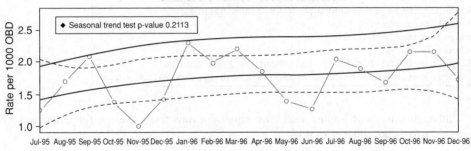

Data gray, fitted GAM thick, 95% CI dashed, control limit black.

Figure 6.20   GAM chart.

control limits using the simple weighted variance (Morton[A] and colleagues). This appears to provide reliable approximate control limits with hospital occupied bed-days denominators that typically do not differ greatly between time periods. Assuming the availability of denominator data, the mean count is $M=\sum X_i/N$ where X_i is the count for the ith month and N is the number of months. The weighted variance is $V=\{1/(N-1)\}\sum\{W_i(X_i/W_i-M)^2\}$ where $W_i=D_i/Dbar$, D_i is the denominator for the ith month and $Dbar=\sum D_i/N$. $S=M^2/(V-M)$. $Pbar=S/(S+M)$. $Cbar=Pbar/(1-Pbar)$. $C_i=Cbar/W_i$. $P_i=C_i/(1+C_i)$. $M^*_i=S\{(1-P_i)/P_i\}$. Shortcuts: $P_i=M/(W_i(V-M)+M)$ and $M^*_i=M\times W_i$.

For the ith month, S corresponds with the number of successes in a series of Bernoulli trials, X_i the number of failures before the Sth success, and P_i is the probability of success for the ith month. P_i differs for each month when the monthly bed-days denominators vary. The negative binomial distribution is equivalent to the Poisson-gamma distribution frequently used to analyse overdispersed count data. (See Chapter 4, section 4.10 and Chapter 6, section 6.13 for further discussion of this distribution.)

To obtain control limits (e.g. the upper 2 SD limit), let $K_i=M^*_i$ rounded upwards. Then for an upper two sigma equivalent control limit, K_i is successively increased by one until (in S language notation) 1-pbeta(P_i,S,K_i)<0.02275. It is then decreased by .001 until 1-pbeta(P_i,S,K_i)>= 0.02275. Other limits are obtained in a similar manner.

```
g.d()# data from datafile monthlymrsa.csv

# mean and weighted variance
m<-mean(datain[,2])
m # mean
#[1] 41.9
dbar<-mean(datain[,3])
dw<-datain[,3]/dbar
v<-sum(dw*(datain[,2]/dw-m)^2/(length(dw)-1)) # weighted variance
v
#[1] 86

#using function runchartdenom(), Figure 6.15
runchartdenom(datain)
```

```
Chart heading.
Enter a heading for the chart
Run chart MRSA colonisations with denominators.
Denominator name.
Enter a denominator name OBD
Y axis heading.
Enter a heading for the Y axis Monthly MRSA Counts
Some increase in rates but seasonal trend test p-value > 0.2
```

Although usually of limited value, we employ a runs test to search for a nonrandom pattern. There is no evidence of this.

```
library(tseries)
d<-rep(0,length(datain[,2]))
d[datain[,2]/datain[,3]>median(datain[,2]/datain[,3])]<-1
runs.test(as.factor(d))$p.value
#
#[1] 0.6270291

# using function do.acf(), Figure 6.16
do.acf(datain[,2]/datain[,3])
#
Enter a heading for the ACF plot MRSA data

#are the data approximately normally distributed
shapiro.test(datain[,2]/datain[,3])$p.value
#
#[1] 0.3109604 (rates appear to be approximately normally distributed

#using function rateewma() with negative binomial limits
rateewma(datain) # Figure 8.17
```

```
The mean count is 41.889.
Do you want to change the mean value (Y/N) n
The mean denominator is 23988.
Do you want to change the mean denominator value (Y/N) n
The weighted variance (V) is 85.954.
Do you want to change V (Y/N) n
Denominators.
Enter name for denominator Bed-days
Denominators.
Per ten thousand (10000), thousand (1000), hundred (100), ten (10), unit (1)
Bed-days 1000
EWMA weight.
Enter weight between 0.2 & 0.8 .2
EWMA control limit.
Enter limit between 2 & 3 2.5
Chart heading.
Enter heading for chart Monthly MRSA Data (Negative Binomial)
```

```
#using function rateewma() with Poisson limits, Figure 6.18
rateewma(datain) # note variance changed to equal mean
```

```
The mean count is 41.889.
Do you want to change the mean value (Y/N) n
The mean denominator is 23988.
Do you want to change the mean denominator value (Y/N) n
The weighted variance (V) is 85.954.
Do you want to change V (Y/N) y
Enter new value for the variance 41.889
Denominators.
Enter name for denominator Bed-days
Denominators.
Per ten thousand (10000), thousand (1000), hundred (100), ten (10),
unit (1) Bed-days 1000
EWMA weight.
Enter weight between 0.2 & 0.8 .2
EWMA control limit.
Enter limit between 2 & 3 2.5
Chart heading.
Enter heading for chart Monthly MRSA Data (Poisson)
```

Figure 6.19 is a Poisson-based chart but with Laney's correction to deal with the excessive variability. It was seen that with the weekly data shown above, Laney's correction failed to deal with the overdispersion. However, with the monthly MRSA data the chart is almost identical to the negative binomial chart. In general it appears to be reliable and is an alternative to the negative binomial chart that is easier to implement and to understand than the latter. Occasionally, winsorising (Spiegelhalter[D]), as discussed in Chapter 5, may result in further improvement. However, with time series data to be displayed in a control chart, it would be preferable to search for predictable data rather than to employ winsorising. When there is severe overdispersion or predictable data are lacking, it will usually be better to use a GAM chart. Laney's correction is available with the function overdispersed(data.frame) and control charts that implement the correction are in rprogs, for example, for the current analysis use rateewmao(datain) where the name of the function ends in o. See the internet Supplement for further discussion.

```
#using Laney's correction
overdispersed(datain)
```

```
Are there denominator data (Y/N) y
Laney's correction 1.392
Spiegelhalter's correction 1.353
```

```
rateewmao(datain)
```

```
The mean count is 41.889.
Do you want to change the mean value (Y/N) n
The mean denominator is 23988.
Do you want to change the mean denominator value (Y/N) n
Enter overdispersion correction 1.39
Denominators.
Enter name for denominator Bed-Days
Denominators.
Per ten thousand (10000), thousand (1000), hundred (100), ten (10),
unit (1) Bed-Days 1000
```

```
EWMA weight.
Enter weight between 0.2 & 0.8 .2
EWMA control limit.
Enter limit between 2 & 3 2.5
Chart heading.
Enter heading for chart Monthly MRSA Data (Laney)
```

```
#using function rategam(), Figure 6.20
rategam(datain) # we do not use rategamauto() as there is no autocorrealtion
```

```
Chart heading.
Enter a heading for the chart GAM Chart Monthly MRSA Data
Denominators.
Enter name for denominator Bed-days
Denominators.
Per ten thousand (10000), thousand (1000), hundred (100), ten (10),
unit (1) Bed-days 1000
Change degrees of freedom (Y/N) n
```

The GAM chart is unremarkable. There is a slight nonsignificant upward trend. The summary (not shown) revealed a dispersion parameter of 2.167 for the quasipoisson glm. The deviance change of 5 on 3 DF is not significant (P=0.17).

The most likely explanation for the large variance is that the outcomes are not independent. If a patient carrying MRSA organisms is admitted to a ward, he or she becomes a potential source of spread of these organisms to other patients. When this happens there is clustering within wards, variation is likely to be excessive, and the Poisson distribution should not be used as a basis for calculating the control limits without, for example, using Laney's correction. In the present case, where the monthly average was over 40, the normal approximation would be satisfactory and the control limits could be found using the calculated standard deviation in an i chart.

When using an i chart to calculate control limits and the number of periods used when calculating the standard deviation is small, it should be divided by a constant C_4 to find the control limits. For a sample of N=18 months, C_4 is 0.9854. For C_4 for above 10 periods the following formula is a suitable approximation for its calculation $C_4=4\times(N-1)/(4\times N-3)$, where N is the number of time periods. For smaller N there are tables in most textbooks on quality statistics and these are included in the ichart() functions that are employed in Chapter 7.

When using the normal approximation to calculate control limits, it is important to determine whether the data are approximately normally distributed. A bar chart is useful for this purpose. The R function shapiro.test() gives p-value=0.31 (see above). This suggests that the data are compatible with having come from a normal distribution.

Count data are positively skewed and are not approximately normally distributed in small samples, for example when mean counts are less than about 10 for potentially overdispersed data. If the test for approximate normality indicates that the data being studied are unlikely to be approximately normally distributed, it is important to determine whether there are two distributions present instead of one. For example, a marked increase in the numbers of events occurring at each time period due to a worsening process or a marked decrease due to a QI activity such as the implementation of the relevant evidence-based bundle may produce data that are not normally distributed because there are two different means present. The EWMA chart is more robust than the Shewhart chart and can often be relied upon when there is a departure from normality. An alternative, which we prefer under these circumstances, is to employ a GAM chart.

When the variance is greater than the mean by more than a few per cent, control limits may be calculated using the negative binomial distribution. Control limits are then obtained from the beta distribution. Approximate negative binomial control limits with varying denominators add to the complexity of the analysis. As we have already noted, maximum likelihood is difficult to implement in a control chart. A linear approximation due to Bissell appears to converge quickly and reliably to a solution but we have employed control limits using the simple weighted variance.

The mean count is $M=\sum X_i/N$ where X_i is the count for the ith month and N is the number of months. The weighted variance is $V=\{1/(N-1)\}\sum\{W_i(X_i/W_i-M)^2\}$ where $W_i=D_i/Dbar$, D_i is the denominator for the ith month and $Dbar=\sum D_i/N$. $S=M^2/(V-M)$, $Pbar=S/(S+M)$, $Cbar=Pbar/(1-Pbar)$, $C_i=Cbar/W_i$, $P_i=C_i/(1+C_i)$.

For the ith month, S corresponds with the number of successes in a series of Bernoulli trials, X_i the number of failures before the Sth success, and P_i is the probability of success for the ith month. P_i differs for each month when the monthly bed-days denominators vary. The negative binomial distribution is equivalent to the Poisson-gamma distribution frequently used to analyse overdispersed count data.

$M^*_i=S\{(1-P_i)/P_i\}$ or equivalently $M^*_i=M\times W_i$. To obtain control limits (e.g. upper 2 SD limit), let $K_i=M^*_i$ rounded upwards. Then for an upper two sigma equivalent control limit K_i is successively increased by one until (in S language notation) 1-pbeta(P_i,S,K_i)< 0.02275. It is then decreased by .001 until 1-pbeta(P_i,S,K_i)>=0.02275. Other limits are obtained in a similar manner.

The Figure 6.17 control limits have been calculated using the negative binomial and not the Poisson distribution; had the latter been used, as shown in Figure 6.18, the count that determined U_2 would have been 57 instead of 64. This is likely to make false positive signals more frequent. Thus using the Poisson distribution could have indicated erroneously that a special cause problem might have been present. If Poisson limits are to be employed, it is wise to include a correction for the large variance such as that described by Laney (Mohammed[A] and Laney). This involves calculating the expected counts and using them to obtain Z-scores (standard normal deviates) by comparing them with the observed counts. Since Z-scores have an expected mean of zero and a standard deviation of one, the Poisson control limits can be corrected by widening them using their standard deviation (Figure 6.19). In some cases, where overdispersion is severe, a GAM chart will be preferable.

The Shewhart and Shewhart/EWMA charts are useful for demonstrating large changes in weekly or monthly counts or rates and the EWMA is useful for predicting changes in its mean. Note again that the negative binomial distribution is more appropriate than the Poisson distribution when the variance exceeds the mean in the absence of some special cause problem that could account for the increased variation. Alternatively Laney's correction may be used but hospital scientists may wish to seek expert advice before using this correction; see the internet Supplement. GAM charts are usually straightforward and the default three degrees of freedom (DF) will usually be satisfactory although sometimes increasing, for example, to five DF will improve the chart by decreasing the amount of smoothing. Autocorrelation must be kept in mind; however with these monthly count and rate data it should be uncommon. Thus the GAM chart is a good general purpose chart for hospital AE data. Splines and generalised additive models are described by Everitt.

6.7   Charts for quarterly data and data without a first date column

In some cases there are insufficient data for monthly display in a control chart and quarterly data may be used provided there are sufficient quarters available (preferably at least 20). In other cases there may not be a first column of dates available for, for example, monthly or quarterly data. In this case it is important that the data are suitably sorted by time and a first column may need to be added such as 1 to 20 for 20 ordered monthly or quarterly (or other time period) rows of data. At the beginning of this chapter, sparse MRSA bacteraemia data were placed in quarterly groupings and saved in the files countquarters.csv and ratequarters.csv and these are now used to illustrate countshewqtr() and rateewmaqtr() respectively. The data in ivdstaphbact.csv and ivstaphbactdenom.csv are also used to illustrate the use of rategamqtr(), see Figure 6.21. For each of the functions already described there is a counterpart, for example, rategamqtr() for rategam().

```
g.d() # countquarters.csv
```

```
Loading data.
Data from clipboard (C) or file (F) c
Do data column(s) have heading(s) (Y/N) y
Is column 1 a date column (Y/N) n
```

```
countshewqtr(datain)
```

```
The mean count is 2.455.
Do you want to change the mean value (Y/N) n
The variance is 2.998 (SD 1.731 ).
Do you want to change the variance (Y/N) n
Chart heading.
Enter heading for chart Quarterly MRSA Bacteraemias
(chart not shown)
```

```
g.d() #ratequarters.csv()
```

```
rateewmaqtr(datain)
```

```
The mean count is 2.455.
Do you want to change the mean value (Y/N) n
The mean denominator is 69790.
Do you want to change the mean denominator value (Y/N) n
The weighted variance (V) is 3.164.
Do you want to change V (Y/N) n
Denominators.
Enter name for denominator OBD
Denominators.
Per ten thousand (10000), thousand (1000), hundred (100), ten (10),
unit (1) OBD 1000
EWMA weight.
Enter weight between 0.2 & 0.8 .2
EWMA control limit.
Enter limit between 2 & 3 2.5
Chart heading.
Enter heading for chart Quarterly MRSA Bacteraemias
(chart not shown)
```

```
g.d() # ivdstaphbact.csv

# monthly counts (can use monthlycounts(datain))
library(chron)
d<-datain[,1]
o<-order(d)
d<-d[o]
fst<-chron("01/01/2004")
lst<-chron("12/31/2008")
s<-seq.dates(from=fst,to=lst,by="months")
k<-NA
for (i in 1:(length(s)-1)){k[i]<-sum(d>=s[i]&d<s[i+1])}
k[length(s)]<-sum(d>=s[length(s)])
s<-chron(s,format="m/d/y",out.format="dd-mmm-yyyy")
dataout<-data.frame(s,k)
names(dataout)<-c("Months","Counts")

#getting denominator data
g.d() # ivdstaphbactdenom.csv

#adding denominator data
ae<-data.frame(dataout,datain[,2])
names(ae)<-c("Months","Counts","Denoms")

#making data quarterly
# can use ratequarters(), output in rateqtr
d<-ae[,1]
e<-ae[,2]
n<-ae[,3]
d<-chron(as.character(d),format="dd-mmm-yyyy",out.format="dd-mmm-yyyy")
Year<-years(d)
m<-as.numeric(months(d))
Qtrs<-rep(0,length(m))
Qtrs[m>=1&m<=3]<-1
Qtrs[m>=4&m<=6]<-2
Qtrs[m>=7&m<=9]<-3
Qtrs[m>=10&m<=12]<-4
Table<-as.data.frame(xtabs(e~Qtrs+Year))
Tablea<-as.data.frame(xtabs(n~Qtrs+Year))
Table<-data.frame(Table,Tablea[,3])
k<-which(Table[,4]==0)
if (length(k)!=0){Table<-Table[-k,]}
Quarter<-paste(Table[,2],"Q",Table[,1],sep="")
Table<-data.frame(Quarter,Table[,-c(1,2)])
names(Table)<-c("Quarter","Count","Denom")
head(Table)
```

	Quarter	Count	Denom
1	2004Q1	10	63714
2	2004Q2	3	66414
3	2004Q3	2	70886
4	2004Q4	5	66279
5	2005Q1	8	65665
6	2005Q2	2	69607

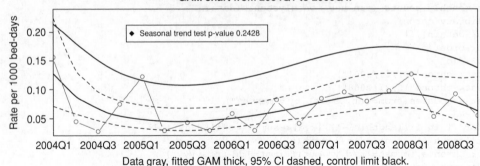

IVD-related Staphylococcus aureus bacteraemias
GAM chart from 2004Q1 to 2008Q4.

Data gray, fitted GAM thick, 95% CI dashed, control limit black.

Figure 6.21   GAM chart, horizontal axis not in date format.

```
# using function rategamqtr(), Figure 6.21
rategamqtr(Table) # rategamqtr(rateqtr) after ratequarters()
```

```
Chart heading.
Enter a heading for the chart
IVD-related Staphylococcus aureus Bacteraemias
Denominators.
Enter name for denominator Bed-Days
Denominators.
Per ten thousand (10000), thousand (1000), hundred (100), ten (10),
unit (1) Bed-Days 1000
Change degrees of freedom (Y/N) n
```

```
Abbreviated summary
                Estimate Std. Error t value Pr(>|t|)
(Intercept)      -8.9727    0.2961 -30.303 1.46e-15 ***
(Dispersion parameter for quasipoisson family taken to be 1.059778)
    Null deviance: 24.065   on 19   degrees of freedom
Residual deviance: 15.697   on 16   degrees of freedom
```

The deviance decreased by 8.368 on three DF suggesting significant nonlinear changes ([1-pchisq(8.368,3)]=0.039) in the quarterly rates although there was no overall trend. The first rate was large and the rate in the first quarter of 2005 may have been an outlier.

6.8   When there are few time periods

Sometimes few time periods are available, for example yearly data may be available for only five or six years. One approach is to calculate confidence intervals for the data for each of the time periods (Figure 6.22). We employ annual *Staphylococcus aureus* bacteraemia data from one hospital. In addition, a control chart using SMRs can be used provided a reference rate is available (Figure 6.23). The reference rate was 0.166 per 1000 bed-days for similar hospitals. Figures 6.22 and 6.23 show that the hospital is similar to the average for comparable hospitals

One hospital in-hospital Staphylococcus aureus bacteraemia rate per 1000 bed-days with 95% and 99.7% confidence intervals.

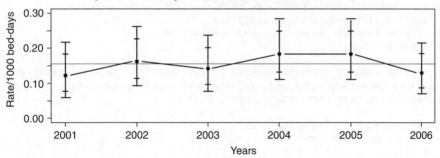

Figure 6.22 Few time periods, confidence intervals.

and has a predictable process. The hospital's average was 0.155 per 1000 bed-days, a little below the overall average of 0.166 but the difference was small.

```
# data with few time periods
Year<-c(2001,2002,2003,2004,2005,2006)
Saureus<-c(23,35,31,42,43,31)
OBD<-c(188514,214805,218009,229590,234446,239160)
Sbact<-data.frame(Year,Saureus,OBD)
#calculates 95% and 99.7% limits per 1000 OBD
n<-length(Sbact[,2])
x<-Sbact[,2]
y<-Sbact[,3]
s<-0;su95<-0;sl95<-0;su997<-0;sl997<-0
up95<-0;lo95<-0;up997<-0;lo997<-0
for (i in 1:n){
if (x[i]==0){lo95[i]<-0;lo997<-0;up95[i]<-qgamma(0.975,x[i]+1,1);
up997[i]<-qgamma(0.9985,x[i]+1,1)
}else{
lo95[i]<-qgamma(0.025,x[i],1);
lo997[i]<-qgamma(0.0015,x[i],1)
up95[i]<-qgamma(0.975,x[i]+1,1);
up997[i]<-qgamma(0.9985,x[i]+1,1)
```

In-hospital Staphylococcus aureus bacteraemias

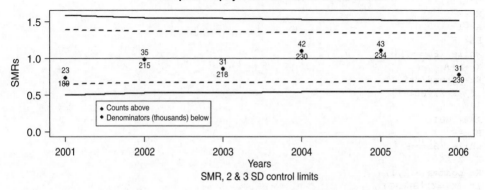

Figure 6.23 Few time periods, control chart for SMR.

```
}
lo95[i]<-lo95[i]/y[i];up95[i]<-up95[i]/y[i];
lo997[i]<-lo997[i]/y[i];up997[i]<-up997[i]/y[i]
s<-c(s,x[i]/y[i]);su95<-c(su95,up95[i]);
sl95<-c(sl95,lo95[i]);su997<-c(su997,up997[i]);
sl997<-c(sl997,lo997[i])
}
s<-s[-1];su95<-su95[-1];sl95<-sl95[-1];su997<-su997[-1];sl997<-sl997[-1]
ss<-data.frame(s*1000,sl95*1000,sl997*1000,su95*1000,su997*1000)
names(ss)<-c("Rate","L95","L997","U95","U997")
#
m<-1000*sum(Sbact[,2])/sum(Sbact[,3])
m #mean rate per 1000 OBDs
#[1] 0.1547726


# Figure 6.22, confidence interval chart
par(xaxs="r")
hdr0<-"One hospital in-hospital Staphylococcus aureus bacteraemia rate"
hdr1<-"\nper 1000 bed-days with 95% and 99.7% Confidence Intervals."
hdr<-paste(hdr0,hdr1,sep="")
plot(ss[,1],type="b",lwd=3,xlab="Years",ylab="Rate/1000 Bed-Days",axes=F,
col="blue",ylim=c(0,.3),
main=hdr)
box()
axis(side=1,labels=Year,at=1:6,tick=T)
abline(h=m)
arrows(1:6,ss[,2],1:6,ss[,4],col="blue",lwd=3,code=3,angle=90,length=.05)
arrows(1:6,ss[,3],1:6,ss[,5],col="blue",lwd=3,code=3,angle=90,length=.1)
axis(side=c(2,3,4))


# control chart using SMR, Figure 6.23
Exp<-Sbact[,3]*.000166
Sbact<-data.frame(Sbact,Exp)
#
O<-Sbact[,2];E<-Sbact[,4];H<-Sbact[,1];D<-Sbact[,3]
TT<-E
AA<-0
U<-0
Z<-.02275
for (i in 1:length(TT)){
M<-TT[i]
X<-M
A<-1
BL<-F
while (BL==F){
X<-X+A
K<-pgamma(M,X,1)
if (K<Z){BL<-T}
}
AA<-.001
BL<-F
while (BL==F){
X<-X-AA
K<-pgamma(M,X,1)
if (K>=Z){BL<-T}
}
```

```
U[i]<-X
}
TT<-E
AA<-0
UU<-0
Z<-.0015
for (i in 1:length(TT)){
M<-TT[i]
X<-M
A<-1
BL<-F
while (BL==F){
X<-X+A
K<-pgamma(M,X,1)
if (K<Z){BL<-T}
}
AA<-.001
BL<-F
while (BL==F){
X<-X-AA
K<-pgamma(M,X,1)
if (K>=Z){BL<-T}
}
UU[i]<-X
}
TT<-E
L<-0
AA<-0
Z<-.02275
for (i in 1:length(TT)){
M<-TT[i]
X<-0
if(1-pgamma(M,X+1,1)>=Z){X<-0}else{
A<-1
BL<-F
while (BL==F){
X<-X+A
K<-1-pgamma(M,X+1,1)
if (K>Z){BL<-T}
}
AA<-.001
BL<-F
while (BL==F){
X<-X-AA
K<-1-pgamma(M,X+1,1)
if (K<=Z){BL<-T}
}
}
L[i]<-X
}
L[L<0]<-0
TT<-E
LL<-0
AA<-0
Z<-.0015
for (i in 1:length(TT)){
```

```
M<-TT[i]
X<-0
if(1-pgamma(M,X+1,1)>=Z){X<-0}else{
A<-1
BL<-F
while (BL==F){
X<-X+A
K<-1-pgamma(M,X+1,1)
if (K>Z){BL<-T}
}
AA<-.001
BL<-F
while (BL==F){
X<-X-AA
K<-1-pgamma(M,X+1,1)
if (K<=Z){BL<-T}
}
}
LL[i]<-X
}
LL[LL<0]<-0
oe<-O/E
plot(oe,ylim=c(0,max(c(oe,UU/E))),axes=F,col="blue",pch=19,
main="In-hospital Staphylococcus aureus Bacteraemias",
xlab="SMR Blue, 2 & 3 SD Control Limits Red",ylab="SMRs")
box()
par(cex=.8)
axis(side=1,labels=H,at=1:length(H))
axis(side=c(2,3,4))
par(cex=1)
lines(U/E,col="red",lty=2,lwd=2)
lines(L/E,col="red",lty=2,lwd=2)
lines(UU/E,col="red",lty=1,lwd=2)
lines(LL/E,col="red",lty=1,lwd=2)
abline(h=1)
par(font=2)
text(oe,labels=as.character(round(O,0)),pos=3,offset=.3,cex=.8,lwd=3,
col="green4")
text(oe,labels=as.character(round(D/1000,0)),pos=1,offset=.3,cex=.8,lwd=3,
col="brown4")
par(font=1)
mtext("Years",side=1,line=2)
legend(locator(1),
legend=c("Counts Green","Denominators(thousands) Brown"),
pch=19,col=c("green4","brown4"),cex=.8)
```

6.9   Cross-tabulation in wide format

Although most users may prefer to perform cross-tabulations in a spreadsheet, it may also be useful to perform them in wide format using the reshape() function in R. The *Staphylococcus aureus* bacteraemia data in the staphbact.csv file are used to illustrate the use of reshape(). Denominators are in staphobd.csv. The data are tabulated by hospitals and by years.

```
# using R for cross-tabulation
g.d() #staphbact.csv
```

```
# denominator data
obds<-read.table("clipboard",T) #staphobd.csv

# tabulation
library(chron)
h<-datain[,1]
d<-chron(as.character(datain[,2]),format="dd-mmm-yyyy",out.format=
"dd-mmm-yyyy")
y<-years(d)
tp<-as.data.frame(table(h,y))
AE<-as.numeric(table(h))
h<-obds[,1]
d<-chron(as.character(obds[,2]),format="d-mmm-yy",out.format="dd-mmm-yyyy")
obd<-obds[,3]
Tot<-tapply(obds[,3],obds[,1],sum)
m<-as.numeric(months(d))
y<-years(d)
bd<-as.data.frame(xtabs(obd~h+y))
All<-data.frame(tp,bd[,3])
names(All)<-c("H","Y","B","D")
rs<-reshape(All,direction="wide",idvar="H",timevar="Y")
q<-dimnames(rs)[[2]]
k<-q[1]
for (i in 2:length(q)){k[i]<-
paste(substr(q[i],1,1),substr(q[i],5,6),sep="")}
dimnames(rs)[[2]]<-k
rs<-data.frame(rs,AE,Tot)
rs
# table in 8 pt to fit page
```

	H	B01	D01	B02	D02	B03	D03	B04	D04	B05	D05	B06	D06	AE	Tot
1	A	1	77795	16	83917	18	83615	8	73998	11	48995	15	99938	69	468258
2	B	15	125841	23	146704	12	174404	16	177675	11	187886	17	184379	94	996889
3	C	6	72562	2	75623	3	76955	0	38303	0	74887	1	78350	12	416680
4	D	24	67283	6	73349	9	74753	7	57907	7	72099	7	69401	60	414792
5	E	6	81249	5	90623	5	83936	7	92989	10	86627	9	94748	42	530172
6	F	23	188514	35	214805	31	218009	42	229590	43	234446	31	239160	205	1324524
7	G	11	118992	18	135263	23	124805	15	127658	16	123388	13	125441	96	755547
8	H	0	42575	4	44337	8	44856	7	46783	4	51408	9	54548	32	284507
9	I	0	0	0	0	34	206280	40	256143	55	266930	61	275760	190	1005113
10	J	16	58285	5	65198	5	65695	5	69523	5	69763	12	76556	48	405020
11	K	16	77212	26	97257	24	104877	35	108771	14	117737	21	122414	136	628268
12	L	0	0	0	20819	3	33008	0	15838	6	32822	6	32847	15	135334
13	M	0	0	2	26812	4	43339	4	50822	2	47827	1	52483	13	221283
14	N	0	0	0	0	0	14688	1	11033	3	24335	1	27338	5	77394
15	O	0	0	4	47674	7	74575	4	78197	2	80610	1	84815	18	365871
16	P	0	0	2	23752	5	35529	3	38040	2	40855	2	41102	14	179278
17	Q	0	0	0	13264	2	18439	3	16434	0	8237	0	18534	5	74908
18	R	0	0	0	10951	1	17190	3	16237	1	18140	3	17576	8	80094
19	S	0	0	1	26194	1	31428	2	25853	1	18842	0	0	3	102317
20	T	0	0	4	41430	5	63090	7	64711	4	63605	7	70754	27	303590
21	U	0	0	0	22993	2	36791	1	36307	3	38203	0	41542	6	175836

```
H=hospital, B=bacteraemias, D=denominators, 01-06=years
AE=bacteraemia totals, Tot=denominator totals
```

```
# tabulation by quarters for one year (2006)
library(chron)
```

```
h<-datain[,1]
d<-chron(as.character(datain[,2]),format="dd-mmm-yyyy",
out.format="dd-mmm-yyyy")
m<-as.numeric(months(d))
y<-years(d)
Qtrs<-rep(0,length(m))
Qtrs[m>=1&m<=3]<-1
Qtrs[m>=4&m<=6]<-2
Qtrs[m>=7&m<=9]<-3
Qtrs[m>=10&m<=12]<-4
Qtrs[Qtrs==1]<-"Jan"
Qtrs[Qtrs==2]<-"Apr"
Qtrs[Qtrs==3]<-"Jul"
Qtrs[Qtrs==4]<-"Oct"
Qtrs<-paste("1-",Qtrs,"-",y,sep="")
Qtrs<-chron(Qtrs,format="dd-mmm-yyyy",out.format="dd-mmm-yyyy")
tp<-table(h,as.Date(Qtrs))
u<-dimnames(tp)[[2]]
u<-chron(u,format="y-m-d",out.format="dd-mmm-yyyy")
u1<-format.Date(u,"%b%y")
dimnames(tp)[[2]]<-as.character(u1)
tp<-as.data.frame(table(h,as.Date(Qtrs)))
h<-obds[,1]
d<-chron(as.character(obds[,2]),format="dd-mmm-yyyy",
out.format="dd-mmm-yyyy")
obd<-obds[,3]
m<-as.numeric(months(d))
y<-years(d)
Qtrs<-rep(0,length(m))
Qtrs[m>=1&m<=3]<-1
Qtrs[m>=4&m<=6]<-2
Qtrs[m>=7&m<=9]<-3
Qtrs[m>=10&m<=12]<-4
Qtrs[Qtrs==1]<-"Jan"
Qtrs[Qtrs==2]<-"Apr"
Qtrs[Qtrs==3]<-"Jul"
Qtrs[Qtrs==4]<-"Oct"
Qtrs<-paste("1-",Qtrs,"-",y,sep="")
Qtrs<-chron(Qtrs,format="dd-mmm-yyyy",out.format="dd-mmm-yyyy")
bd<-as.data.frame(xtabs(obd~h+as.Date(Qtrs)))
All<-data.frame(tp,bd[,3])
names(All)<-c("H","Dt","AE","Dn")
rs<-reshape(All,direction="wide",idvar="H",timevar="Dt")
q<-dimnames(rs)[[2]]
a<-substr(q,9,10)
a[a=="01"]<-"1"
a[a=="04"]<-"2"
a[a=="07"]<-"3"
a[a=="10"]<-"4"
b<-substr(q,6,7)
k<-paste("Y",b,"Q",a,sep="")
k[1]<-"H"
dimnames(rs)[[2]]<-k
bactstaph06<-rs[,c(1,42:49)] # 2006 data
AE<-apply(bactstaph06[,c(2,4,6,8)],1,sum)
Tot<-apply(bactstaph06[,c(3,5,7,9)],1,sum)
```

```
bactstaph06<-data.frame(bactstaph06,AE,Tot)
names(bactstaph06)<-
c("H","Q1B","Q1D","Q2B","Q2D","Q3B","Q3D","Q4B","Q4D",
"AE","Tot")
bactstaph06
```

	H	Q1B	Q1D	Q2B	Q2D	Q3B	Q3D	Q4B	Q4D	AE	Tot
1	A	1	24705	7	25240	4	26237	3	23756	15	99938
2	B	5	49862	2	50555	3	51679	7	32283	17	184379
3	C	0	18529	1	19887	0	21051	0	18883	1	78350
4	D	1	17236	1	17774	4	17920	1	16471	7	69401
5	E	0	22518	3	23591	3	24714	3	23925	9	94748
6	F	6	58006	9	60984	12	62329	4	57841	31	239160
7	G	2	28862	5	31021	4	34552	2	31006	13	125441
8	H	2	12570	2	14538	4	13802	1	13638	9	54548
9	I	18	66040	11	70168	19	72085	13	67467	61	275760
10	J	4	18404	2	18363	2	20065	4	19724	12	76556
11	K	3	29610	6	30818	7	32193	5	29793	21	122414
12	L	0	7607	4	8266	1	8575	1	8399	6	32847
13	M	0	10758	1	12854	0	14392	0	14479	1	52483
14	N	0	6396	0	6882	1	7066	0	6994	1	27338
15	O	0	20664	0	21384	1	22290	0	20477	1	84815
16	P	0	10176	0	10891	1	10132	1	9903	2	41102
17	Q	0	3851	0	4711	0	5641	0	4331	0	18534
18	R	1	4548	0	4376	1	4593	1	4059	3	17576
19	S	0	0	0	0	0	0	0	0	0	0
20	T	2	16573	2	17752	1	18509	2	17920	7	70754
21	U	0	9995	0	10267	0	11007	0	10273	0	41542

Q=quarters, other headings as above

```
# further use of reshape to cross-tabulate.
#using data.frame All
#expected derived from hospital levels
level<-read.table("clipboard",T) # data from levels.csv

# make sure level is in order
o<-order(level[,1])
level<-level[o,]


# 2006 data for selected hospitals
Counts<-tapply(All[,3],All[,1],sum)
Denoms<-tapply(All[,4],All[,1],sum)
levels<-data.frame(level,Counts,Denoms)
N<-tapply(levels[,3],levels[,2],sum)
M<-tapply(levels[,4],levels[,2],sum)
NM<-N/M
E<-0
for (i in 1:length(levels[,1]))
{E[i]<-NM[as.numeric(names(NM))==levels[i,2]]}
levels<-data.frame(levels,E)
o<-order(All[,1])
All1<-All[o,]
row.names(All1)<-1:length(All1[,1])
Ex<-rep(E,each=24) # 24 quarters 2001-06
Exp<-Ex*All1[,4]
All1<-data.frame(All1,Exp)
```

```
names(All1)<-c("H","DT","SB","DN","Exp")
d<-data.frame(rep(All1[,1],3),rep(All1[,2],3))
s<-stack(All1[,c(3,4,5)])
e<-data.frame(d,s)
names(e)<-c("Hosp","Qtr","Dta","Cat")
f<-reshape(e,direction="wide",timevar="Qtr",idvar=c("Hosp","Cat"))
a<-f[f[,1]==f[1,1],]
for (i in 2:21){a<-rbind(a,f[f[,1]==f[i,1],])} # 21 hospitals
Tot<-0
for (i in 1:63){Tot[i]<-sum(a[i,3:26])} # 3 by 21 hospitals
aa<-a
aa<-data.frame(aa,Tot)
Tot<-round(Tot,0)
a[,3:26]<-round(a[,3:26],0) #26 columns in a
row.names(a)<-NULL
names(a)<-c("Hosp","Cat","Y1Q1","Y1Q2","Y1Q3","Y1Q4","Y2Q1","Y2Q2","Y2Q3",
"Y2Q4","Y3Q1","Y3Q2","Y3Q3","Y3Q4","Y4Q1","Y4Q2","Y4Q3","Y4Q4","Y5Q1","Y5Q2",
"Y5Q3","Y5Q4","Y6Q1","Y6Q2","Y6Q3","Y6Q4")
a<-data.frame(a,Tot)
staphbact06<-aa[,c(1,2,23:26)]
#selected hospitals
sel<-staphbact06[staphbact06[,1]=="A"|staphbact06[,1]=="B"|
staphbact06[,1]=="F"|staphbact06[,1]=="I",]
Tot<-0
for (i in 1:12){Tot[i]<-sum(sel[i,3:6])}
Tot<-round(Tot,0)
sel[,3:6]<-round(sel[,3:6],0)
sel<-data.frame(sel,Tot)
names(sel)<-c("Hosp","Cat","Y6Q1","Y6Q2","Y6Q3","Y6Q4","Tot")
row.names(sel)<-NULL
sel
```

	Hosp	Cat	Y6Q1	Y6Q2	Y6Q3	Y6Q4	Tot
1	A	SB	1	7	4	3	15
2	A	DN	24705	25240	26237	23756	99938
3	A	Exp	2	2	2	2	9
4	B	SB	5	2	3	7	17
5	B	DN	49862	50555	51679	32283	184379
6	B	Exp	4	4	5	3	16
7	F	SB	6	9	12	4	31
8	F	DN	58006	60984	62329	57841	239160
9	F	Exp	10	10	10	10	40
10	I	SB	18	11	19	13	61
11	I	DN	66040	70168	72085	67467	275760
12	I	Exp	11	12	12	11	46

SB staphylococcus aureus bacteraemia
DN OBD denominator, Exp expected.

Note that the expected values in the table above are integers whereas their values are not. They may not add up exactly in the total column. This has been done because the other data in the columns are integers.

In the first table of this section the bacteraemia and denominator data have been cross-tabulated by years and hospitals. When quarters or months are required it becomes more complicated because the process converts data especially dates to factors or strings. Also the headings provided by reshape may be unsatisfactory and may need to be changed and the width of the table may make its study difficult. Using s.d(rs) and the clipboard to transfer the table to a spreadsheet for further formatting may be desirable. There are further examples later in the chapter.

6.10   Uncommon count data AEs

On some occasions, the average of the required counts will be quite low, for example one or two each month. When this occurs, Shewhart/EWMA charts are less informative. In addition, when control limits are calculated using the customary large sample normal approximations, the results can be unsatisfactory due to the discrete nature of the data and the skewness of the Poisson and negative binomial distributions. When events are uncommon, it may be preferable to employ a CUSUM and cumulative O-E chart similar to those described in Chapter 3. Spiegelhalter[E] and colleagues describe a suitable Poisson CUSUM. Although a negative binomial approach is possible, these uncommon events will usually occur independently when behaving predictably so the Poisson CUSUM should be suitable.

The formula for the Poisson log-likelihood weight is $W=O\times\log_e(R)-E\times(R-1)$, where E is the expected value for the time period, O is the observed value and R is the increase to be detected (the corresponding negative binomial formula is $W=O\times\log((1-P_1)/(1-P_0))-S\times\log(P_0/P_1)$ where O is the observed count, $S=M^2/(V-M)$, $P_0=S/(S+M)$, $P_1=S/(S+R\times M)$, M and V are the mean and variance, and R is the rate increase to be detected). When E is small it has been found empirically that $R=2$ is often suitable. Suppose E is known to be one outcome per month on average for line related bacteraemias during periods when predictable AE rates and monthly values are observed, then $[W=O\times\{\log_e(2)\}-1=O\times0.69-E]$ when $E=1$ and $R=2$. However, although these data are often grouped, for example, by months, we have employed daily rates, and we have assumed a single average daily rate. It should be borne in mind that daily rates will vary slightly as activity on weekdays is greater than at weekends, and some correction for this may prove to be desirable. For grouped data, see the internet Supplement.

The CUSUM (cumulative sum of the weights) required for a signal will depend on the false positive and false negative balance that is required. Since our main interest is in anticipating and if possible preventing an outbreak, we set the decision interval h to a low level, for example 2.5 or 3. We find that it is relatively easy for an infectious diseases physician to detect a false positive signal in hospital (but usually not community) data and false negative states that go undetected can be potentially dangerous. A suitable value for the CUSUM signal h can be determined by simulation. The file mrsabacts.csv contains MRSA bacteraemia data and ivdstaphbact.csv contains intravenous line-related *Staphylococcus aureus* bacteraemia data. The former has an expected value of approximately one per month (about 0.03 per day) and the latter approximately three every two months (approximately 0.05 per day). Figures 6.24 and 6.25 are the corresponding cumulative observed–expected plus CUSUM [(O-E)/CUSUM] charts using function countoecusum().

```
g.d() # mrsabact.csv

# using poiarl() to get ARL
poiarl()
```

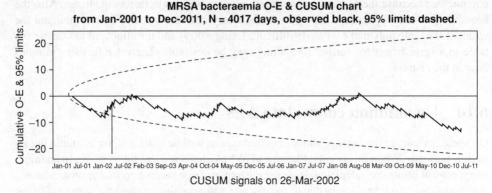

Figure 6.24 Count data cumulative observed minus expected (O-E)/CUSUM chart for uncommon count data AEs.

```
Enter the expected count .03
Enter the observed count .03
Enter the value for h 3
The ARL is 2006.81.
```

```
poiarl()
```

```
Enter the expected count .03
Enter the observed count .06
Enter the value for h 3
The ARL is 185.55.
```

Although simulated values vary, they provide reasonable approximations. There would be, at least approximately, a false signal in six to seven years. With just doubling of the rate a signal could be expected in about six months.

```
# using function countoecusum()
countoecusum(datain)
```

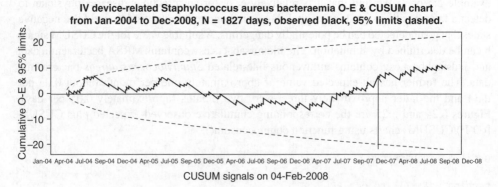

Figure 6.25 Similar type of chart to Figure 6.24.

```
The first date is 06-Feb-2001
Is an earlier date required (Y/N) y
Enter the new starting date 1-Jan-2001
The last date is 30-Dec-2011
Is a later date required (Y/N) y
Enter the new finishing date 31-Dec-2011
The mean outcome rate is  0.028
Do you wish to enter another value (Y/N) y
Enter the required value .03
Cumulative sum alert.
Enter the Cumulative sum (CUSUM) alert value 3
Chart heading.
Enter a heading for the chart MRSA Bacteraemia
```

g.d() # ivdstaphbact.csv, Figure 6.25

countoecusum(datain)

```
The first date is 14-Jan-2004
Is an earlier date required (Y/N) y
Enter the new starting date 1-Jan-2004
The last date is 07-Dec-2008
Is a later date required (Y/N) y
Enter the new finishing date 31-Dec-2008
The mean outcome rate is  0.055
Do you wish to enter another value (Y/N) y
Enter the required value .05
Cumulative sum alert.
Enter the Cumulative sum (CUSUM) alert value 3.5
Chart heading.
Enter a heading for the chart
IVD-related Staphylococcus aureus Bacteraemia
```

An issue with these charts is that they provide a CUSUM signal if there is a significant run of AEs and a cumulative count. While both are very useful, clinicians may ask for the current rate. We suggest two possible approaches. Cook and colleagues have proposed using an EWMA chart for ICU and CCU mortality data. While these are for risk-adjusted binary data with average outcome rates often exceeding 10%, the idea can be employed with these uncommon count data AEs. We illustrate with Figure 6.26. While Cook and colleagues advocate the method with ICU mortality data and include variance based limits, we feel that the method requires more evaluation when employed with uncommon binary and count data outcomes. We outline a possible approach to obtaining precision limits for binary data in the appendix to Chapter 3 and a similar approach may be feasible with count data. An alternative, that we feel could be useful for clinicians, is to employ quarterly counts.

g.d() # mrsabact.csv

countewmacusum(datain)

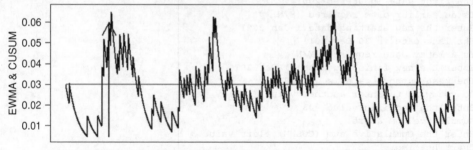

MRSA bacteraemias from Jan-2001 to Dac-2011.

CUSUM signals on 26-Mar-2002
EWMA expected gray, EWMA observed black, CUSUM signal arrow

Figure 6.26   EWMA plus CUSUM chart for uncommon AEs.

```
The first date is 06-Feb-2001
Is an earlier date required (Y/N) y
Enter the new starting date 1-Jan-2001
The last date is 30-Dec-2011
Is a later date required (Y/N) y
Enter the new finishing date 31-Dec-2011
The mean outcome rate is  0.028
Do you wish to enter another value (Y/N) y
Enter the required value .03
Cumulative sum alert.
Enter the Cumulative sum (CUSUM) alert value 3
EWMA weight .01
Enter a heading MRSA Bacteraemias
```

```
# Figure 6.27. quarterly data with precision limits
library(chron)
d<-datain[,1]
o<-order(d)
d<-d[o]
fst<-chron("01/01/2001")
lst<-chron("12/31/2011")
s<-seq.dates(from=fst,to=lst,by="months")
k<-NA
for (i in 1:(length(s)-1)){k[i]<-sum(d>=s[i]&d<s[i+1])}
k[length(s)]<-sum(d>=s[length(s)])
s<-chron(s,format="m/d/y",out.format="dd-mmm-yyyy")
dataout<-data.frame(s,k)
names(dataout)<-c("Months","Counts")
d<-dataout[,1]
e<-dataout[,2]
d<-chron(as.character(d),format="dd-mmm-yyyy",out.format="dd-mmm-yyyy")
Year<-years(d)
m<-as.numeric(months(d))
Qtrs<-rep(0,length(m))
Qtrs[m>=1&m<=3]<-1
```

```
Qtrs[m>=4&m<=6]<-2
Qtrs[m>=7&m<=9]<-3
Qtrs[m>=10&m<=12]<-4
Table<-as.data.frame(xtabs(e~Qtrs+Year))
Qtrs<-paste(Table[,2],"Q",Table[,1],sep="")
Tables<-data.frame(Qtrs,Table$Freq)
names(Tables)<-c("Qtrs","Freq")
library(exactci)
U<-0
L<-0
U1<-0
L1<-0
q<-paste("MRSA bacteraemias from ",Tables[1,1]," to ",
Tables[length(Tables[,1]),1],sep="")
for (i in 1:length(Tables[,1]))
{U[i]<-poisson.exact(Tables[i,2])$conf.int[2];
L[i]<-poisson.exact(Tables[i,2])$conf.int[1]}
for (i in 1:length(Tables[,1]))
{U1[i]<-poisson.exact(Tables[i,2],conf.level=.997)$conf.int[2];
L1[i]<-poisson.exact(Tables[i,2],conf.level=.997)$conf.int[1]}
m<-median(Tables[,2])
par(xaxs="r")
plot(Tables[,2],axes=F,col="blue",lwd=2,main=q,xlab="Quarters",
ylab="Counts",ylim=c(0,max(U1)))
box()
axis(side=1,labels=Tables[,1],at=1:length(Tables[,1]))
axis(side=c(2,3,4))
abline(h=m,lwd=2,col="red")
points(U,lwd=2,col="blue",pch="-",cex=1.5)
points(L,lwd=2,col="blue",pch="-",cex=1.5)
arrows(1:length(Tables[,1]),L1,1:length(Tables[,1]),U1,angle=90,code=3,
lwd=2,col="blue",length=.05)
mtext("Data, 95% & 99.7% CIs blue, Expected red",side=1,line=2)
text(Tables[,2],labels=as.character(Tables[,2]),pos=4,
offset=.3,cex=.8,lwd=3)
```

While Figure 6.27 would give clinicians a good idea of counts of uncommon AEs at various times, the 95% precision (confidence) limits should be viewed with caution; they are better thought of as indicating the precision of the quarterly counts. The CUSUM will usually signal promptly when there is a run of AEs that indicate an unpredictable system. However, a quarterly count with a lower confidence limit that exceeds the expected value would indicate that further study was warranted, especially if this were the case with the 99% or 99.7% (approximate 2.5 standard deviation or 3 standard deviation equivalent) confidence limit.

Displaying prediction limits, for example, in a quarterly data control chart may be an alternative if there are sufficient data, for example, at least four years. Figure 6.28 is a Shewhart/EWMA chart using the function countewmaqtr() that shows the upper 2 SD control limit exceeded in the first quarter of 2002. Other count data functions for quarterly or other data lacking dates in the first column include countshewqtr() and countgamqtr().

```
# quarterly data with prediction limits
g.d() # mrsabacts.csv

# monthly data (or use monthlycounts(datain))
```

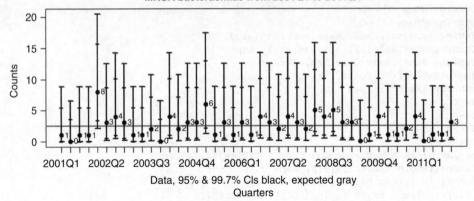

Figure 6.27   Quarterly counts with confidence intervals.

```
library(chron)
d<-datain[,1]
o<-order(d)
d<-d[o]
fst<-chron("01/01/2001")
lst<-chron("12/31/2011")
s<-seq.dates(from=fst,to=lst,by="months")
k<-NA
for (i in 1:(length(s)-1)){k[i]<-sum(d>=s[i]&d<s[i+1])}
k[length(s)]<-sum(d>=s[length(s)])
s<-chron(s,format="m/d/y",out.format="dd-mmm-yyyy")
dataout<-data.frame(s,k)
names(dataout)<-c("Months","Counts")

# quarterly data without denominators
# use dataout (monthly data) from above
# or use countquarters(dataout) with data in countqtr
d<-dataout[,1]
```

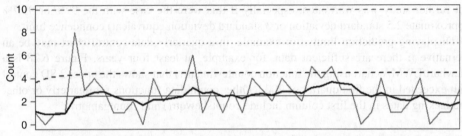

Figure 6.28   Shewhart/EWMA chart quarterly data, uncommon AEs.

```
e<-dataout[,2]
d<-chron(as.character(d),format="dd-mmm-yyyy",out.format="dd-mmm-yyyy")
Year<-years(d)
m<-as.numeric(months(d))
Qtrs<-rep(0,length(m))
Qtrs[m>=1&m<=3]<-1
Qtrs[m>=4&m<=6]<-2
Qtrs[m>=7&m<=9]<-3
Qtrs[m>=10&m<=12]<-4
Table<-as.data.frame(xtabs(e~Qtrs+Year))
q<-F
while(q==F){
if (Table[length(Table[,1]),3]==0){Table<-Table[-
length(Table[,1]),]}else{q<-T}
}
Table1<-Table
Qtr<-paste(Table1[,2],"Q",Table1[,1],sep="")
Table2<-data.frame(Qtr,Table1[,3])
names(Table2)<-c("Quarters","Counts")

# using countewmaqtr()
countewmaqtr(Table2) # or countewmaqtr(countqtr)
```

```
The mean count is 2.455.
Do you want to change the mean value (Y/N) n
The variance is 2.998 (SD 1.731 ).
Do you want to change the variance (Y/N) n
Chart heading.
Enter heading for chart MRSA bacteraemias
EWMA weight.
Enter weight between 0.2 & 0.8 .2
EWMA control limit.
Enter limit between 2 & 3 2.5
```

6.11   Additional scripts for tabulations and charts

Here we refer to some additional scripts that may prove to be of value when summarising count data in tables. The following example shows the tabulation of three years (2008–2010) of criterion 1 (definite) bacteraemias and new isolates of hospital-acquired organisms by source with row and column totals and by quarters. In the first case, modification would be required for different years. Tabulation can also be by organisms, wards or units.

```
g.d() # counttabulate.xls (cr1bacts)

#yearly tabulations by source
Source<-datain[,2]
Counts<-rep(1,length(datain[,1]))
Years<-years(datain[,1])
Rates<-as.data.frame(xtabs(Counts~Source+Years))
RatesRes<-reshape(Rates,direction="wide",timevar="Years",idvar="Source")
L<-length(RatesRes[1,])
Tl<-0
```

```
for (i in 1:length(RatesRes[,1])){Tl[i]<-sum(RatesRes[i,2:L])}
RatesRes1<-data.frame(RatesRes,Tl)
row.names(RatesRes1)<-1:length(RatesRes1[,1])
l<-length(RatesRes1[,1])
Tc<-0
for (i in 2:length(RatesRes1[1,])){Tc[i]<-sum(RatesRes1[1:l,i])}
Tc<-Tc[-1]
Tc1<-c("Tc",Tc)
x<-data.frame(t(Tc1))
names(RatesRes1)<-c("Source","Y8","Y9","Y10","Tr")
names(x)<-c("Source","Y8","Y9","Y10","Tr")
RatesRes2<-rbind(RatesRes1,x)
RatesRes2
```

	Source	Y8	Y9	Y10	Tr
1	bone.and.joint	1	2	0	3
2	cardiac	5	2	0	7
3	central.nervous.system	1	0	2	3
4	gastrointestinal	0	2	5	7
5	head.and.neck	0	1	0	1
6	hepatobiliary	16	28	14	58
7	intra-abdominal	8	11	9	28
8	Intravascular.catheter	81	88	67	236
9	Neutropaenic.Sepsis	9	14	6	29
10	other	3	0	1	4
11	respiratory.tract	10	10	12	32
12	skin.and.soft.tissue	11	8	13	32
13	surgical.site	22	5	10	37
14	Unknown.or.Disseminated	31	10	11	52
15	urinary.tract	37	45	43	125
16	Tc	235	226	193	654

```
#mros (multiple antibiotic-resistant organisms) worksheet
g.d() # counttabulate.xls (mros)


# yearly tabulations by organism
Orgs<-datain[,2]
Counts<-rep(1,length(datain[,1]))
Years<-years(datain[,1])
Rates<-as.data.frame(xtabs(Counts~Orgs+Years))
RatesRes<-reshape(Rates,direction="wide",timevar="Years",idvar="Orgs")
L<-length(RatesRes[1,])
Tl<-0
for (i in 1:length(RatesRes[,1])){Tl[i]<-sum(RatesRes[i,2:L])}
RatesRes1<-data.frame(RatesRes,Tl)
row.names(RatesRes1)<-1:length(RatesRes1[,1])
l<-length(RatesRes1[,1])
Tc<-0
for (i in 2:length(RatesRes1[1,])){Tc[i]<-sum(RatesRes1[1:l,i])}
Tc<-Tc[-1]
Tc1<-c("Tc",Tc)
x<-data.frame(t(Tc1))
names(RatesRes1)<-c("Orgs","Y8","Y9","Y10","Tr")
names(x)<-c("Orgs","Y8","Y9","Y10","Tr")
RatesRes2<-rbind(RatesRes1,x)
```

RatesRes2

	Orgs	Y8	Y9	Y10	Tr
1	Clostridium.difficile	28	25	41	94
2	K.pneumoniae.(ESBL)	19	17	6	42
3	MRAB	6	0	2	8
4	Multiresistant.MRSA	82	119	65	266
5	Non-multiresistant.MRSA	56	59	71	186
6	UK.EMRSA-15	25	43	26	94
7	VRE.Van.A	0	1	0	1
8	VRE.Van.B	39	72	181	292
9	Tc	255	336	392	983

```
#tabulations by quarters
g.d() # counttabulate.xls (cr1bacts)

# tabulations by source and quarters, first 6 rows shown
Source<-datain[,2]
Counts<-rep(1,length(datain[,1]))
Years<-years(datain[,1])
Months<-as.numeric(months(datain[,1]))
Qtrs<-rep(0,length(Months))
Qtrs[Months>=1&Months<=3]<-1
Qtrs[Months>=4&Months<=6]<-2
Qtrs[Months>=7&Months<=9]<-3
Qtrs[Months>=10&Months<=12]<-4
Rates<-as.data.frame(xtabs(Counts~Source+Qtrs+Years))
RatesRes<-reshape(Rates,direction="wide",timevar="Qtrs",idvar=c("Source",
"Years"))
Tl<-0
for (i in 1:length(RatesRes[,1])){Tl[i]<-sum(RatesRes[i,3:6])}
RatesRes1<-data.frame(RatesRes,Tl)
o<-order(RatesRes1[,1])
RatesRes1<-RatesRes1[o,]
names(RatesRes1)<-c("Source","Years","Q1","Q2","Q3","Q4","TR")
RatesRes1<-RatesRes1[RatesRes1<-RatesRes1[,7]!=0,]
l<-length(RatesRes1[,1])
TC<-0;TC[2]<-0
for (i in 3:length(RatesRes1[1,])){TC[i]<-sum(RatesRes1[1:l,i])}
TC<-TC[-c(1,2)]
TC1<-c("AllTotals","",TC)
x<-data.frame(t(TC1))
names(x)<-c("Source","Years","Q1","Q2","Q3","Q4","TR")
RatesRes2<-rbind(RatesRes1,x)
row.names(RatesRes2)<-1:length(RatesRes2[,2])
Totals<-as.data.frame(xtabs(RatesRes1[,3]~RatesRes1[,1]))
X<-data.frame(rep("Total",length(Totals[,1])))
Totals<-cbind(Totals[,1],X,Totals[,2])
for (i in 4:7){X<-as.data.frame(xtabs(RatesRes1[,i]~RatesRes1[,1]));Totals<-
cbind(Totals,X[,2])}
names(Totals)<-c("Source","Years","Q1","Q2","Q3","Q4","TR")
y<-rbind(RatesRes1,Totals)
o<-order(y[,1])
y<-y[o,]
Totals<-as.data.frame(xtabs(RatesRes1[,3]~RatesRes1[,2]))
```

```
X<-data.frame(rep("Total",length(Totals[,1])))
Totals<-cbind(X,Totals[,1],Totals[,2])
for (i in 4:7){X<-as.data.frame(xtabs(RatesRes1[,i]~RatesRes1[,2]));Totals<-
cbind(Totals,X[,2])}
names(Totals)<-c("Source","Years","Q1","Q2","Q3","Q4","TR")
y1<-rbind(y,Totals)
RatesRes3<-rbind(y1,x)
row.names(RatesRes3)<-1:length(RatesRes3[,1])
head(RatesRes3)
```

	Source	Years	Q1	Q2	Q3	Q4	TR
1	bone.and.joint	2008	0	1	0	0	1
2	bone.and.joint	2009	0	0	2	0	2
3	bone.and.joint	Total	0	1	2	0	3
4	cardiac	2008	0	2	2	1	5
5	cardiac	2009	0	0	1	1	2
6	cardiac	Total	0	2	3	2	7

```
tail(RatesRes3) # last 6 rows
```

	Source	Years	Q1	Q2	Q3	Q4	TR
52	urinary.tract	2010	16	9	10	8	43
53	urinary.tract	Total	41	29	23	32	125
54	Total	2008	60	72	60	43	235
55	Total	2009	63	55	46	62	226
56	Total	2010	59	38	40	56	193
57	AllTotals		182	165	146	161	654

There are a large number of potentially useful tabulations and only a small selection is shown, in particular to illustrate the use of the R functions xtabs() and reshape() and stack(). There are additional examples in the R code file on the internet.

6.12   Intervals between uncommon count data events

We discuss the analysis of intervals between uncommon binary data AEs in Chapter 3. Similar methods may be applied to time between rare events as the exponential and geometric distributions are similar for these types of events (Figures 6.29 to 6.32). MRSA bacteraemias in the file mrsabacts.csv occurred predictably at one hospital approximately once per month. Interval charts may be useful if there is a fall in the MRSA bacteraemia rate and a consequent increase in the intervals between these bacteraemias. Alternatively, a sustained increase in their frequency would result in a run of short intervals. The charts for the mrsabacts.csv data show several periods when intervals were longer and one when intervals appeared to become shorter than expected. Ideally, one might preferably be able to use data from a larger series, as was possible with the binary data, to obtain the mean and standard deviation for the transformed data. The final interval with no AE at its end is very short and is removed.

```
g.d() # mrsabact.csv

# run chart Figure 6.29
d<-datain[,1]
```

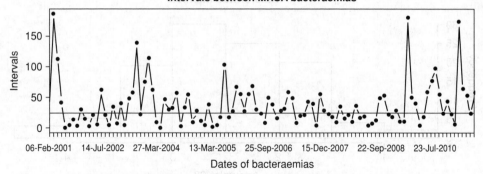

Figure 6.29   Run chart, intervals between uncommon AEs.

```
Start<-chron("1/1/2001",format="m/d/y",out.format="dd-mmm-yyyy")
End<-chron("12/31/2011",format="m/d/y",out.format="dd-mmm-yyyy")
da<-c(Start,d,End)
d1<-0
for (i in 1:(length(da)-1)){d1[i]<-da[i+1]-da[i]}
d1[d1==0]<-.5 # two on the one day, if 3 use e.g. 0.33
l<-length(d1)
d1[l] # short open last interval, remove
#[1] 1
d1<-d1[-l]
mean(d1)
#[1] 37.18519
1/mean(d1)
#[1] 0.02689243
qexp(.5,1/mean(d1))
#[1] 25.77481
db<-c(d,End)
db<-db[-1]
plot(d1,type="b",axes=F,col="blue",lwd=2,pch=19,
main="Intervals between MRSA bacteraemias",
xlab="Dates of bacteraemias",ylab="Intervals")
box()
axis(side=1,labels=db,at=1:length(db))
abline(h=24.5,col="red",lwd=2)
axis(side=c(2,3,4))


# Weibull transformation Figure 6.30
dd<-d1^.28
hist(dd,main="Transformed intervals",xlab="Intervals^.28")


qqnorm(dd)
qqline(dd)
shapiro.test(dd)$p.value # distribution approximately normal Figure 6.31
#[1] 0.3662093
mean(dd)
#[1] 2.521157
sd(dd)
#[1] 0.7056607
```

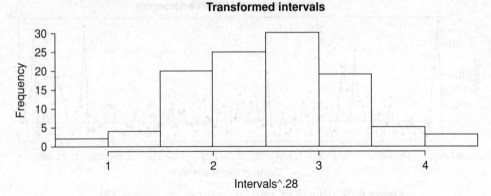

Figure 6.30   Histogram, normal distribution of transformed intervals.

```
iewmachart(data.frame(db,dd)) # Figure 6.32
```

```
Chart heading.
Enter a heading for the chart Transformed interval chart MRSA bacteraemias
Y axis heading.
Enter a heading for the Y axis Transformed intervals
The mean value is 2.52116.
Do you want to change the mean value (Y/N) n
The standard deviation is 0.70566.
Do you want to change it (Y/N) n
EWMA weight.
Enter weight between 0.2 & 0.8 .2
EWMA control limit.
Enter limit between 2 & 3 2.5
```

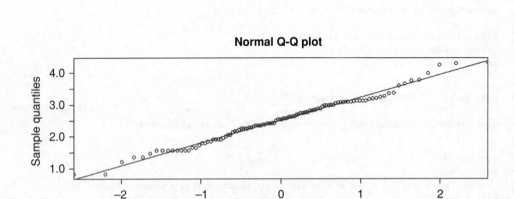

Figure 6.31   Q-Q plot of transformed intervals.

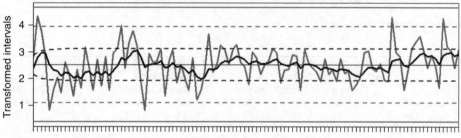

Transformed interval chart MRSA bacteraemias
Shewhart/EWMA i chart from Feb-01 to Dec-11.

Feb-01 Feb-02 Jun-02 Oct-02 Jan-04 Jul-04 Jan-05 Apr-05 Jan-06 Nov-06 Jun-07 Jan-08 Apr-08 Sep-08 Aug-09 Jul-10 Jun-11

Data, 2 & 3 sigma control limits gray, EWMA thick & control limit dashed.

Figure 6.32   Shewhart/EWMA chart of transformed intervals.

6.13   Note on calculation of negative binomial parameters for control charts when denominators vary

6.13.1   Simple weighted variance

The mean count is $M=\sum X_i/N$ where X_i is the count for the ith month and N is the number of months. The weighted variance is $V=\{1/(N-1)\} \sum\{W_i \cdot (X_i/W_i-M)^2\}$ where $W_i=D_i/Dbar$, Di is the denominator for the ith month and $Dbar=\sum D_i/N$. $S=M^2/(V-M)$, $Pbar=S/(S+M)$, $Cbar=Pbar/(1-Pbar)$, $C_i=Cbar/W_i$, $P_i=C_i/(1+C_i)$. $M^*_i=S\cdot((1-P_i)/P_i)$. Simplifying, $P_i=M/((W_i \times (V-M)+M))$ and $M^*_i=M \times W_i$.

6.13.2   Linear approximation (Bissell)

$Y=\sum((X_i-M \times W_i)^2/W_i)$
$C=M/((Y/(N-1))-M)$

Repeat five times (may need more if very variable denominators)
$M=\sum(X_i/(C+W_i))/\sum(W_i/(C+W_i))$
$T=(C/(M \times (N-1))) \times \sum((X_i-M \times W_i)^2/(W_i \times (C+W_i)))$
$C=C/(C \times T+T-C)$
End repeat

$C_i=C/W_i$
$M^*_i=M \times W_i$
$S=C \times M$

6.13.3 Comparison of simple weighted variance and Bissell's linear approximation

Example (monthlymrsa.csv).

	Monthly New MRSA Isolates & Bed-Days		Weighted Variance		Linear Approximation	
Times	Counts	Denominators	P_i	M^*_i	P_i	M^*_i
01-Jul-1995	32	25683	0.47	44.85	0.47	44.84
01-Aug-1995	43	25497	0.47	44.52	0.47	44.52
01-Sep-1995	50	23971	0.49	41.86	0.49	41.85
01-Oct-1995	33	24192	0.49	42.24	0.49	42.24
01-Nov-1995	24	23911	0.49	41.75	0.49	41.75
01-Dec-1995	31	21738	0.51	37.96	0.51	37.96
01-Jan-1996	52	22720	0.50	39.67	0.50	39.67
01-Feb-1996	48	24035	0.49	41.97	0.49	41.97
01-Mar-1996	55	25058	0.48	43.76	0.48	43.75
01-Apr-1996	42	22795	0.50	39.81	0.50	39.80
01-May-1996	34	24397	0.48	42.60	0.48	42.60
01-Jun-1996	30	23686	0.49	41.36	0.49	41.36
01-Jul-1996	51	25005	0.48	43.66	0.48	43.66
01-Aug-1996	48	25412	0.47	44.38	0.47	44.37
01-Sep-1996	39	23266	0.49	40.63	0.50	40.62
01-Oct-1996	53	24631	0.48	43.01	0.48	43.01
01-Nov-1996	51	23700	0.49	41.39	0.49	41.38
01-Dec-1996	38	22092	0.51	38.58	0.51	38.57

```
g.d() # monthlymrsa.csv

# datain[,1] dates, datain[,2] counts, datain[,3] denominators
# Bissell's approximation
x<-datain[,2]
d<-datain[,3]
xt<-mean(datain[,2])
l<-length(datain[,2])
w<-d/mean(d)
ysq<-sum((x-xt*w)^2/w)
c1<-xt/((ysq/(l-1))-xt)
for (i in 1:5){
x2<-sum(x/(c1+w))/sum(w/(c1+w))
t1<-(c1/(x2*(l-1)))*sum(((x-x2*w)^2)/(w*(c1+w)))
c1<-c1/(c1*t1+t1-c1)
i<-i+1
}
S<-c1*x2
S
#[1] 39.94706
ci<-c1/w
mi<-x2*w
pi<-ci/(1+ci)
print(pi)
print(mi)
```

```
# using weighted variance
d1<-datain[,2]
d2<-datain[,3]
m<-mean(d1)
dbar<-mean(d2)
dw<-d2/dbar
v<-sum(dw*(d1/dw-m)^2/(length(dw)-1))
S<-m^2/(v-m)
S
#[1] 39.81985
Mi<-m*dw
Pi<-m/((dw*(v-m)+m))
print(Mi)
print(Pi)
```

For an upper two sigma equivalent control limit we successively increase a counter K_i starting at M^*_i, until we find pbeta$(P_i,S,M^*_i+K_i)==.97725$. To achieve this, K_i is successively increased by one until pbeta$(P_i,S,M^*_i+K_i)>.97725$ (or 1-pbeta$(P_i,S,M^*_i+K_i)<.02275$) and K_i is then decreased by .001 until pbeta$(P_i,S,M^*_i+K_i)<.97725$ (or 1-pbeta$(P_i,S,M^*_i+K_i)>.02275$). $M^*_i+K_i$ is then the approximate upper two sigma control limit for the ith monthly count. The other control limits are calculated in a similar way.

There is a potential difficulty with using Bissell's approximation: when the negative binomial parameters are obtained from a predictable subset of the data it is difficult to implement the analysis in a single simple function. There are two functions in rprogs, getnegbinparams() and ratenegbin() that enable the parameters and the chart to be obtained separately. However, the informal comparison shown above suggests that the simple weighted variance should be sufficiently accurate for calculating control limits in the Shewhart/EWMA charts that we use. The maximum likelihood calculations would improve accuracy further but implementation in a control chart has proved difficult and the difference in the P_i and M^*_i values shown above appear small, at least with the fairly limited range of denominators that are typical of most hospital count AE data. Unfortunately, so far as we are aware, no R library currently contains a function for implementing negative binomial maximum likelihood in a suitable way when there are differing denominators. Further work may clarify this situation but it appears that the simple weighted variance provides sufficient accuracy for practical purposes with MRSA new isolate data, a common situation for the use of negative binomial control limits. However, as we have observed, this may reflect the fact that hospital denominator data usually do not differ markedly. When denominators differ greatly, for example, funnel plot data in Chapter 5, the simple weighted variance may prove less satisfactory. However, when denominators differ greatly the reason needs to be understood and any sequential analysis may need to be re-started. Moreover, for sequential data, a GAM chart can be employed. We prefer the latter approach.

```
getnegbinparams(datain)
```

```
The mean count is 41.889.
The mean denominator is 23988.
The weighted variance (V) is 85.954.
S=39.94706, Cbar=0.9537518, Pbar=0.4881643, Mean=41.88413
```

```
ratenegbin(datain) # chart not shown
```

```
Enter S 39.95
Enter Cbar .95
Enter Mean 41.88
Denominators.
Enter name for denominator Bed-days
Denominators.
Per ten thousand (10000), thousand (1000), hundred (100), ten (10), unit (1)
Bed-days 1000
Chart heading.
Enter heading for chart Monthly New MRSA Isolates
```

7

Miscellaneous AEs

In this chapter we describe some further miscellaneous AEs. First, we deal with multiple antibiotic-resistant organism (MRO) prevalence (burden) that typically has no predictable mean value in sequential data and that can display considerable autocorrelation. Similar remarks apply to antibiotic usage and may be relevant to some other drug usage. For these we employ spline regression although loess regression may be a useful alternative. We will refer to the chart using splines as a GAM (generalised additive model) chart.

Some data may display marked skewness (long right tails), and at least approximately, distributions like fractal power law distributions. Some preliminary analysis suggests that in some cases these may include length of stay (LOS) in hospital, or ICU or time on a ventilator (and possibly also cost of stay), waiting times (Papadopoulos and colleagues), severity of medication errors, possibly severity of some other AEs and some risk-adjustment scores. Analysis of these data must depend on the purpose of the analysis. For example, many operations have fairly stable postoperative LOS and the occurrence of excess numbers exceeding a median value derived from a group of hospitals may be a cause for concern. These data can therefore be dichotomised and, if a suitable risk adjustment tool or some covariate information is available, they can then be risk adjusted, in the latter case using logistic regression. In other cases, interest may be in the long right tails of the distributions. A simple approach would be to employ a high percentile (e.g. the 90th) of the data from a reference group of hospitals and dichotomise the data from the hospital of interest at that value. As with the median, the data can then be risk-adjusted, for example, using logistic regression if suitable covariate information is available, or a risk adjustment tool like the EuroSCORE may be suitable with re-calibration. The power law issue is of great interest but detailed consideration is currently beyond the scope of these notes.

Other numerical data of interest include ward, theatre or other resource utilisation. These can usually be handled with conventional Shewhart charts for numerical data. Occasionally, data in ordered categories are of interest and a control chart based on RIDITs can be employed.

Statistical Methods for Hospital Monitoring with R, First Edition. Anthony Morton, Kerrie Mengersen, Michael Whitby and George Playford.
© 2013 John Wiley & Sons, Ltd. Published 2013 by John Wiley & Sons, Ltd.

To aid in the selection of suitable control chart methods, there is an appendix Control Chart Menu at the end of the Introduction. In addition, there is a corresponding function CCMenu() in rprogs.

7.1   MRO prevalence

It is useful to monitor prevalence of MRO colonisation (MRO Burden) as increasing prevalence will promote enhanced transmission to new patients and thus the possible occurrence of new colonisations and infections. This may then result in the emergence of an outbreak. It is also important for determining screening, isolation and cohorting requirements and can indicate the need to improve environmental cleaning (especially of high-touch surfaces), and hand hygiene, and to gain better control of staff-patient networks. Burden data can display autocorrelation or trends that may be real or the wandering of a tine-series. By far the most common type of autocorrelation (AR1 or first-order autoregressive) occurs when today's prevalence is more like yesterday's than it would be if each day's data were independent. When this occurs statistical analysis that assumes independence will usually display a spuriously large number of abnormal results. Analysis with conventional control charts is usually not advisable (the moving average EWMA chart developed for this purpose and described by Montgomery can be difficult for hospital scientists to implement and to interpret). A run chart may be employed with suitable smoothing, for example using the R function smooth.spline().

The R spline library is useful for analysing potentially trended and autocorrelated time series data for QI; an alternative is to use the more advanced and complex mgcv library but we have found that the simpler spline library suffices. Infectious disease physicians should be alerted if there is new evidence of unusual prevalence of any organism of interest such as *Acinetobacter* sp., vancomycin-resistant *Enterococcus* (VRE), ESBL-*Klebsiella pneumoniae*, *Clostridium difficile* or methicillin-resistant *Staphylococcus aureus* (MRSA), especially if the unusual level is sustained for several days and if there is difficulty with isolating or cohorting carriers.

Montgomery suggests statistical process control (SPC) methods for dealing with autocorrelation. These include employing the exponentially weighted moving average (EWMA) method (see sections 3.20.2 and 6.5.1) with the EWMA weight that minimises the sum of the squared one-ahead forecast errors and to employ the latter in a Shewhart chart that is called a Moving Average EWMA or MAEWMA chart. However, as we have indicated, hospital staff may have difficulty with MAEWMA charts. A further method is to use unweighted batch means in an i chart (Runger and Willemain). We concentrate on average daily numbers per month that is equivalent to using unweighted batch means and autocorrelation is usually greatly diminished or eliminated. However, we prefer a GAM (spline regression) chart to a MAEWMA chart or i chart as the MAEWMA chart can be difficult to interpret and the i chart requires data from which a stable mean can be calculated (Morton[B] and colleagues). Trends can be monitored using a seasonal Mann-Kendall test from the R Kendall library.

Daily MRSA prevalence data in a hospital are in the data file mrsaburden.csv. The R time series functions acf() and pacf() show evidence of marked autocorrelation (Figure 7.1). The usual pattern is an AR1 or first-order autoregressive process where contiguous results are more alike than they would be if independent. The ACF chart typically shows a large spike at lag 1 with exponentially decreasing spikes thereafter and the partial autocorrelation function (PACF) a single large spike at lag 1. The latter shows the influence of autocorrelation

Daily MRSA Burden, ACF Chart.

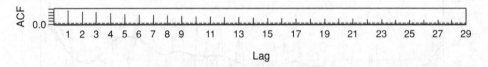

Daily MRSA Burden, PACF Chart.

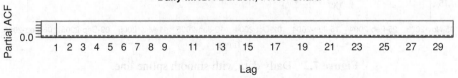

Figure 7.1   ACF/PACF chart showing autocorrelation.

between time periods while controlling for other time periods. However, the presence of a trend may suggest that autocorrelation is present. If a trend is present it is important to run a test, for example by creating a time-series object with a lag, and testing for its significance, for example in a GAM analysis.

In practice, although monitoring daily burden may be desirable and surveillance staff will be aware of daily numbers as they juggle isolation bed usage, it is usually more practicable to employ charts with monthly data.

```
g.d() #mrsaburden.csv
#
```

```
Loading data.
Data from clipboard (C) or file (F) c
Do data column(s) have heading(s) (Y/N) y
Is column 1 a date column (Y/N) y
Date format.
 5-Nov-03
Date format.
Enter the required date format d-mmm-yy
```

```
# using function do.acf()
do.acf(datain[,2])
```

```
Enter a heading for the ACF plot Daily MRSA Burden
```

```
#creating time-series object, assessing autocorrelation
library(splines)
a<-datain[,2]
a1<-ts(a)
id<-1:length(a);id1<-ts(id)
tg<-ts.union(a1,id1,a2=lag(a1,-1))
mg<-glm(a1~a2+bs(id1),data=tg,family=poisson)
summary(mg) # a2, the lag variable, is highly significant
```

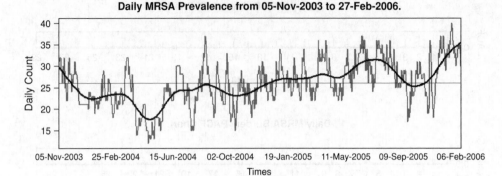

Figure 7.2   Daily data with smooth spline line.

```
Abbreviated summary
                Estimate    Std.Error    z value    Pr(>|z|)
(Intercept)     2.361989    0.050898     46.407     < 2e-16    ***
a2              0.034116    0.001622     21.038     < 2e-16    ***
 Null deviance: 844.94 on 798 degrees of freedom
Residual deviance: 148.92 on 794 degrees of freedom
AIC: 4214.7
```

Figure 7.2 and 7.3 are charts employing the R function smooth.spline() and a glm involving the splines library (GAM chart), the latter incorporating an autocorrelation term. In Figure 7.3, note that the lines on either side of the prediction line indicate the precision of the generalised additive model predictions; they have no relationship to the individual data values. The upper black line is equivalent to two standard deviations above the smoothed prediction line. It shows, approximately, those individual observations that may be too large to fit the pattern of the time series, analogous to a warning control limit on a control chart. Although requiring rigorous evaluation, this is motivated by the Poisson outbreak detection (POD) method proposed by Pelecanos and colleagues. It may help detect time periods when the data values are not typical of the time-series.

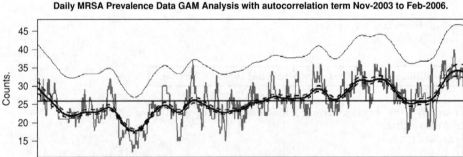

Figure 7.3   GAM chart of daily autocorrelated data.

```
# smooth.spline Figure 7.2
d<-datain[,1]
a<-datain[,2]
d<-chron(as.character(d),format="dd-mmm-yyyy",out.format="dd-mmm-yyyy")
par(xaxs="i")
plot(a,type="l",col="dark blue",lwd=2,axes=F,xlab="Times",ylab="Daily
Count",main="Daily MRSA Prevalence from 05-Nov-2003 to 27-Feb-2006.")
box()
axis(side=1,labels=d,at=1:length(d),tick=F)
axis(side=c(2,3,4))
lines(smooth.spline(a,spar=.7),col="red",lwd=2)
abline(h=median(a))

# GAM chart Figure 7.3
library(chron)
library(splines)
d<-datain[,1]
d<-chron(as.character(d),format="dd-mmm-yyyy",out.format="dd-mmm-yyyy")
a<-datain[,2]
o<-order(d)
d<-d[o]
a<-a[o]
dd<-as.Date(d,"%d-%b-%Y")
ddd<-format.Date(dd,"%b%y") # dates in  small format for horizontal
# axis of chart
a1<-ts(a)
id<-1:length(a);id1<-ts(id)
tg<-ts.union(a1,id1,a2=lag(a1,-1))
mg<-glm(a1~a2+bs(id1),data=tg,family=poisson)
mgp<-predict(mg,se=T)
u<-0
TT<-exp(mgp$fit)
AA<-0
U<-0
Z<-.02275
for (i in 1:length(TT)){
M<-TT[i]
X<-M
A<-1
BL<-F
while (BL==F){
X<-X+A
K<-pgamma(M,X,1)
if (K<Z){BL<-T}
}
if (M<=2){AA<-.001}
if (M>2 & M<=5){AA<-.01}
if (M>5){AA<-.1}
BL<-F
while (BL==F){
X<-X-AA
K<-pgamma(M,X,1)
if (K>=Z){BL<-T}
}
U[i]<-X
}
```

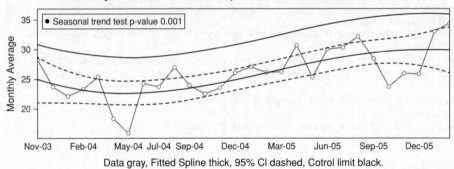

Figure 7.4 GAM chart monthly data.

```
u<-smooth.spline(U,spar=.6)
par(xaxs="i")
hdr0<-"Daily MRSA Prevalence Data GAM Analysis"
hdr1<-"\nwith autocorrelation term Nov 2003 to Feb 2006."
hdr2<-"Data blue, GAM red, 95% CI brown,"
hdr3<-" Upper 2 sigma-equivalent control limit black, Median green."
hdr<-paste(hdr0,hdr1,sep="");hdr4<-paste(hdr2,hdr3,sep="")
plot(a1[-1],type="l",lwd=2,col="blue",axes=F,
ylim=c(min(a1[-1]),max(u$y)),ylab="Counts.",
xlab=hdr4,main=hdr)
box()
axis(side=1,tick=F,labels=as.character(ddd[-1]),at=id[-length(id)])
axis(side=c(2,3,4))
k<-exp(mgp$fit)
lines(smooth.spline(k,spar=.6),lwd=2,col="red")
abline(h=median(a),lwd=2,col="green4")
up<-exp(mgp$fit+1.96*mgp$se.fit)
lo<-exp(mgp$fit-1.96*mgp$se.fit)
lines(smooth.spline(up,spar=.6),lwd=2,col="brown")
lines(smooth.spline(lo,spar=.6),lwd=2,col="brown")
lines(u,col="black",lty=1)
```

Figure 7.4 is a GAM chart of the monthly average values and Figure 7.5 is a GAM chart of the weekly average values. With these averages we use lm() in R instead of glm(). Although

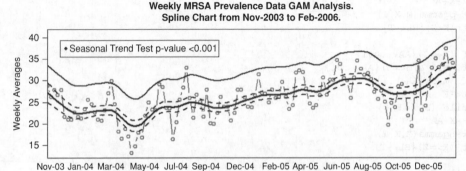

Figure 7.5 GAM chart weekly autocorrelated data.

it may at times be possible to use a Shewhart i chart with monthly averages that are often free of autocorrelation, these data usually display trends. Because there is so often no predictable mean value available, the latter analysis is often difficult to recommend. For example, the mean value of the data in Figure 7.3 is 25.9 and the median is 26. These are typical of a few of the data values.

```
# monthly averages
# using function monthlyaverage()
monthlyaverage(datain) # data in dataout

#using function numgamauto(), figure not shown
numgamauto(dataout) #includes autocorrelation term
```

```
Chart heading.
Enter a heading for the chart Monthly MRSA Prevalence Data
Y axis heading.
Enter a heading for the Y axis Monthly Average
Change degrees of freedom (Y/N) n
```

The P-value for the autocorrelation term (a2) was 0.2 so the inference is that there is not significant autocorrelation in this series. The residual standard error was 3.074 on 22 degrees of freedom and the multiple R-squared $= 0.5364$ (adjusted $= 0.4521$). The F-statistic was 6.364 on 4 and 22 DF (p-value $= 0.001466$). These terms are interpreted in the usual manner for a regression analysis (Crawley). When the chart appears, the pointer is a +; position it in clear area and press the left mouse button to place the Mann-Kendall time-series trend test result. We repeat the analysis without the autocorrelation term.

```
#using function numgam(), Figure 7.4
numgam(dataout)
```

```
Chart heading.
Enter a heading for the chart Monthly MRSA Prevalence Data
Y axis heading.
Enter a heading for the Y axis Monthly Average
Change degrees of freedom (Y/N) n
```

The residual standard error was 3.169 on 24 degrees of freedom and the multiple R-squared was 0.4682 (adjusted R-squared $= 0.4018$). The F-statistic value was 7.044 on 3 and 24 DF (p-value $= 0.001469$). The trend test result is highly significant (p-value $= .001$).

```
#weekly counts
#find beginning and end of series
#start on Sunday, finish on Saturday
library(chron)
d<-datain[,1]
d<-chron(d,format="dd-mmm-yyyy",out.format="dd-mmm-yyyy")
m<-datain[,2]
o<-order(d)
d<-d[o]
m<-m[o]
#finding start
fst<-chron(d[1])
weekdays(fst)
```

```
#
#[1] Wed
#Levels: Sun < Mon < Tue < Wed < Thu < Fri < Sat

k<-as.numeric(weekdays(fst))
k
#[1] 4
fst<-fst-k+1 # find Sunday
weekdays(fst)
#[1] Sun
#Levels: Sun < Mon < Tue < Wed < Thu < Fri < Sat
chron(fst,out.format="dd-mmm-yyyy")
#[1] 02-Nov-2003
#finding end
lst<-chron(d[length(d)])
weekdays(lst)
#
#[1] Mon
#Levels: Sun < Mon < Tue < Wed < Thu < Fri < Sat

k<-as.numeric(weekdays(lst))
k
#[1] 2
lst<-lst-k+7
chron(lst,out.format="dd-mmm-yyyy")
#1] 04-Mar-2006
weekdays(lst)
#[1] Sat
#Levels: Sun < Mon < Tue < Wed < Thu < Fri < Sat

#finding weekly sequence
s<-seq.dates(from=fst,to=lst,by="weeks")
#finding counts for each week
#weekly averages, imputing data in weeks with no data
k<-NA
for (i in 1:(length(s)-1)){k[i]<-mean(m[d>=s[i]&d<s[i+1]])}
k[length(s)]<-mean(m[d>=s[length(s)]])
nak<-which(is.na(k)) # week with no data
nak
#[1] 110

#imputing week with no data
k[nak]<-(k[nak-1]+k[nak+1])/2
k[nak]
#[1] 27.08333

dm<-data.frame(s,k)
dm[1,1]<-d[1] # adjust first day of series
names(dm)<-c("Weeks","Averages")

# using numgamauto(), Figure 7.5
# change date format
d<-as.character(dm[,1])
d<-chron(d,format="m/d/y",out.format="dd-mmm-yyyy")
a<-dm[,2]
numgamauto(data.frame(d,a))
```

```
Chart heading.
Enter a heading for the chart Weekly MRSA Prevalence Data GAM Analysis.
Y axis heading.
Enter a heading for the Y axis Weekly averages
Change degrees of freedom (Y/N) n
```

The autocorrelation term a2 (P-value<.001) was highly significant. The residual standard error was 3.207 on 116 degrees of freedom with two observations deleted due to missingness (creating the time series object) and the multiple R-squared was 0.5654 (adjusted R-squared = 0.5504). The F-statistic value was 37.73 on 4 and 116 DF (p-value < 2.2e-16). The trend test result was highly significant (p-value<.001). It is clear that it is an irregular time series unsuited to standard control chart analysis.

7.2   Antibiotic usage

Like MRO burden, antibiotic usage tends to display as a nonstationary time-series without an identifiable mean value that makes using conventional control charts difficult (Morton[B] and colleagues). It is worth emphasising again that it is the employment of the best currently available evidence that is the key to optimum usage. Although sequential statistical analysis is valuable, control of usage of powerful antibiotic drugs by infectious diseases physicians, audit of compliance with guidelines and feedback are necessary. Pharmacists play a crucial role in this process.

Due to the nonstationary nature of these data when examined sequentially, we employ a GAM for their analysis. We illustrate the analysis with monthly carbapenem usage in defined daily doses (DDDs) per 1000 occupied bed-days (OBDs) in the file carbapenem.csv (Figure 7.6). If DDDs and OBDs are in separate columns, it is necessary to multiply the former for example, by 1000 and divide by the latter, for example, dataout<-data.frame(datain[,1],datain[,2]*1000/datain[,3]). In some cases, OBDs may not be available; if so one can just use the DDDs. Daily usage data and corresponding OBDs can be aggregated by months using the function monthlynumbers().

```
# loading carbapenem data
g.d() # carbapenem.csv (dates in first column)

#testing for autocorrelation
library(splines)
a<-datain[,2]
a1<-ts(a)
id<-1:length(a);id1<-ts(id)
tg<-ts.union(a1,id1,a2=lag(a1,-1))
mg<-lm(a1~a2+bs(id1),data=tg)
summary(mg) #the autocorrelation term a2 is not significant (P-value=0.15)
#using function numgam(), Figure 7.6
numgam(datain)
```

```
Chart heading.
Enter a heading for the chart Monthly Carbapenem Usage.
Y axis heading.
Enter a heading for the Y axis DDD per 1000 OBDs
Change degrees of freedom (Y/N) n
```

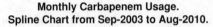

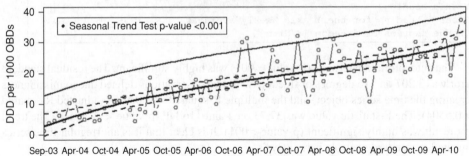

Data gray, Fitted Spline thick, 95% CI dashed, Control limit black.

Figure 7.6   GAM chart, antibiotic usage.

The residual standard error was 5.081 on 80 degrees of freedom and the multiple R-squared was 0.6753 (adjusted R-squared = 0.6632). The F-statistic was 55.47 on 3 and 80 DF (P-value $< 2.2e\text{-}16$). When the chart appears, the pointer is a +, position it in a clear area and press left mouse button to place the Mann-Kendall time-series trend test result that is highly significant (P-value $< .001$). As well as a prominent trend, there were three monthly values that are possible outliers.

7.3   Spurious proportions, some blood culture data

When confronted with data that have outcomes in the numerator and procedures in the denominator, it is natural to consider using a binomial control chart. However, there are situations where this approach is unwise. If the monthly grouped data have markedly differing rates, use of the binomial distribution is likely to be incorrect. One situation where this occurs is illustrated by the data in bloodcult.csv where the numerator is blood cultures that were positive and the denominator is blood specimens taken. (We thank Dr Graeme Nimmo for the use of these data.) Since patients differ in the probability of having a bacteraemia and some patients have multiple tests, these data are not independent and homogeneous. In addition, there was a change in the processing of these specimens so that a single mean value is not present. We illustrate the use of a Shewhart i control chart using a run of the data values that displayed predictability to determine the mean value, and a GAM chart to further analyse the data.

```
g.d() # bloodcult.csv (first column dates in d/m/y format)

#using function runchart(), Figure 7.7
runchart(datain)
```

```
Chart heading.
Enter a heading for the chart Positive Blood Culture Data
Y axis heading.
Enter a heading for the Y axis Proportions Positive
```

There appears to be a change point about June 1996 with data values becoming lower. Before proceeding further, it is necessary to define the extent of the earlier predictable data

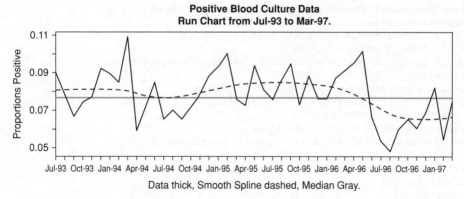

Figure 7.7   Run chart blood culture data.

using the locator() function. Use the left mouse button to define the start and end of this and then right click to return to the R prompt. The predictable data ended about month 35, May 1996.

```
# using locator()
locator()

#$x

#[1]  35.00479
#$y
#[1]  0.1009057

# mean and sd of predictable data
m<-mean(datain[1:35,2])
std<-sd(datain[1:35,2])
m
#[1]  0.08242857
std
#[1]  0.01161947
```

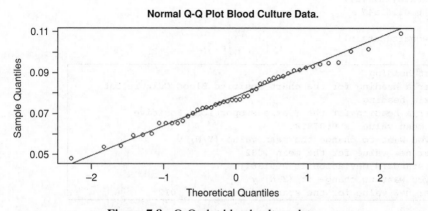

Figure 7.8   Q-Q plot blood culture data.

```
#look for normal distribution, important for i chart
shapiro.test(datain[,2])
#          Shapiro-Wilk normality test
#W = 0.9898, p-value = 0.9588
qqnorm(datain[,2],main="Normal Q-Q Plot Blood Culture Data.")
qqline(datain[,2])
#data are compatible with normal distribution
#however, there appear to be two distributions
# testing predictable data
shapiro.test(datain[1:35,2])$p.value
#[1] 0.8062321 (compatible with normal distribution)

#look for autocorrelation
library(splines)
a<-datain[,2]
a1<-ts(a)
id<-1:length(a);id1<-ts(id)
tg<-ts.union(a1,id1,a2=lag(a1,-1))
mg<-lm(a1~a2+bs(id1),data=tg)
summary(mg) #the autocorrelation term a2 is not significant (P-value=0.13)

#test for change point in May 1996
n<-length(datain[,1])-35
x<-c(rep(0,35),rep(1,n))
y<-1:length(datain[,1])
l<-lm(datain[,2]~x+bs(y)) # using a GAM with a dummy variable
summary(l) #change in mean level of x, high significance of x
# (P-value=.0001)
#test for change point using Wilcoxon's test (Pettitt)
wilcox.test(datain[,2]~x)
# P-value=.0002
```

These data can be analysed using a Shewhart i chart that employs the mean and standard deviation of the first 35 months' data.

```
#using function ishewchart(), Figure 7.9
mean(datain[1:35,2])
#[1] 0.08242857
var(datain[1:35,2])
#[1] 0.0001350121
sd(datain[1:35,2])
#[1] 0.01161947

ishewchart(datain)
```

```
Chart heading.
Enter a heading for the chart Positive Blood Culture Data
Y axis heading.
Enter a heading for the Y axis Proportions Positive
The mean value is 0.07818.
Do you want to change the mean value (Y/N) y
Enter new value for the mean .082
The standard deviation is 0.01381.
Do you want to change it (Y/N) y
Enter new value for the standard deviation .012
```

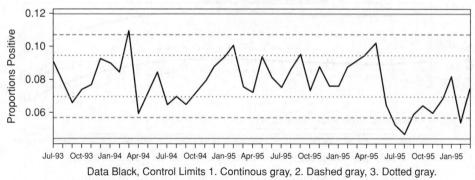

Data Black, Control Limits 1. Continous gray, 2. Dashed gray, 3. Dotted gray.

Figure 7.9   Shewhart i chart blood culture data.

```
#Shewhart/EWMA i chart, Figure 7.10
#using function iewmachart()
iewmachart(datain)
```

```
Chart heading.
Enter a heading for the chart Positive Blood Culture Data
Y axis heading.
Enter a heading for the Y axis Proportions Positive
The mean value is 0.07818.
Do you want to change the mean value (Y/N) y
Enter new value for the mean .082
The standard deviation is 0.01381.
Do you want to change it (Y/N) y
Enter new value for the standard deviation .012
EWMA weight.
Enter weight between 0.2 & 0.8 .2
EWMA control limit.
Enter limit between 2 & 3 2.5
```

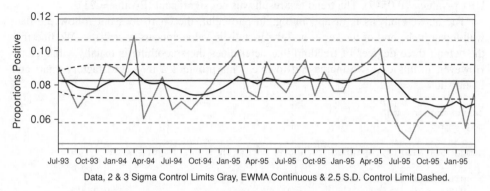

Data, 2 & 3 Sigma Control Limits Gray, EWMA Continuous & 2.5 S.D. Control Limit Dashed.

Figure 7.10   Shewhart/EWMA i chart blood culture data.

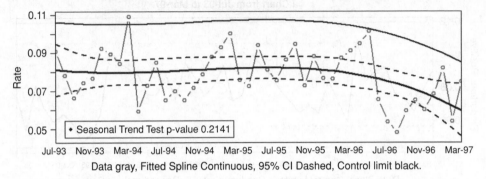

Figure 7.11   GAM chart, blood culture data, 3 degrees of freedom.

The i chart may be useful for single observation numerical data that display approximate normality when in a predictable state. Although it was possible to identify a suitable run of predictable data, a substantial change occurred after the 35th observation. An alternative is to employ a GAM chart. In some cases, approximate normality may be achieved by using a transformation. It is then a good idea to add a run chart of the un-transformed data. Staff in the wards tend not to be impressed with charts of for example, the log or square root of the AE data.

```
#using function numgam(), Figure 7.11
numgam(datain)
```

```
Chart heading.
Enter a heading for the chart Monthly blood culture data
Y axis heading.
Enter a heading for the Y axis Rate
Change degrees of freedom (Y/N) n
```

The residual standard error was 0.01306 on 41 degrees of freedom and the multiple R-squared was 0.1677 (adjusted R-squared = 0.1068). The F-statistic was 2.753 on 3 and 41 DF (p-value = 0.0547). The trend test result was not significant (P-value=.21).

The above analysis is disappointing. In particular, the chart does not follow the data well towards the end of the series and the F-statistic value appears unrealistic. We find that the default three degrees of freedom that determines the smoothing is usually satisfactory. However, in this case we increase it to five. This provides a more satisfactory chart and F-statistic.

```
#save mmg in mmg0
mmg0<-mmg
```

```
numgam(datain) # repeated as above but with 5 DF, Figure 7.12
```

```
# using anova to compare models
anova(mmg0,mmg)
```

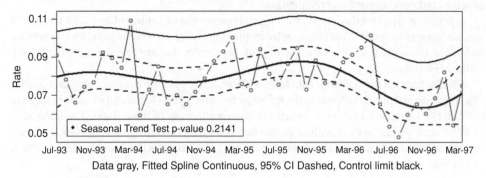

Figure 7.12   GAM chart, blood culture data, 5 degrees of freedom.

```
Analysis of Variance Table
Model 1: a ~ bs(id, df = df1)
Model 2: a ~ bs(id, df = df1)
Res.Df        RSS Df   Sum of Sq        F   Pr(>F)
1      41 0.0069889
2      39 0.0061699   2 0.00081904  2.5886  0.08798 .
```

Although the anova F test result is not conventionally statistically significant so that using 5 DF does not appear to explain the variation in the data better, comparison of Figure 7.12 with Figure 7.11 indicates that the former chart is superior. In addition, with the 5 DF analysis, the overall test results are improved. Residual standard error: 0.01258 on 39 degrees of freedom, Multiple R-squared: 0.2652, Adjusted R-squared: 0.171, F-statistic: 2.815 on 5 and 39 DF, P-value: 0.02897.

7.4   RIDIT charts, ECG data

There may be potential for increased use of ordered categorical data methods in hospital QI. The airline industry has, as an important part of its safety measures, mechanisms for reporting near misses. When these are analysed and appropriate process and system adjustments are subsequently made, serious problems can often be averted.

The same principle could be applied in the hospital. For example, as described by Pearse and others, increasing postoperative mortality rates may be preceded or accompanied by an increasing number of complications such as unplanned returns to the operating theatre, unplanned admissions to special care units, or increasing lengths of stay. By collecting data on the latter as well as on mortality and using ordered categorical data methods for their examination, a more powerful analysis might be possible making earlier intervention potentially practicable.

Other possible outcomes of this kind include increasing use of intra-operative and postoperative blood transfusions preceding a serious postoperative haemorrhage necessitating return to theatre, increasing use of antibiotics postoperatively preceding a potentially preventable case of life-threatening postoperative sepsis, and increasing evidence of postoperative fluid imbalance, disturbance of renal or cardiac function, or pulmonary congestion preceding cases of acute cardio-pulmonary and renal failure.

A simple general method exists for the implementation of control charts with these data that are often analysed in Xbar charts or by employing the all-or-none approach advocated by Nolan and Berwick. It involves the use of rank percentiles that are calculated by the RIDIT method (Fleiss).

We illustrate the method with data from 6326 admissions to the coronary care unit (CCU) of a large regional public hospital in the 6.5 years from mid-1984 to the end of 1990 in the data file ridit.csv (we thank Professor Annette Dobson for the use of these data). The admission ECG of each patient was classified as Normal (954 cases), Ischaemia only (1600 cases), Injury pattern (2359 cases) and Infarction pattern (1413 cases). RIDIT scores are calculated as follows:

1. Normal $(954 \div 2) \div 6326 = 0.0754$,

2. Ischaemia $(954 + 1600 \div 2) \div 6326 = 0.2773$,

3. Injury $(954 + 1600 + 2359 \div 2) \div 6326 = 0.5902$ and

4. Infarction $(954 + 1600 + 2359 + 1413 \div 2) \div 6326 = 0.8883$.

In the first month there were 14 admissions, 1 in the first category, 2 in the second, 9 in the third and 2 in the fourth. In the second month the numbers were 8, 18, 33 and 18, and in the final month they were 7, 21, 22 and 16. For the first month the mean RIDIT was $(1 \times 0.0754 + 2 \times 0.2773 + 9 \times 0.5902 + 2 \times 0.8883)/14 = 0.55$. The second month's mean RIDIT was 0.53 and for the final month the mean RIDIT value was 0.50. The approximate standard deviation for calculating the control limits is $\sqrt{[1/(12 \times N_i)]}$, where N_i is the number of admissions in the month i. For the first month SD$=\sqrt{[1/(12 \times 14)]} = 0.0772$. The analysis in i charts is shown in Figures 7.13 and 7.14. There is a marked trend. At the beginning of the series there were presumably fewer CCU beds and the evidence of infarction before admission needed to be stronger. An alternative analysis involves using a GAM (Figure 7.16). There is a suggestion of autocorrelation but it fails to reach conventional statistical significance.

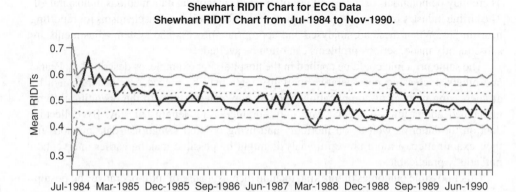

Figure 7.13 Shewhart RIDIT chart.

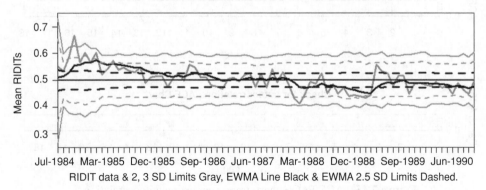

Figure 7.14 Shewhart/EWMA RIDIT chart.

```
g.d() # ridit.csv (dates in first column, format d/m/y)

#using function riditshew(), Figure 7.13
riditshew(datain)
```

```
Chart heading.
Enter heading for chart Shewhart RIDIT Chart for ECG Data
```

```
#using function riditewma()
riditewma(datain)
```

```
EWMA weight.
Enter weight between 0.2 & 0.8 .2
EWMA control limit.
Enter limit between 2 & 3 2.5
Chart heading.
Enter heading for chart Shewhart/EWMA RIDIT Chart of ECG Data
```

It is noteworthy in this case that the EWMA limits are not, as is usual, narrower at the beginning of the series. At the beginning, there were smaller numbers of patients. See RIDIT section internet file ChaptersR.

```
#checking for autocorrelation
#first convert to RIDITs
library(chron)
da<-datain[,1]
da<-chron(as.character(da),format="day-month-year",
out.format="day-mon-year")
o<-order(da);da<-da[o];datain<-datain[o,]
datain1<-datain[,-1]
a0<-as.numeric(apply(datain1,2,sum))
b0<-as.numeric(apply(datain1,1,sum))
q<-sum(a0)
n<-length(datain1[,1])
a1<-a0/2
```

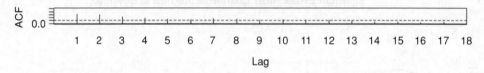

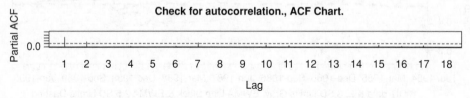

Figure 7.15   ACF/PACF chart, trend suggesting autocorrelation.

```
a2<-c(0,cumsum(a0))
a2<-a2[-length(a2)]
a3<-a1+a2
a4<-a3/q
d<-0
for (j in 1:n){
s<-as.numeric(datain1[j,])
d[j]<-sum(s*a4)
}
a<-d/b0
dataout<-data.frame(da,a)

#check for autocorrelation using do.acf()
do.acf(dataout[,2]) #ACF and PACF chart Figure 7.15
```

```
Enter a heading for the ACF plot. Check for autocorrelation.
```

Figure 7.15 suggests the presence of autocorrelation but there is a trend. This is a trap as the presence of a trend can suggest autocorrelation. We perform a further check using a lag (a2)

```
library(splines)
a<-dataout[,2]
a1<-ts(a)
id<-1:length(a);id1<-ts(id)
tg<-ts.union(a1,id1,a2=lag(a1,-1))
mg<-lm(a1~a2+bs(id1),data=tg)
summary(mg) # not shown
#
# a2 p-value = .065
# a2 is borderline but not significant at the .05 level

# GAM chart
numgam(dataout)
```

**Severity of ECG Changes CCU Admission.
Spline Chart from Jul-1984 to Nov-1990.**

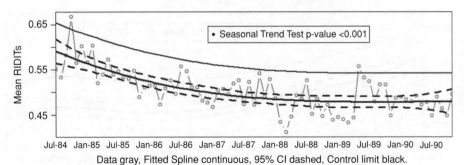

Data gray, Fitted Spline continuous, 95% CI dashed, Control limit black.

Figure 7.16   GAM chart of RIDITs, 3 degrees of freedom.

```
Chart heading.
Enter a heading for the chart Severity of ECG Changes CCU Admission.
Y axis heading.
Enter a heading for the Y axis Mean RIDITs
Change degrees of freedom (Y/N) n
```

The residual standard error was 0.03218 on 73 degrees of freedom and the multiple R-squared was 0.5145 (adjusted R-squared = 0.4946). The F-statistic was 25.79 on 3 and 73 DF (P-value = 1.752e-11). There is a pronounced downward trend. We repeat the analysis using 5 DF. There appears to be little difference between the models but the 5 DF chart (Figure 7.17) appears slightly better. See RIDIT section of internet file ChaptersR.

```
# save model summary for anova test
mmg0<-mmg
numgam(dataout)
```

```
Chart heading.
Enter a heading for the chart Severity of ECG Changes CCU Admission.
Y axis heading.
Enter a heading for the Y axis Mean RIDITs
Change degrees of freedom (Y/N) y
Enter degrees of freedom 5 (note change to 5 DF)
```

The residual standard error was 0.03225 on 71 degrees of freedom and the multiple R-squared was 0.5259 (adjusted R-squared = 0.4925). The F-statistic was 15.75 on 5 and 71 DF (p-value = 2.064e-10). There is a pronounced trend: tau = -0.465, pvalue = 2.2082e-09.

```
anova(mmg0,mmg)
```

```
Analysis of Variance Table
Model 1: a ~ bs(id, df = df1)
Model 2: a ~ bs(id, df = df1)
  Res.Df      RSS Df Sum of Sq      F Pr(>F)
1     73 0.075605
2     71 0.073835  2 0.0017703 0.8512 0.4312
```

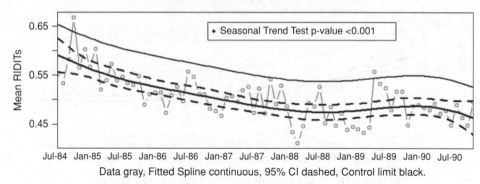

**Severity of ECG Changes CCU Admission.
Spline Chart from Jul-1984 to Nov-1990.**

Data gray, Fitted Spline continuous, 95% CI dashed, Control limit black.

Figure 7.17   GAM chart of RIDITs, 5 degrees of freedom.

7.5   Numerical data – theatre utilisation

The next type of chart we describe is the Shewhart Xbar chart and its accompanying standard deviation S chart (Montgomery). Commonly the latter, a chart of the variability of the data, is calculated from the ranges of the data values and it is then called an R chart. However, the availability of computers makes it no longer necessary to use ranges, and assessment of variation using methods based on the standard deviation may be preferable (Ryan).

These charts can be useful for displaying aspects of resource usage such as ward occupancy and theatre utilisation. It is often valuable to record some aspect of usage for each day of the week, so that the N_i for the groups will be 7, or 5 for weekdays. However, it is necessary to be careful when grouping data in this way. If the pattern of utilisation is different on some days, for example at weekends, they should not be grouped with weekdays. We illustrate the methods with data from an operating theatre utilisation study.

The nursing directors of the operating theatres of a hospital were concerned that utilisation was too high and too variable for optimum performance. They wanted the hospital administration to appreciate this problem that caused serious difficulty, for example with rosters, overtime and staff performance, in a climate of financial restraint. In order to do this they collected data on utilisation of the operating theatres for 20 weeks.

If a three-hour operating session was fully used, they counted utilisation as 100%. If less than full utilisation occurred, they recorded it as a proportion of 3 hours, and if a session went over time they recorded a utilisation of greater than 100%. For example, if the session went over by 30 minutes this was counted as $(3.5 \div 3) \times 100 = 117\%$. They recorded the data for each weekday and having obtained the data, they sought a method for their presentation that would deliver their message to the hospital administration. The data are in the data file theateruse.csv. Figure 7.18 is an S chart, Figure 7.19 a Shewhart chart and Figure 7.20 a Shewhart/EWMA chart.

The first step is to calculate the means (Xbars) and standard deviations (S) for each week. Then the average of the Xbars and the average of the standard deviations (Sbar) are calculated; the former becomes the centre-line (CL) of the Xbar chart. For the Xbar chart the control

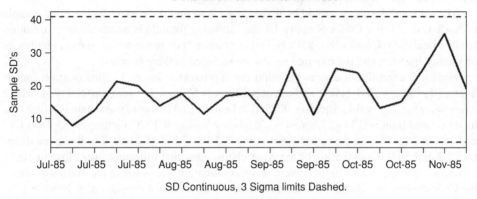

Theater Utilization
S chart from Jul-1985 to Nov-1985.

SD Continuous, 3 Sigma limits Dashed.

Figure 7.18   Sbar chart for numerical data variation.

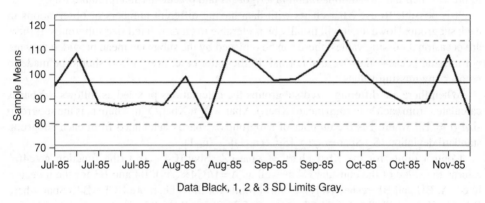

Theater Utilization
Shewhart chart from Jul-1985 to Nov-1985.

Data Black, 1, 2 & 3 SD Limits Gray.

Figure 7.19   Shewhart Xbar chart.

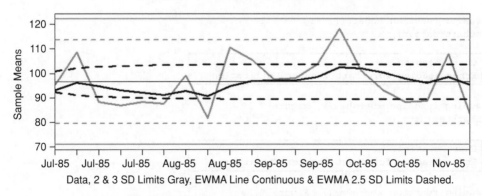

Theater Utilization
Shewhart/EWMA chart from Jul-1985 to Nov-1985.

Data, 2 & 3 SD Limits Gray, EWMA Line Continuous & EWMA 2.5 SD Limits Dashed.

Figure 7.20   Shewhart/EWMA Xbar chart.

limits are then $CL+Z\times Sbar/(C4\times\sqrt{N})$, where for the number of observations per week N=5, C4=0.94 and for 2 sigma 'warning' control limits, Z=2.

The standard deviation should be divided by C4 to find the control limits. For a sample of N=5, C4=.94. For C4 for N above 10, the following formula is a suitable approximation for its calculation: $C4=4\times(N-1)/(4\times N-3)$. For smaller N there are tables in most text books on quality statistics and the required values are included in these functions.

For the S chart that monitors variation the approximate lower 3 sigma control limit is $Sbar\times\sqrt{[\chi^2_{0.0015,N-1}/(N-1)]}/c4$, and the upper limit is $Sbar\times\sqrt{[\chi^2_{0.9985,N-1}/(N-1)]}/c4$, where $c4_4=.94$. $\chi^2_{0.0015,4}$ is 0.11 (qchisq(.0015,4)=.11 and $\sqrt{(.11/4)}=.17$). As sbar is 17.89, the lower control limit is $0.17\times17.89/.94=3.2$. Also, $\chi^2_{0.9985,4}$ is 17.57 (qchisq(.9985,4)=17.57 and $\sqrt{(17.57/4)}=2.1$) so the upper control limit is $2.1\times17.89/.94=39.9$. The limits are therefore 3.2 and 39.9. Examination of the Xbar charts show that utilisation was close to 100% and between weeks 9 and 16 there were seven consecutive weeks where the mean was above the CL including one above U_2 at the 14th week. There is also a run-sum of 4. However, the EWMA chart does not reach the 2.5 SD limit. This has an ARL of approximately 100. The S chart remains in control. One concludes that there was overall excessive utilisation. Using these charts and others for individual theatres and surgeons, the nursing directors were able to present their data to administration in a rigorous and practically interpretable way.

It is possible to use Xbar charts with data having different numbers of observations in each subgroup. However, it will usually be preferable to employ fixed size subgroups. If there are occasional missing values, these can be replaced by the subgroup mean provided they are not missing because they were abnormal. In the latter case, every effort should be made to recover any missing values.

When there are differing sized subgroups the calculations proceed as follows – Xbar is calculated from each subgroup mean $(Xbar_i)$. $Xbar = \sum n_i Xbar_i / \sum n_i$ where n_i is the subgroup size ($i = 1..I$ where I is the number of subgroups). Sbar is calculated from each subgroup standard deviation (S_i) $Sbar = \sqrt{(\sum[S_i^2\times(n_i-1)]/\sum(n_i-1))}$.

Control limits for the Xbar chart $= Xbar\pm Z\times Sbar/(C4\times\sqrt{n_i})$ (the function getc4(n) returns the value of the constant C4 as well as $A=1/(C4\times\sqrt{n_i})$, B4 and B3 for the n vector, in c4, A, BU and BL respectively). Control limits for the S chart are UCL=B4×Sbar where $B4 = 1+Z\times\sqrt{(1-C4^2)}/C4$ and LCL = max(0,B3×Sbar) where $B3 = 1-Z\times\sqrt{(1-C4^2)}/C4$. For three sigma limits Z = 3.

```
g.d() # theateruse.csv (the first column contains dates in d/m/y format)

#using function schart(), Figure 7.18
schart(datain)
```

```
Chart heading.
Enter heading for chart Theater Utilization
```

```
#using function xbarshew(), Figure 7.19
xbarshew(datain)
```

```
Chart heading.
Enter heading for chart Theater Utilization
```

```
#using function xbarewma(), Figure 7.20
xbarewma(datain)
```

```
EWMA weight.
Enter weight between 0.2 & 0.8 .2
EWMA control limit.
Enter limit between 2 & 3 2.5
Chart heading.
Enter heading for chart Theater Utilization
```

7.6   Length of stay (LOS) data

Time to event data are frequently of interest. For example, time requiring mechanical ventilation, time in ICU and length of stay in hospital each has information about recovery from
medical and surgical treatment. Length of time in surgery is one of the variables used in determining the NNIS SSI risk index. These data tend to have skewed distributions with 'thick'
right tails that make them difficult to model using conventional statistical distributions. In
addition, it is possible that costs of stay may have similar distributions.

Recent interest in fractal (power law) distributions suggests that they may offer new ways
of analysing hospital time to event data (Papadopoulos and colleagues). Hospital length of
stay data for then ANDRG 252 (Heart failure and shock) during 1994–95 are in the file
losdata.csv. There were 4180 lengths of stay in chronological order in the state reference
data base and the median LOS was five days. Their distribution is summarised in Figure 7.21
and 7.22.

```
g.d() # losdata.csv, column A

# Figure 7.21
d<-datain[,1]
z<-c(0,10,20,30,40,50,60,70,80,90,100,1000)
k<-cut(d,z)
tk<-as.numeric(table(k))
tk<-tk[1:10] # removes 16 > 100 days (0.38% of the data)
kk<-c(5,15,25,35,45,55,65,75,85,95)
par(xaxs="r")
```

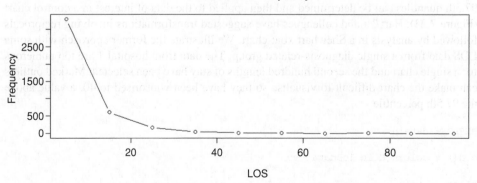

Figure 7.21 Plot of length of stay versus frequency.

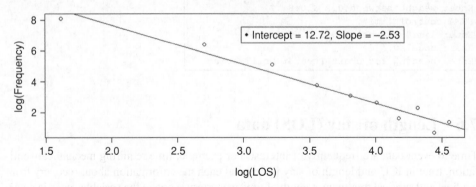

Figure 7.22 Fractal, power law plot, length of stay.

```
plot(tk~kk,main="Plot LOS v Frequency.",type="b",xlab="LOS days"
,ylab="Frequency")

# demonstrating possible approximate fractal (power law) distribution,
# Figure 7.22
d<-datain[,1]
z<-c(0,10,20,30,40,50,60,70,80,90,100,1000)
k<-cut(d,z)
tk<-as.numeric(table(k))
tk<-tk[1:10]
kk<-c(5,15,25,35,45,55,65,75,85,95)
par(xaxs="r")
plot(log(tk)~log(kk),main="Fractal Plot of LOS.",xlab="log(LOS)"
,ylab="log(Frequency)")
l<-lm(log(tk)~log(kk))
abline(a=l$coef[1],b=l$coef[2])
Z1<-round(l$coef[1],2);Z2<-round(l$coef[2],2)
legend(locator(1),
legend=paste("Intercept = ",Z1,",  Slope = ",Z2,sep=""),
pch=19,cex=.8)
```

Faced with data that may not have a practically useful average, there are several potential approaches to their analysis. If a large reference database is available, the 50th, 84th and 97.5th quantiles can be determined and then applied to the data of interest in a control chart (Figure 7.23). Hart [B,C] and colleagues have suggested transformations involving reciprocals followed by analysis in a Shewhart xbar chart. We illustrate the former approach with some LOS data from a single diagnosis-related group. The data from hospital 1 are too numerous for a single chart and the second hundred lengths of stay have been selected. Marked outliers can make the chart difficult to visualise so they have been winsorised to 40, a value above the 97.5th percentile.

```
REFLOS<-datain

g.d() # column C in losdata.csv

h1los<-datain
m<-median(REFLOS[,1]) # Figure 7.23
```

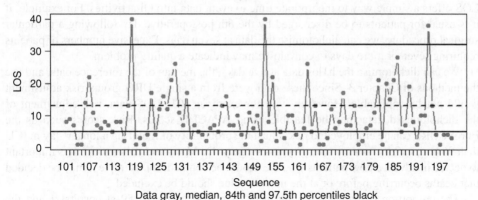

Figure 7.23   Length of stay run chart with quantiles.

```
m
#
#[1] 5
u1<-quantile(REFLOS[,1],.84)
u1
#
#84%
# 13
u2<-quantile(REFLOS[,1],.975)
u2
#
#97.5%
#    32

d<-as.numeric(h1los[,1])
d[d>40]<-40 # large outliers winsorised in order to see data clearly
plot(d[101:200],type="b",axes=F,main="Hospital 1 LOS",
xlab="Data blue, 84th and 97.5th percentiles red",
ylab="LOS",pch=19,col="blue",lwd=2)
box()
axis(side=1,labels=101:200,at=1:100)
axis(side=c(2,3,4))
abline(h=m)
abline(h=u1,lwd=2,col="red",lty=2)
abline(h=u2,lwd=2,col="red")
mtext("Sequence",side=1,line=2)
```

The chart shows three points above the reference 97.5th percentile value of 32 days, a run of 7 above the median at 169 to 175 and a run-sum of 4 at numbers 183 to 186.

```
d[169:175]
#
#[1] 12   6   8 17   7   7 13
#
d[183:186]
#[1] 20 15 21 28
```

Determining the proportion of patients requiring recovery times that exceed the median LOS offers a simple way to incorporate time to event data into QI activities. For example, if it is usual for patients to be discharged by the 6th postoperative day following a particular surgical procedure, we can dichotomise the data at seven days. Excessive numbers of patients requiring seven or more days to convalesce may indicate a quality problem.

We can dichotomise the h1los data at five days, the median of the reference data, and use the methods of Chapter 3. Since these data were from a single DRG group, risk adjustment would not be applicable. However, with for example, ICU LOS data, risk adjustment of the dichotomised data may be feasible using APACHE scores. Risk scores such as the EuroSCORE can be employed to risk-adjust the probability of requiring a longer stay in ICU than 96 hours after coronary artery bypass surgery (De Maria and colleagues). It is important to decide in advance how patients who die should be counted; for example it may be decided that deaths occurring before or at the median value should be excluded.

The proportion of patients staying more than five days was .59 at hospital 1 and the reference value was .49. Thus, hospital 1 had more long stay patients than the average. However, there are many possible reasons for this. Some hospitals have special facilities for diagnosis and treatment and this may prolong LOS. Moreover, patients who are more difficult to treat may be referred to these institutions. If hospital 1 had suitable discharge planning and a run of predictable data, it would be preferable to use their median value. Use of the cumulative O-E/CUSUM would then give warning should a problem with discharge planning occur. The following charts (Figures 7.24 to 7.27) suggest a predictable process.

```
LOS<-rep(0,length(h1los[,1]))
LOS[h1los[,1]>m]<-1
mean(LOS) # .59
head(LOS)

# [1] 1 0 1 1 0 1

# cumulative O-E/CUSUM (Figure 7.24)
d<-1:length(LOS)
a<-LOS
mm<-sum(REFLOS[,1]>5)/length(REFLOS[,1]) # reference value .49
p<-rep(mm,length(d))
h<-5 # large h value as proportions are large
hd<-"Hospital 1 LOS > reference median"
nm<-paste(hd,"\nCumulative O - E and CUSUM chart.",sep="")
Observed<-cumsum(a)
Procedures<-1:length(Observed)
Expected<-cumsum(p)
O<-Observed/Procedures
E<-Expected/Procedures
n<-Procedures
L2<-0
for (i in 1:length(n)){
Z<-.02275;P<-E[i];N<-n[i]
X<-0
if (1-pbeta(P,X+1,N-X)>=Z){X<-0}else{
X<-P*N
A<-1
bl<-F
while (bl==F){
```

```
X<-X-A
K<-1-pbeta(P,X+1,N-X)
if (K<=Z){bl<-T}
}
A<-.01
bl<-F
while (bl==F){
X<-X+A
K<-1-pbeta(P,X+1,N-X)
if (K>=Z){bl<-T}
}
}
L2[i]<-X/n[i]
}
U2<-0
for (i in 1:length(n)){
Z<-.02275;P<-E[i];N<-n[i]
X<-N
if (pbeta(P,X,N-X+1)>=Z){X<-N}else{
X<-N*P
A<-1
bl<-F
while (bl==F){
X<-X+A
K<-pbeta(P,X,N-X+1)
if (K<Z){bl<-T}
}
A<-.01
bl<-F
while (bl==F){
X<-X-A
K<-pbeta(P,X,N-X+1)
if (K>=Z){bl<-T}
}
}
U2[i]<-X/n[i]
}
On<-O*n
En<-E*n
Un<-U2*n
Ln<-L2*n
On<-On-En
Un<-Un-En
Ln<-Ln-En
w<-log((a+1)/(1+p)) # formula when OR=2
ju<-0
su<-0
su1<-0
gu<-w[1]
if (gu<0){gu<-0}
if (gu>=h){su<-c(su,Procedures[1]);su1<-c(su1,d[1]);gu<-0}
ju<-gu
for (i in 2:length(w)){
gu[i]<-ju+w[i]
ju<-gu[i]
if (gu[i]<0){gu[i]<-0;ju<-0}
```

```
if (gu[i]>=h){su<-c(su,Procedures[i]);su1<-c(su1,d[i]);ju<-0}
}
su<-su[-1]
su1<-su1[-1]
su1<-chron(su1,out.format="dd-mmm-yyyy")
ma<-max(c(On,Un))
mi<-min(c(On,Ln))
c2<-rep(0,length(d))
for (i in 1:length(d)){if (i%%50==0){c2[i]<-ma/20}}
tv<-"Cumulative O - E."
z1<-"Observed Blue, 95% Limits Red, Arrows CUSUM Signals,"
z2<-" Tick Marks Every 50 Units."
th<-paste(z1,z2,sep="")
par(xaxs="i")
plot(On,col="blue",lwd=2,type="l",ylim=c(mi,ma),main=nm,ylab=tv,xlab="",
axes=F)
box()
par(cex=.7)
axis(side=1,tick=F,labels=d,at=Procedures)
axis(side=c(2,3,4))
par(cex=1)
lines(Un,col="red",lwd=2)
lines(Ln,col="red",lwd=2)
lines(c2,type="l",col="green4",lwd=2)
mtext(text=th,side=1,line=2)
if (length(su)>0){
arrows(su,mi,su,On[su],lwd=3,col="black")
if (length(su)>0 & length(su)<6){
w0<-d[su[1]]
if (length(su)>1){
for (i in 2:length(su)){w0<-paste(w0,d[su[i]])}
}
w0<-paste("Signals at",w0)
mtext(w0,side=1,line=3)
}
cat("Cusum h = ",h,"\n",sep="")
cat("Cusum signals at numbers\n")
qu<-d[su]
print(qu)
}


# hospital 1 data dates
g.d() # column E of losdata.csv (select n for order dates)

datain<-data.frame(datain,LOS)
# convert to monthly data
binmonths(datain)
# monthly rates with CIs Figure 7.25
library(exactci)
Rate<-dataout[,2]/dataout[,3]
Expected<-.485
M<-0
L<-0
U<-0
L0<-0
U0<-0
```

Hospital 1 LOS > reference median
Cumulative O-E and CUSUM chart.

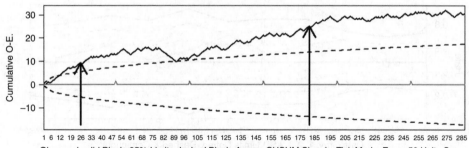

Observed solid Black, 95% Limits dashed Black, Arrows CUSUM Signals, Tick Marks Every 50 Units Gray.
Signals at observations 26 181

Figure 7.24 Cumulative observed minus expected (O-E)/CUSUM chart length of stay above reference median.

```
LL<-length(dataout[,1])
for (i in 1:LL){M<-binom.exact(dataout[i,2],dataout[i,3])$conf.int;U[i]<-
M[2];L[i]<-M[1]}
for (i in 1:LL)
{M<-binom.exact(dataout[i,2],dataout[i,3],conf.level=.99)$conf.int;
U0[i]<-M[2];L0[i]<-M[1]}
mx<-max(U0)
ma<-("Proportion of LOS values > reference median")
par(xaxs="r")
plot(Rate,ylim=c(0,mx),col="blue",lwd=2,pch=19,axes=F,main=ma,ylab="Rate",
xlab="Months")
box()
axis(side=1,labels=as.character(dataout[,1]),at=1:LL)
axis(side=c(2,3,4))
abline(h=Expected,col="red")
arrows(1:LL,L0,1:LL,U0,angle=90,code=3,col="blue",length=.1,lwd=2)
points(L,lwd=2,pch="-",col="blue",cex=1.75)
points(U,lwd=2,pch="-",col="blue",cex=1.75)
mtext("Monthly rate, 95% & 99% CIs blue, Expected red",side=1,line=2)
```

Proportion of LOS values > reference median

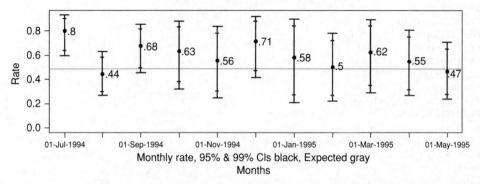

Monthly rate, 95% & 99% CIs black, Expected gray
Months

Figure 7.25 Proportions above reference median with confidence intervals, monthly data.

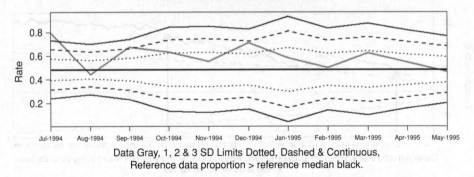

Figure 7.26 Shewhart chart length of stay above reference median, monthly data.

```
text(Rate,labels=substr(as.character(round(Rate,2)),2,4),pos=4,offset=.3,
cex=.8,lwd=3)

# Shewhart chart Figure 7.26 (or use bshew(dataout))
library(chron)
da<-dataout[,1]
da<-chron(as.character(da),format="dd-mmm-yyyy",out.format="dd-mmm-yyyy")
d1<-dataout[,2]
d2<-dataout[,3]
o<-order(da)
da<-da[o];d1<-d1[o];d2<-d2[o]
d6<-d1/d2
d7<-sum(d1)/sum(d2)
s1<-paste(months(min(da)),years(min(da)))
s2<-paste(months(max(da)),years(max(da)))
da1<-paste(months(da),years(da))
p0<-.485 # Reference data proportion exceeding the reference median
eh<-"Proportion of LOS values exceeding reference median"
eh<-paste(eh,"\nfrom ",s1," to ",s2,", N=",sum(d2),".",sep="")
ei1<-"Data Blue, 1, 2 & 3 SD Limits Orange, Brown & Red,"
ei2<-"\nReference data proportion > reference median black."
ei<-paste(ei1,ei2,sep="")
ej<-"Rate"
p<-rep(p0,length(da))
n<-d2
L1<-0;L2<-0;L3<-0
for (I in 1:3){
if (I==1){Z<-.15866}
if (I==2){Z<-.02275}
if (I==3){Z<-.00135}
L0<-0
for (i in 1:length(n)){
P<-p[i];N<-n[i]
X<-0
if (1-pbeta(P,X+1,N-X)>=Z){X<-0}else{
X<-P*N
A<-1
bl<-F
while (bl==F){
```

```
X<-X-A
K<-1-pbeta(P,X+1,N-X)
if (K<=Z){bl<-T}
}
A<-.01
bl<-F
while (bl==F){
X<-X+A
K<-1-pbeta(P,X+1,N-X)
if (K>=Z){bl<-T}
}
}
L0[i]<-X/n[i]
}
if (I==1){L1<-L0}
if (I==2){L2<-L0}
if (I==3){L3<-L0}
}
U1<-0;U2<-0;U3<-0;UE<-0
for (I in 1:3){
if (I==1){Z<-.15866}
if (I==2){Z<-.02275}
if (I==3){Z<-.00135}
U0<-0
for (i in 1:length(n)){
P<-p[i];N<-n[i]
X<-N
if (pbeta(P,X,N-X+1)>=Z){X<-N}else{
X<-N*P
A<-1
bl<-F
while (bl==F){
X<-X+A
K<-pbeta(P,X,N-X+1)
if (K<Z){bl<-T}
}
A<-.01
bl<-F
while (bl==F){
X<-X-A
K<-pbeta(P,X,N-X+1)
if (K>=Z){bl<-T}
}
}
U0[i]<-X/n[i]
}
if (I==1){U1<-U0}
if (I==2){U2<-U0}
if (I==3){U3<-U0}
}
L1[L1<0]<-0
L2[L2<0]<-0
L3[L3<0]<-0
ej<-"Rate"
plot(d6,type="l",pch=20,lwd=3,col="blue",axes=F,ylim=c(min(c(L3,d6)),
max(c(U3,d6))),xlab=ei,ylab=ej,main=eh)
```

```
box()
par(cex=.7)
axis(side=1,tick=T,labels=as.character(da1),at=1:length(da1))
axis(side=c(2,3,4))
par(cex=1)
abline(h=p0,lwd=3)
lines(U1,lwd=2,lty=1,col="orange")
if (min(L1)>0){lines(L1,lwd=2,lty=1,col="orange")}
lines(U2,lwd=2,lty=1,col="brown")
if (min(L2)>0){lines(L2,lwd=2,lty=1,col="brown")}
lines(U3,lwd=2,lty=1,col="red")
if (min(L3)>0){lines(L3,lwd=2,lty=1,col="red")}

# GAM chart Figure 7.27 (or use bgam(dataout))
library(chron)
library(splines)
library(Kendall)
da<-dataout[,1]
d1<-dataout[,2]
d2<-dataout[,3]
mm<-sum(d1)/sum(d2)
d3<-mm*d2
o<-order(da)
da<-da[o]
d1<-d1[o]
d2<-d2[o]
d3<-d3[o]
s1<-paste(months(min(da)),years(min(da)))
s2<-paste(months(max(da)),years(max(da)))
id<-1:length(d1)
ebar<-sum(d3)/sum(d2)
pd<-d1*ebar/d3
a<-d1*ebar*d2/d3
df1<-3
mg<-glm(a/d2~bs(id,df=df1),weight=d2,family=binomial)
mgp<-predict(mg,se=T)
b<-mgp$fit;e<-mgp$se.fit
v1<-exp(b)/(1+exp(b))
p<-as.numeric(v1);n<-d2
U2<-0
Z<-.02275
U0<-0
for (i in 1:length(n)){
P<-p[i];N<-n[i]
X<-N
if (pbeta(P,X,N-X+1)>=Z){X<-N}else{
X<-N*P
A<-1
bl<-F
while (bl==F){
X<-X+A
K<-pbeta(P,X,N-X+1)
if (K<Z){bl<-T}
}
A<-.01
bl<-F
```

```
while (bl==F){
X<-X-A
K<-pbeta(P,X,N-X+1)
if (K>=Z){bl<-T}
}
}
U0[i]<-X/n[i]
}
up<-U0
eh<-"Proportion of LOS Values > Reference Median"
eh<-paste(eh,"\nfrom ",s1," to ",s2,", N=",sum(d2),".",sep="")
ei<-"Data blue, Fitted GAM red, 95% CI brown, Control limit black,
Reference Data Proportion > Reference Median gray."
ej<-"Rate"
k<-format.Date(da,"%b%y")
v2<-exp(b+1.96*e)/(1+exp(b+1.96*e));v3<-exp(b-1.96*e)/(1+exp(b-1.96*e))
x1<-min(c(pd,v3))
x2<-max(c(pd,v2,up))
par(xaxs="i")
plot(pd,axes=F,ylim=c(x1,x2),type="b",main=eh,ylab=ej,xlab=ei,col="blue",
lwd=2)
box()
axis(side=1,tick=F,labels=k,at=id)
axis(side=c(2,3,4))
abline(h=.486,col="gray60",lwd=2)
lines(v1,lwd=2,col="red")
lines(v2,lwd=2,lty=1,col="brown")
lines(v3,lwd=2,lty=1,col="brown")
lines(smooth.spline(up,spar=.6),lwd=2)
s<-SeasonalMannKendall(ts(pd))
ss<-0
if(s$sl<.001){ss<-"<0.001"}else{ss<-as.character(round(s$sl,4))}
msg2<-paste("Seasonal Trend Test p-value ",ss,sep="")
legend(locator(1),legend=msg2,pch=19,col="brown4",cex=.8)
```

7.7   Changepoint

When studying a series of data values, for example, in a GAM chart, Shewhart chart or cumulative O-E chart, there is interest in knowing whether there are one or more outlier values, one or more trends or a change in the location of the data distribution (a changepoint). More generally we wish to determine whether there is a change from a predictable state to an unpredictable one or vice versa. The GAM analysis provides an approximate significance test that can be helpful. However, although it can indicate the presence of significant variation, the detailed nature of this variation can be difficult to determine (GAM analyses of numerical data provide an F test and those of attribute data a change in deviance (ΔD) and degrees of freedom (ΔDF) that can be analysed approximately by a chi-squared test, for example, 1-pchisq($\Delta D,\Delta DF$)). As we have already described, the GAM chart we employ also has an additional line the equivalent of two standard deviations above the predicted GAM line that may help to identify outlier values. This is motivated by the Poisson outbreak detection (POD) method proposed by Pelecanos and colleagues. A seasonal MannKendall trend test is also provided.

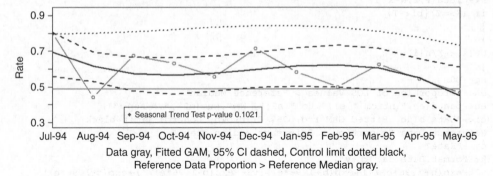

Figure 7.27   GAM chart length of stay above reference median, monthly data.

Additional support in determining whether a distribution change may have occurred may be provided by identifying two predicted values where there are stable values before and after an expected change point, for example, using the locator() function. Then one can use these values and their confidence intervals or standard errors to perform an approximate Z-test eg $Z=(D1-D2)/\sqrt{(SE1^2+SE2^2)}$, where D1 and D2 are the data points of interest and SE1 and SE2 their standard errors. If 95% confidence intervals are used, $SE\approx(U-L)/(2\times1.96)$, where U and L are the relevant upper and lower 95% confidence limits. An alternative would be to use Newcombe's method described in section 1.4.1 of Chapter 1 (Newcombe, Zou and Donner). However, it is necessary to be cautious when such changes are suggested by the data. We again emphasise Montgomery's advice to know the process, for example, has a change been made to it and, if so, when? We should also consider employing the Benjamini-Hochberg procedure for multiple comparisons as previously described. The spline GAM analysis has a predict function that provides GAM predicted values and their standard errors. With attribute data these are on a log or logit scale and their use will enhance accuracy as these values will usually be approximately normally distributed. A dummy variable can be employed in the GAM analysis to indicate a possible change point. An alternative is to use a Bayesian approach (Assareh and Mengersen).

It is important to be wary of analyses suggested by the data. However, such statistically significant results may focus on areas for more detailed study, for example, by M&M audit or systems analysis (Vincent). In addition, a change that occurs after a system review and that is sustained is important to document. It is also necessary to be wary of doing multiple significance tests, for example, if several data points are used to perform Z-tests or if just two points suggested by the data are used among a series of points, a correction should be applied for multiple testing such as the Benjamini-Hochberg procedure.

An additional procedure that may be useful is Pettitt's change point test described in Siegel and Castellan. There are several change point tests described in R libraries but Pettitt's test uses a Wilcoxon test for numerical and count data and a Kolmogorov-Smirnov test for binary data. For the latter we substitute a Fisher exact test. It is important to realise that the rank Wilcoxon test is not truly 'distribution free' as it requires the shapes of the distributions of the two sets of data being compared to be similar, a requirement that will often be met in this situation. It also requires the data to be independent so it should not be used in the presence of autocorrelation or a seasonal effect.

The presence of risk-adjustment is a further complication with some binary data such as ICU mortality. Conversion to risk-adjusted rates may be feasible (Hart[A] and colleagues).

We provide three examples. The first involves the weekly bacteraemia data from section 6.5 of Chapter 6 (Figures 6.1 to 6.7).There were changes in infection control practices during the year so the presence of a change might have been expected although its position in this case is suggested by the data. The data in bactdata.csv were saved in weeklybacts.csv. There were only 15 weeks before the supposed change point so assessing the distributions before and after it is difficult but the distributions are probably similar. It was noted in section 6.5 of Chapter 6 that there was an overall trend whereas the trend test for the predictable data from after the supposed change point did not suggest a trend. The Wilcoxon test comparing the before and after data was highly significant. A median test was made difficult by the presence of many ties at the median value but was also significant. It is worth emphasising again that the Wilcoxon test is not distribution free; the data before and after the putative change point should have similar distributions (Figure 7.28) and dispersions. In addition, we can repeat the countgam() analysis and include a dummy variable.

```
g.d() #  weeklybacts.csv

# comparison of the two distributions Figure 7.28
n1<-"Before supposed change."
n2<-"After supposed change."
l<-length(datain[,1])
h<-hist(datain[,2],xlab="",ylab="")

h1<-hist(datain[1:15,2],xlab="",ylab="",freq=T)

h2<-hist(datain[16:l,2],xlab="",ylab="",freq=T)

q<-max(c(h1$counts,h2$counts))
mz<-matrix(1:2,1,2)
layout(mz,1,c(1:1))
h1<-hist(datain[1:15,2],main=n1,freq=T,ylim=c(0,q),xlab="",col="gray70")
h2<-hist(datain[16:l,2],main=n2,freq=T,ylim=c(0,q),xlab="",col="gray70")
mz<-matrix(1:1,1,1)
layout(mz)
#distributions probably similar
#difficult to judge distributions due to small samples
```

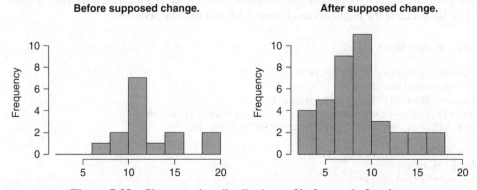

Figure 7.28 Change point, distributions of before and after data.

```
#test for dispersion
#Fligner-Killeen rank dispersion test
#distributions have similar dispersions
w<-datain[,2]
a<-rep(0,1)
a[1:15]<-1
a[16:1]<-2
flg<-fligner.test(w,a)
flg1<-flg$p.value
k9<-paste("Fligner-Killeen dispersion test p-value = ",round(flg1,5),sep="")
cat (k9,"\n")
#[[1] Fligner-Killeen dispersion test p-value = 0.68789

#test for change point using spline regression with a dummy variable
library(splines)
n<-length(datain[,1])-15
x<-c(rep(0,15),rep(1,n))
y<-1:length(datain[,1])
l<-glm(datain[,2]~x+bs(y),family=quasipoisson) # using a GAM with a dummy
# variable
summary(l) #change in mean level of x is significant (P-value=.0175)
```

```
Coefficients:
            Estimate Std. Error t value Pr(>|t|)
(Intercept)   2.1636     0.1847  11.717  1.1e-15 ***
x            -0.5205     0.2114  -2.462   0.0175 *
(Dispersion parameter for quasipoisson family
taken to be 1.144076)
    Null deviance: 78.486  on 52  degrees of freedom
Residual deviance: 55.137  on 48  degrees of freedom
1-pchisq(78.486-55.137,52-48), P< 0.001
```

Faced with these and similar data, it may be difficult using simple methods to say with assurance that there was a change point. However, the analysis of section 6.5 of Chapter 6 together with Figures 6.5 and 6.7 strongly suggest a change from elevated unpredictable data to data that have become predictable at a lower level. This is the most important finding.

Example 2 involves the blood culture data of section 7.3 of this chapter (Figure 7.7 to 7.12). These data have already undergone analysis suggesting a change point. However, their distribution was not assessed. There only 10 data values after the putative change point so histograms are likely to be of little use. However, there is clearly a location difference (Figure 7.29). We examine the distributions (Figure 7.30) and their dispersions.

```
g.d() # bloodcult.csv

# location difference Figure 7.29
l<-length(datain[,1])
boxplot(datain[1:35,2],datain[36:l,2],
main="Blood culture data location difference",ylab="Mean")
axis(side=1,labels=c("Before","After"),at=1:2)

# distributions, Figure 7.30
graphics.off()
mz<-matrix(1:2,1,2)
```

Blood culture data location difference

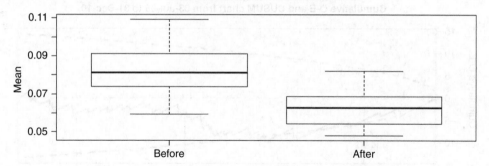

Figure 7.29   Change point, box plots before and after data.

```
layout(mz,1,c(1:1))
h1<-c(qqnorm(datain[1:35,2],main="Pre Changepoint Data",
xlab="",col="gray70"),qqline(datain[1:35,2]))
h2<-c(qqnorm(datain[36:1,2],main="Post Changepoint Data",
xlab="",col="gray70"),qqline(datain[36:1,2]))
mz<-matrix(1:1,1,1)
layout(mz)

shapiro.test(datain[1:35,2])$p.value
# [1] 0.8062321

shapiro.test(datain[36:1,2])$p.value
# [1] 0.9325415

#test for dispersion
#Fligner-Killeen rank dispersion test
#distributions have similar dispersions
w<-datain[,2]
a<-rep(0,1)
a[1:35]<-1
a[36:1]<-2
flg<-fligner.test(w,a)
flg1<-flg$p.value
k9<-paste("Fligner-Killeen dispersion test p-value = ",round(flg1,5),sep="")
```

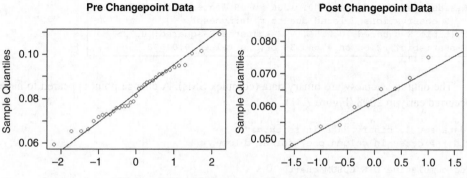

Figure 7.30   Change point data, Q-Q plots.

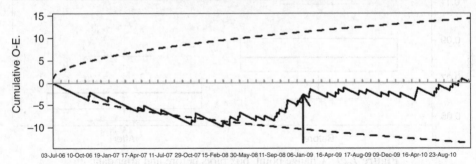

Figure 7.31 Cumulative observed – expected/CUSUM chart for complex surgical site infections.

```
cat (k9,"\n")
#[[1] Fligner-Killeen dispersion test p-value = 0.40704
```

Although there are few data values after the putative change point, these data appear to differ only in their location. There is probably a definite change point. However, we should check for the presence of autocorrelation and be aware of the possibility of seasonal effects.

```
# looking for autocorrelation
a<-datain[,2]
id<-1:length(a);id1<-ts(id)
a1<-ts(a)
tg<-ts.union(a1,id1,a2=lag(a1,-1))
mg<-lm(a1~a2+bs(id1),data=tg)
summary(mg) # a2 is not significant
```

```
Coefficients:
            Estimate Std. Error t value Pr(>|t|)
(Intercept) 0.056553  0.015700   3.602 0.000881 ***
a2          0.245028  0.157737   1.553 0.128408
Residual standard error: 0.01286 on 39 degrees of freedom
  (2 observations deleted due to missingness)
Multiple R-squared: 0.2156,     Adjusted R-squared: 0.1351
F-statistic:  2.68 on 4 and 39 DF,  p-value: 0.04569
```

The data in ssicp.csv are binary data (complex SSIs). A change point appeared to have occurred early in 2008 (Figure 7.31).

```
#data set 3, binary data in ssicp.csv
g.d() # dates in column one, format d-mmm-yy
```

```
#do cumulative O-E/CUSUM chart
boecusum(datain) # Figure 7.31
```

```
Date format.
  03-Jul-2006
Date format.
Enter the required date format dd-mmm-yyyy
Do you have risk-adjusted data (Y/N) n
The mean outcome rate is  0.018
Do you wish to enter another value (Y/N) n
Cumulative sum alert.
Enter the Cumulative sum (CUSUM) alert value 3
Chart heading.
Enter heading for chart Complex Surgical Site Infections
```

There is a CUSUM signal in January 2009. The cumulative O − E chart suggests that the distribution before 2008 may have differed from that after 2008. The average rate prior to 2008 was mean(datain[years(datain[,1])<.2008,2]) = .01 and after 2008 mean(datain[years(datain[,1])>2008,2]) = .02.

```
#using locator() function to find lowest cumulative O-E value
locator()
#$x
#[1] 1043.212
datain[1043,]
#
#              d d0
#1043 14-Mar-2008   0
# suggests possible changepoint in March 2008
which(datain[,1]=="02-Mar-2008") #no procedure on 1st March
#[1] 1025
d1<-datain[1:1024,2]
d2<-datain[1025:length(datain[,1]),2]
rbind(table(d1),table(d2))
```

```
         0    1
[1,]  1015    9
[2,]  1500   37
```

```
fisher.test(rbind(table(d1),table(d2)))$p.value
#[1] 0.003717281
#suggests that a change in the distribution occurred about March 2008.
```

Although the result of this analysis suggests a changepoint, some further analysis indicates that the relationship may be more complex. First, the data can be grouped by quarters using binqtrs(datain) and the resulting output in the data.frame qtrs can then be analysed for example, in bgamqtr(qtrs).

```
binqtrs(datain) # output in qtrs
head(qtrs)
```

	Quarters	Counts	Totals
1	06Q3	0	149
2	06Q4	2	147
3	07Q1	1	179
4	07Q2	2	169
5	07Q3	1	138
6	07Q4	3	143

```
bgamqtr(qtrs)   # chart not shown
```

```
Do you have risk-adjusted data (Y/N) n
Change degrees of freedom (Y/N) n
Chart heading.
Enter heading for the chart Quarterly Complex SSI Data
```

```
The model is in mmg.
Type summary(mmg)/predict(mmg,se=T) to see.
tau = 0.475, 2-sided pvalue =0.0063
Coefficients:
                Estimate Std. Error z value Pr(>|z|)
(Intercept)       -5.962      0.922   -6.47    1e-10 ***
      Null deviance: 18.9001  on 17  degrees of freedom
Residual deviance:  9.6129  on 14  degrees of freedom
AIC: 64.42
```

```
l<-1:length(qtrs[,1]) # first quarter in 2008 is 7th
s<-c(rep(1,7),rep(2,l[length(l)]-7))
g<-glm(qtrs$AEs/qtrs$Denoms~s+bs(l),family=binomial,weight=qtrs$Denoms)
summary(g)
```

```
Coefficients:
            Estimate Std. Error z value Pr(>|z|)
(Intercept)   -6.555      0.963   -6.81  9.8e-12 ***
s              0.908      0.715    1.27     0.20
      Null deviance: 18.9001  on 17  degrees of freedom
Residual deviance:  7.9502  on 13  degrees of freedom
AIC: 64.76
```

The dummy variable s for after the first quarter of 2008 is clearly not significant. The MannKendall trend test result suggests an upward trend (P-value=.006). The chart produced by bgamqtr(qtrs) (not shown) together with the MannKendall result suggests an uneven upward trend that was showing signs of levelling off rather than a changepoint. When suspecting the presence of a changepoint, for example, in response to an M&M audit and system review, a hospital scientist may wish to seek expert advice.

7.8   Assessing agreement

QI work often involves staff reading hospital records to extract evidence of adverse outcomes. In addition, IM staff must make judgements about whether or not there is an SSI or other nosocomial infection. It is important that there are carefully standardised definitions of the adverse occurrences and other events to be detected, and that the people doing the assessment are able to agree about their presence or absence.

Agreement has conventionally been assessed by the Kappa statistic (Fleiss). However, as described by Grant, the proportion of agreement for both normal and abnormal assessments may be preferable although it is probable that the exercise of performing a formal assessment of agreement is much more important than the statistic used to estimate the ability of observers to agree. We illustrate the method using the hypothetical data in Grant's paper shown in the table.

```
ObserverA<-c(rep("Abnormal",18),rep("Normal",32))
ObserverB<-c(rep("Abnormal",16),"Normal","Normal",rep("Normal",28),rep
("Abnormal",4))
table(ObserverA,ObserverB)
```

	ObserverB	
ObserverA	Abnormal	Normal
Abnormal	16	2
Normal	4	28

For these data the proportion of agreement for abnormality is AA/(AA+AN+NA)=16/22=0.74, and the proportion of agreement for normality is NN/(NN+AN+NA)=28/34=0.82, where AA=16, AN=2, NA=4 & NN=28. Approximate confidence intervals for these proportions can be calculated using the methods of Chapter 1. The 95% limits are 0.5 to 0.89 and 0.65 to 0.93 respectively.

Grant has emphasised the importance of obtaining samples of sufficient size and, if the proportion of abnormal results occurring naturally is small, selecting samples for testing that contain a higher proportion of abnormal findings. This would be easy to do when documentation is to be assessed but more difficult with an infrequently occurring nosocomial infection. Grant has stated that the proportions of agreement that are considered satisfactory will differ depending on the subject, but that a confidence interval including 50% agreement will generally be inadequate provided samples of sufficient size are employed. The method can be extended to the assessment of multiple observers as described in Grant's paper.

An important aspect is the assessment of observer bias, which is illustrated in the next table. In this case there are the same number of disagreements as before but they all occur when Observer A indicates a normal and Observer B an abnormal result. The probability of getting such a result by chance is $2/2^6=0.032$ for a two tailed test. Since this is unlikely, it is probable that the two observers are making systematically different assessments of patients who may be borderline, and that further training is required to improve overall assessment capability.

```
ObserverA<-c(rep("Abnormal",16),rep("Normal",34))
ObserverB<-c(rep("Abnormal",16),rep("Normal",28),rep("Abnormal",6))
table(ObserverA,ObserverB)
```

	ObserverB	
ObserverA	Abnormal	Normal
Abnormal	16	0
Normal	6	28

Two then medical students (McGrath and Morton) undertook as their Social and Preventative Medicine project a study of postoperative respiratory complications. This involved searching patients' files for evidence of such a complication. In order to assure themselves that they were doing this properly they first performed an independent retrospective assessment of 82 patient files to determine whether a respiratory complication existed. The result of their study is shown in the following table.

```
ObserverA<-c(rep("Abnormal",20),rep("Normal",62))
ObserverB<-c(rep("Abnormal",18),"Normal","Normal",rep("Normal",60),
rep("Abnormal",2))
table(ObserverA,ObserverB)
```

```
          ObserverB
ObserverA  Abnormal   Normal
Abnormal         18        2
Normal            2       60
```

For these data the proportion of agreement for normality was 0.94 (95% confidence interval 0.85 to 0.98) and the proportion of agreement for abnormality was 0.82 (95% confidence interval 0.60 to 0.95). They concluded that their level of agreement was satisfactory and thus were able to proceed with their study.

7.8.1   Numerical data agreement

When dealing with numerical data, for example to assess two sets of risk-adjustment values, correlation coefficients are frequently and erroneously employed. The intraclass correlation is a generalisation of kappa that gives a truer picture than a conventional correlation coefficient; its value usually needs to be at least 0.7 for worthwhile agreement to be judged present. It is available in the R psy library. A Bland-Altman plot described in Kirkwood and Sterne that displays the differences between the methods and their mean is probably the best way to analyse these data. When outcome data with risk adjustment are available, the methods for assessing calibration and discrimination described in Chapter 2 may be applied, with the method displaying the highest AUC value and the better calibration being preferred.

We illustrate the intraclass correlation and Bland-Altman plot with risk adjustment scores for a group of surgical site infections. The risk adjustment had been performed by two methods labelled RIONE and RITWO (Figure 7.32). There were noticeable differences between the risk scores but little difference between the expected counts. The discrimination of RITWO as measured by AUC described in Chapter 2 was slightly superior although their discriminative ability was little better than chance.

```
g.d() #data from ricomp.xls (no dates in first column)

#using a correlation coefficient
#incorrect method of assessing agreement
cor(datain[,1],datain[,2])
#[1] 0.8822201
#this above approach is incorrect

#employing the correct intraclass correlation
library(psy)
ICC<-icc(datain)
ICC$icc.agreement
#[1] 0.8687921

#Bland-Altman method
```

Comparison of risk-adjustment scores

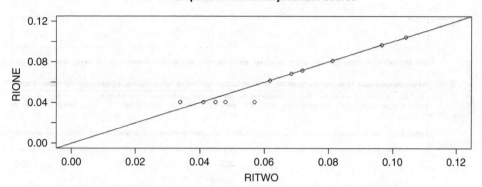

Figure 7.32   Comparison of SSI predictions by two methods.

```
d<-datain[,1]-datain[,2]
m<-mean(d)
m #mean difference between the methods
#[1] -0.002408731
s<-sd(d)
u<-m+2*s
u
#[1] 0.01172174
l<-m-2*s
l
#[1] -0.01653920
#plot of differences
plot(datain[,1]~datain[,2],main="Comparison of risk-adjustment scores",
ylab="RIONE",xlab="RITWO",ylim=c(0,.12), xlim=c(0,.12))
abline(coef=c(0,1))

#Bland-Altman plot
plot(d,axes=F,ylim=c(-.02,.02),main="Comparison of risk-adjustment scores",
ylab="Differences",xlab="Sequence")
box()
abline(h=m)
abline(h=u,lty=2)
abline(h=l,lty=2)
axis(side=1)
axis(side=2)

# Bland-Altman plot of grouped data
par(xaxs="r")
mm<-(datain[,1]+datain[,2])/2
plot(d~mm,axes=F,ylim=c(-.02,.02),
main="Comparison of risk-adjustment scores",
ylab="Differences",pch=19, xlab="Averages")
box()
abline(h=m)
abline(h=u,lty=2)
abline(h=l,lty=2)
axis(side=1)
axis(side=2)
```

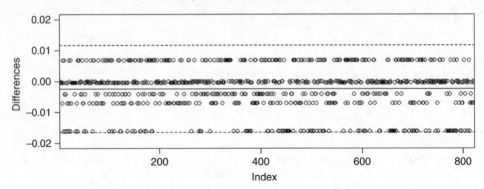

Figure 7.33   Bland-Altman plot with many ties.

```
# counting largest negative differences
dmin<-d[d==min(d)]
length(dmin)
#[1] 115
```

There were 823 procedures illustrated but only 10 groups as many of the procedure and risk index combinations were repeated. It can be seen that 115 of the RITWO minus RIONE differences were close to the lower confidence limit as shown in Figures 7.33 and 7.34.

7.9   Making decisions (decision analysis)

It is often important to determine whether some actions such as employing screening tests should be incorporated into a process. For example, should otherwise well patients undergoing relatively minor surgery such as hernia repair or excision of skin lesions be required to have

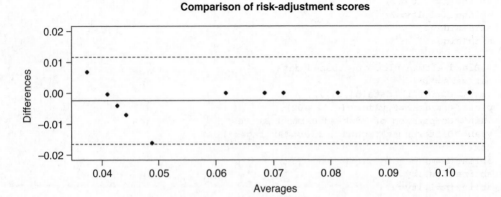

Figure 7.34   Bland-Altman plot with ties removed.

a preoperative chest X-ray? Some people may consider such investigations important for medico-legal reasons.

Suppose that a preoperative test has a sensitivity of 95% and a specificity of 95%. Thus if the patient has a lesion there would be 95 chances in 100 that it will be detected. Similarly, if there is no lesion, there are 95 chances in 100 that the test will be negative. Suppose also that, in this group of patients, the probability of a lesion being present is 1 in 200.

From these data we can say that the probability of the lesion is 0.005 and the probability of a positive test in its presence is $0.005 \times 0.95 = 0.00475$. Similarly the probability of no lesion is 0.995 and the probability of a positive test in the absence of a lesion is $0.995 \times (1-0.95) = 0.04975$. From these figures the probability of a positive test is $0.04975 + 0.00475 = 0.05425$ and the probability of a lesion when the test is positive is $0.00475/0.05425 = 0.088$. Thus only $0.088 \times 100 \approx 9$ in every 100 positive tests (about 1 in 11) will signify the presence of a definite lesion and the remaining 91 will ultimately be shown to be false positive results.

These calculations, called Bayes' Rule, illustrate the importance of the prevalence of the condition in question in determining the usefulness of the test. Thus if 200 tests are taken there will be about 11 positive results (0.05425×200), only 1 of which would represent the presence of a lesion and the remainder would be false positives.

In addition, one negative result is likely to occur in the presence of the lesion (false negative result) in every 20 groups of 200 tests performed $0.00025/(0.94525+0.00025) \approx 1/4000)$.

Although such testing is not necessarily wrong, it is important to understand what it costs and also what further costs are generated in investigating the false positive results to establish that no lesion exists. Often these investigations can be quite invasive and there may be risk of harm, including unfounded anxiety and inconvenience, as well as added cost.

Furthermore, it should be determined what the result would be if this money were spent differently. For example, if it were used to improve IM systems and processes it might be possible to prevent three or four hospital acquired infections that might be more serious and costly than the one lesion that the test finds.

Two further concepts of importance are the disutility of missing the lesion and the sensitivity of the decision analysis. If the lesion were to cause death in the postoperative period it would be much more serious than if it simply had a low probability of causing a minor postoperative complication. In the former case its disutility would be measured at 100% (or its utility zero), and in the latter case its disutility might be estimated as 10%. Thornton and Lilford show how to incorporate disutility, or its opposite utility, in a decision analysis.

The baseline probabilities of the presence of disease that are used in the decision analysis may not be known precisely and it may be necessary to estimate them. Because of this a range of probabilities can be selected and the outcome of the analysis determined for each of them. By doing this it is possible to judge which course of action would be appropriate in a particular set of circumstances. For example, the sensitivity analysis may indicate that the same course of action is appropriate over a wide range of probabilities of disease presence, and this would add to confidence in the analysis. Alternatively, there may be a cut-off point where each course of action is equally appropriate. Thus on one side of this threshold, for example when the probability of disease in the population is below a certain level, the test would not be indicated, whereas if it were above this level, the test should be performed.

7.10   Investigating outbreaks, further analysis of stratified data

There are excellent descriptions of outbreak investigations available (Giesecke, Ostrowsky and Jarvis). *Principles of Epidemiology in Public Health Practice* 3rd Edition (www.cdc.gov/training/products/ss1000/ss1000-ol.pdf), Myatt M *'Open Source Solutions–R'* and Quigley M and Myatt M *'Don't Panic'* (http://www.brixtonhealth.com) are good sources of relevant information. Reingold's *'Outbreak Investigations-A Perspective'* summarizes the required approach. This includes case definition and confirmation, checking the background rate, case finding, descriptive epidemiology including graphs of epidemic curves and tabulations of age, sex and location, attack rates, environmental investigation including collecting required specimens for analysis, generating and testing hypotheses, control measures, and interacting with the authorities, the public and the press.

A brief summary of how outbreak investigation relates to in-hospital events follows. Statistical methods that may aid in the analysis of hospital outbreaks, for example Mantel-Haenszel analysis and logistic regression are described. Since all or most of the potential explanatory variables and the outcome variable are dichotomous, a multivariate analysis, that is in fact rarely required for hospital outbreak data, should usually be technically uncomplicated.

Determining the causes of within hospital outbreaks is frequently straightforward. For example excess falls, medication errors or pressure ulcers are frequently due to failure to follow evidence-based systems embodied in bundles and checklists. Other common situations are increases of device-related bacteraemias, urosepsis and pneumonias due to failure to adhere to evidence-based systems (e.g. bundles and checklists) for the care of intravenous devices, urinary catheters or ventilation equipment respectively. Increases in new MRSA or VRE isolates occur when hand hygiene, cleaning of high-touch surfaces or isolation practices are inadequate and increases in infections due to hospital-acquired organisms generally are related to antibiotic misuse, poor hygiene and inadequate cleaning, overcrowding with numerous outlier patients and attendant staff-patient contact networks, understaffing or poor surveillance systems and inadequate isolation resources. Excess surgical site infections are usually related to sub-optimal wound care, postoperative oxygenation or thermal or glucose regulation, or failure with antibiotic prophylaxis. Outbreaks due for example, to norovirus infection are not uncommon in hospitals.

It will rarely be necessary to resort to a multivariate analysis. However, there are frequent meetings of various groups in hospitals and these commonly occur at meal times so the potential for food borne infection exists. We therefore include an example of the analysis of these data.

Notwithstanding the above, it is increasingly being recognised that hospitals are complex systems that are characterised by emergent behaviour and self-organisation. Outbreaks can occur without apparent cause and generic defences are important. Outbreaks may be due to defective systems in which a number of interacting agents precipitate a transition from an endemic to an epidemic state (see The Hospital as a Network in section 8.16 of Chapter 8). It is well known that surveillance of adverse events and feedback of the data often result in their reduction, and this is frequently called a Hawthorne effect (section 6.4 of Chapter 6. It is probably related to subtle improvements in a number of potential causative agents that, interacting together, result in more satisfactory emergent behaviour in a complex system. This should warn us to be wary of the reliance of QI on the Pareto Principle that ascribes most risk to a small number of major causes and on root cause analysis. There may be no straightforward root cause, instead increases in AEs may sometimes be the result of complex system emergent behaviour. If subtle changes in many interacting agents can result in improved emergent behaviour, it is reasonable to hypothesise that, in an unhappy environment in which violations are occurring (see section 8.3.1 of Chapter 8), equally subtle changes in many interacting agents may result in unfavourable emergent behaviour that may precipitate a change from a predictable system to one exhibiting unpredictable behaviour.

Uncommonly, detailed statistical analysis may be required to identify the causes of an outbreak and worked examples using hypothetical data and well known public health data are presented.

A hospital-acquired infection epidemic is defined as an increase in incidence over expected rates. If a surveillance programme is in progress, the increase may be readily apparent; otherwise alert hospital or microbiology staff may detect its presence. For infections included in a surveillance programme, statistical process control methods may aid in its prompt identification. A single case due to an unusual organism or an unusual infection by a common organism may constitute an epidemic.

An important issue is the early detection of an outbreak. Infection control surveillance staff in their rounds of the wards will often be the first to detect an unusual pattern requiring attention. For example, if one MRSA bacteraemia is expected on average every 40 days, a microbiology report of 3 MRSA bacteraemias in three or four days would alert them to begin investigation of a possible outbreak. A useful approach with uncommon events is to count the intervals between them. This is what infection control surveillance staff would have been doing informally in the MRSA bacteraemia example.

The presence of the outbreak needs to be confirmed, for example by an infectious diseases physician. Rare but serious adverse events all require detailed individual attention and an independent audit may sometimes be desirable. Shewhart/EWMA control charts and GAM charts are useful with more common count data AEs such as new MRSA isolates and CUSUM and cumulative observed minus expected analysis when the data are binary or counts that are usually very low for example with MRSA bacteraemias. However, statistical analysis may not provide an early warning.

Systematic investigation of the outbreak is required and one of the first things is to look to previously identified cases and their causes.

A case definition is required. This states:

1. Who had the findings including ages, sex, co-morbidities and other relevant data,

2. The time period when the illnesses occurred, and

3. The ward or wards involved.

A gantt chart that displays the patients' ward and bed number within the ward, dates of confirmation of AE status, for example carrier of a multiple-antibiotic resistant organism, date of transfer, for example to an isolation bed, and date of discharge may be useful for displaying interrelationships between person, time and place. Gantt chart software is mainly designed for project management so, provided large numbers of patients are not involved, manual entry of the data, for example in a spreadsheet, may be the most suitable approach. Recent work has emphasised the importance of understanding the network of patient and staff contacts that have occurred (Ueno and Masuda, Temime and colleagues).

At the same time there should be a careful search for all cases. When the outbreak involves person-to-person spread, contacts of cases such as patients occupying adjacent beds, or relevant staff, may need to be identified, screened and in extreme cases isolated. Treatment regimes including antibiotic usage should be reviewed. Susceptible patients and carriers may need to be isolated.

This is followed by the drawing of an epidemic curve that may help differentiate between point source outbreaks (e.g. a norovirus outbreak in a ward) when an index case may be identified that helps define the incubation period, continuous source outbreaks (e.g. when there is continuing contamination or re-contamination of patient-care equipment) and propagated outbreaks associated with person-to-person spread where a serial interval may be identified.

From the patients' hospital documents and other relevant sources, a line listing is created of the characteristics of the affected patients that may be important including times, places, ages, sex, severity of illness and relevant clinical data. These data need to be entered into a suitable data table in a spreadsheet or database programme. Interviews with relevant staff and patients may follow and a careful review of microbiology isolates and other possible sources of information is required.

Calculation of attack rates may be useful. Attack rates are illustrated using the widely used Oswego data (www.cdc.gov/excite/classroom/outbreak/steps.htm). Source: Centers for Disease Control and Prevention Epidemiology Program Office, Case Studies in Applied Epidemiology No.401-303. Oswego – An Outbreak of Gastrointestinal Illness Following a Church Supper.

Oswego Data

Vanilla ice cream	No vanilla ice cream
Ill 43	Ill 3
Total 54	Total 21
Attack rate 80%	Attack rate 14%
Difference 66%	

Males
Vanilla ice cream	No vanilla ice cream
Ill 16	Ill 0
Total 23	Total 8
Attack rate 70%	Attack rate 0%
Difference 70%	

Females
Vanilla ice cream	No vanilla ice cream
Ill 27	Ill 3
Total 31	Total 13
Attack rate 87%	Attack rate 23%
Difference 64%	

Male/Female difference
Vanilla ice cream 17%   No vanilla ice cream 13%
Vanilla ice cream/No vanilla ice cream difference
Males 70%   Females 66%

Analysis using logistic regression (section 7.7.2 of this chapter) suggests that vanilla ice cream was the cause of the gastroenteritis outbreak. However, there was a statistically significant difference between females and males. The attack rate tables show that the attack rate for vanilla ice cream was high and that for no vanilla ice cream low. The difference was large. The sex difference was small. The attack rate differences for vanilla ice cream within the sex groups were large and for the sex differences within the vanilla ice cream groups were small. The vanilla ice cream is clearly implicated.

At this stage a working hypothesis is formed and further preventive and control measures instituted. If required, the outbreak should be reported to the relevant health authorities. Occasionally, statistical analysis using Mantel-Haenszel tests and/or logistic regression and possibly including a case-control study may be needed to throw further light on the causes of the outbreak.

7.10.1   Reviewing stratified data analysis

Example 1. Hypothetical data to illustrate Mantel-Haenszel analysis (Rosner). The data are in the file example1.csv. The stratum column appears ordered. This could be unusual in practice but could represent a variable such as age group or ordered risk categories such as low risk, medium risk and high risk. The remaining columns contain hypothetical data representing exposure and outcome. We illustrate a random effects analysis that assumes the stratifying variable can be regarded as a random variable and there is appreciable variation among the strata. This would not be appropriate if the stratifying variable were for example, sex, an item of potentially contaminated food or if the strata were ordered. If the individual stratum effects differ, it is usual to recommend that the data be examined within the individual strata. If the stratifying agent can be regarded as a random variable that may differ among the strata, a random effects analysis may be appropriate to deal with the variability among the strata. This mostly occurs in meta-analysis that is not dealt with in these notes. However, Spiegelhalter[D] has introduced the use of a derSimonian-Laird random effects analysis to cope with excessive variability among hospitals when displaying AE data from several hospitals in funnel plots, and we illustrate the calculations involved. This is an important issue when analysing data from groups of hospitals, for example, in funnel plots in Chapters 2 and 5, and we refer to it also in Chapters 1 and 4.

```
g.d()#example1.csv, first column not dates

attach(datain)
table(exposure,outcome)
```

```
          outcome
exposure   0     1
0         26    14
1         15    60
```

```
fisher.test(table(exposure,outcome))
```

```
Fisher's Exact Test for Count Data
data:  table(exposure, outcome)
p-value = 3.675e-06
alternative hypothesis: true odds ratio is not equal to 1
95 percent confidence interval:
2.895024 19.266722
sample estimates:
odds ratio
7.271667
```

```
table(exposure,outcome,stratum)

, , stratum = 0

        outcome
exposure  0  1
       0  5  4
       1  4  2

, , stratum = 1

        outcome
exposure  0  1
       0  6  5
       1  4 21

, , stratum = 2

        outcome
exposure  0  1
       0 15  5
       1  7 37
```

```
# tidier display
ftable(exposure,outcome,stratum)
```

```
                 stratum  0   1   2
exposure  outcome
       0        0         5   6  15
                1         4   5   5
       1        0         4   4   7
                1         2  21  37
```

```
ftable(stratum,exposure,outcome)
```

```
                      outcome  0   1
stratum   exposure
      0          0             5   4
                 1             4   2
      1          0             6   5
                 1             4  21
      2          0            15   5
                 1             7  37
```

```
mantelhaen.test(table(exposure,outcome,stratum))
```

```
        Mantel-Haenszel chi-squared test with continuity correction
data:   table(exposure, outcome, stratum)
Mantel-Haenszel X-squared = 18.2942, df = 1, p-value = 1.893e-05
alternative hypothesis: true common odds ratio is not equal to 1
95 percent confidence interval:
  2.507172 13.972983
sample estimates:
common odds ratio
         5.918841
```

There appears to be a strong exposure–outcome association and the relationship appears to persist after stratification.

```
# tests for exposure/stratum differences
exp0<-exposure[stratum==0];outc0<-outcome[stratum==0]
exp1<-exposure[stratum==1];outc1<-outcome[stratum==1]
exp2<-exposure[stratum==2];outc2<-outcome[stratum==2]
ta<-table(exp0,outc0)
ta
```

```
       outc0
 exp0   0   1
 0      5   4
 1      4   2
```

```
fisher.test(ta)
```

```
Fisher's Exact Test for Count Data
data:  ta
p-value = 1
alternative hypothesis: true odds ratio is not equal to 1
95 percent confidence interval:
0.03851115 7.90017915
sample estimates:
odds ratio
0.6448271
```

```
tb<-table(exp1,outc1)
tb
```

```
       outc1
 exp1   0    1
 0      6    5
 1      4   21
```

```
fisher.test(tb)
```

```
Fisher's Exact Test for Count Data
data:  tb
p-value = 0.03904
alternative hypothesis: true odds ratio is not equal to 1
95 percent confidence interval:
0.9851765 41.7820773
sample estimates:
odds ratio
5.912998
```

```
tc<-table(exp2,outc2)
tc
```

```
       outc2
 exp2    0    1
 0      15    5
 1       7   37
```

```
fisher.test(tc)
```

```
Fisher's Exact Test for Count Data
data:  tc
p-value = 7.836e-06
alternative hypothesis: true odds ratio is not equal to 1
95 percent confidence interval:
3.738592 71.899569
sample estimates:
odds ratio
14.91094
```

```
#Woolf stratified odds ratio plus homogeneity and trend tests
#description in Chapter 1
lor<-0
vlor<-0
x<-0
ta1<-ta # add .5 if any zeros
or1<-ta1[1]*ta1[4]/(ta1[2]*ta1[3])
lor[1]<-log(or1)
vlor[1]<-sum(1/ta1)
x[1]<-1
tb1<-tb # add .5 if any zeros
or2<-tb1[1]*tb1[4]/(tb1[2]*tb1[3])
lor[2]<-log(or2)
vlor[2]<-sum(1/tb1)
x[2]<-2
tc1<-tc # add .5 if any zeros
or3<-tc1[1]*tc1[4]/(tc1[2]*tc1[3])
lor[3]<-log(or3)
vlor[3]<-sum(1/tc1)
x[3]<-3
#
alor<-sum(lor/vlor)/sum(1/vlor)
valor<-1/sum(1/vlor)
OR<-exp(alor)
L95<-exp(alor-1.96*valor^.5)
U95<-exp(alor+1.96*valor^.5)
Z.score<-alor/valor^.5
P.value<-2*(1-pnorm(Z.score))
cat("Woolf OR=",round(OR,2),"\nL95=",round(L95,2),"\nU95=",round(U95,2),
"\nZ-score=",round(Z.score,2),"\nP-value=",round(P.value,5),"\n",sep="")
```

```
Woolf OR=6.56
L95=2.64
U95=16.32
Z-score=4.05
P-value=5e-05
```

```
ch<-sum((1/vlor)*(lor-alor)^2)
ch # Homogeneity test (Woolf)
#[1] 6.392962
1-pchisq(ch,2) # P-value
#[1] 0.0409059
```

If the stratifying agent is exchangeable (e.g. it might be hospitals or units within hospitals), a trend analysis would usually be inappropriate. If a trend is expected to exist among the strata, for example, age groupings, they would not be exchangeable and a random effects analysis would not be performed.

```
# Trend test
w<-1/vlor
a<-sum(w*x*lor);b<-sum(w*lor);d<-sum(x*w);e<-sum(w);f<-sum(w*x^2)
Lxy<-a-b*d/e
Lxx<-f-d^2/e
ch.sq<-Lxy^2/Lxx
ch.sq # trend using weighted regression (Rosner)
#[1] 5.944605
1-pchisq(ch.sq,1) # P-value
#[1] 0.0147624
```

If the stratifying agent is not exchangeable, for example, it is something like sex or age group, we should not proceed to the random effects analysis. The within stratum analyses should be examined. Since there is an obvious trend among the strata, it seems unlikely that they could be regarded as random agents. We nevertheless continue to use them to illustrate the methods involved.

```
#derSimonian-Laird random effects
# assuming strata are exchangeable
w<-1/vlor
W<-sum(w)-(sum(w^2)/sum(w))
Q<-max(0,ch-length(w)+1)
Q/W # random effects variance
#
#[1] 1.537931

rvlor<-vlor+Q/W
w1<-1/rvlor
rlor<-sum(w1*lor)/sum(w1)
vrvlor<-1/sum(w1)
L<-exp(rlor-1.96*vrvlor^.5)
U<-exp(rlor+1.96*vrvlor^.5)
Z<-rlor/vrvlor^.5
P<-2*(1-pnorm(rlor/vrvlor^.5))
cat("Adjusted OR=",round(exp(rlor),2),"\nL95=",round(L,2),"\nU95=",
round(U,2),"\nZ-score=",round(Z,2),"\nP-value=",round(P,5),"\n",sep="")
```

```
Adjusted OR=4.74
L95=0.86
U95=26.02
Z-score=1.79
P-value=0.07308
```

```
detach(datain)
```

There is evidence of heterogeneity, especially a trend associated with the stratum level, so the Mantel-Haenszel test may not be suitable. Because of this interaction it is difficult to assess the exposure-outcome association. However, the within-stratum analyses (fisher.test for ta, tb and tc) show no association at the first stratum level but definite association at the middle level and a strong association at the third level. The derSimonian-Laird random effects analysis suggests that significance is at most borderline but, in this instance, its use would be questionable as data in ordered categories are unlikely to be exchangeable. However, if the stratifying agent were for example, hospitals and there was no reason to expect any trend, the random effects analysis could be appropriate. It is instructive to see how much difference can occur when there is a random stratifying agent, inhomogeneity and a random effects analysis can be used to account for among stratum variability.

As a check we employ the analysis in the library rmeta. There is clear evidence of a trend among the strata. If this possibility could have been anticipated before the analysis, for example the strata could have been age groups, a random effects analysis would have been inappropriate. It would appear wise to analyse these data in their separate strata.

The calculations for the Woolf odds ratio, heterogeneity tests and random-effects analysis are described in Chapter 1. Here the rmeta library is also employed. Another approach is to use the spreadsheet provided by derSimonian and Kacker (www.niaid.nih.gov/about/organization/dcr/BRB/staff/Pages/rebecca.aspx). There is a large random effects variance.

```
# using library rmeta
#the data in the data.frame datain, must be re-arranged as follows
for (i in 1:3){A<-datain[datain[,1]==i-1,];if (i==1){A0<-c(sum(as.numeric
(A[,2])==0),sum(A[,3]==1&A[,2]==0),sum(as.numeric(A[,2])==1),sum(A[,3]==1
&A[,2]==1))}else{A0<-rbind(A0,c(sum(as.numeric(A[,2])==0),sum(A[,3]==1
&A[,2]==0),sum(as.numeric(A[,2])==1),sum(A[,3]==1&A[,2]==1)))}}
A0
```

	[,1]	[,2]	[,3]	[,4]
A0	9	4	6	2
	11	5	25	21
	20	5	44	37

```
library(rmeta)
MMH<-meta.MH(A0[,3],A0[,1],A0[,4],A0[,2])
summary(MMH) #similar to mantelhaen.test result
```

```
Fixed effects ( Mantel-Haenszel ) meta-analysis
Call: meta.MH(ntrt=A0[,3],nctrl=A0[,1],ptrt=A0[,4],pctrl=A0[,2])
       OR (lower  95% upper)
[1,]  0.62   0.07       5.35
[2,]  6.30   1.28      31.12
[3,] 15.86   4.34      57.89
Mantel-Haenszel OR =5.92 95% CI ( 2.51,13.97 )
Test for heterogeneity: X^2( 2 ) = 6.44 ( p-value 0.0399 )
```

```
#Z-score and P-value (Bland and Altman)
SE<-(log(13.97)-log(2.51))/(2*1.96)
Z<-log(5.92)/SE
P<-exp(-0.717*Z-0.416*Z^2)
Z;P
#[1] 4.060911
#[1] 5.703032e-05
```

```
#derSimonian-Laird
MDSL<-meta.DSL(A0[,3],A0[,1],A0[,4],A0[,2])
summary(MDSL)
```

```
Random effects ( DerSimonian-Laird ) meta-analysis
Call: meta.DSL(ntrt=A0[,3],nctrl=A0[,1],ptrt=A0[,4],pctrl=A0[,2])
       OR (lower  95% upper)
[1,]  0.62    0.07       5.35
[2,]  6.30    1.28      31.12
[3,] 15.86    4.34      57.89
SummaryOR= 4.74  95% CI ( 0.86,26.02 )
Test for heterogeneity: X^2( 2 ) = 6.39 ( p-value 0.0409 )
Estimated random effects variance: 1.54
```

```
#Z-score and P-value
SE<-(log(26.02)-log(.86))/(2*1.96)
Z<-log(4.74)/SE
P<-exp(-0.717*Z-0.416*Z^2)
Z;P
#[1] 1.788922
#[1] 0.07324414
```

```
#random effects logistic regression
library(hglm)
h<-hglm(fixed=outcome~exposure,random=~exposure|stratum,family=binomial
(link=logit),data=datain,fix.disp=1)
summary(h) #abbreviated output
```

```
Summary of the fixed effects estimates:
          Estimate Std. Error t-value Pr(>|t|)
(Intercept)  -0.6190      0.3315  -1.867    0.0645 .
exposure      1.6507      0.7578   2.178    0.0315 *
Summary of the random effects estimates:
                            Estimate Std. Error
exposure:as.factor(stratum)0  -1.0415      0.7639
exposure:as.factor(stratum)1   0.4937      0.7143
exposure:as.factor(stratum)2   0.5479      0.6996
Dispersion parameter for the random effects: 1.084
```

It has been assumed here that the stratifying variable is not a fixed effect. In the presence of heterogeneity, it can be seen that the Mantel-Haenszel analysis may mislead by suggesting a difference exists when this may not be the case. Also, the derSimonian-Laird analysis appears conservative while the random effects logistic regression appears to suggest a much more conservative P-value for exposure than the Mantel-Haenszel analysis. The random effects variance estimated by hglm() is smaller than that estimated by the derSimonian-Laird analysis.

7.10.2   Outbreak investigation example

Example 2. The Oswego data set (www.cdc.gov/excite/classroom/outbreak/steps.htm, Gross, Centers for Disease Control and Prevention Epidemiology Program Office, Case Studies in Applied Epidemiology No.401-303. Oswego – An Outbreak of Gastrointestinal Illness Following a Church Supper) describes a gastroenteritis outbreak following a supper in 1940; it is in the file oswego.csv. This represents an outbreak of food poisoning and includes information about possible causes. We approach the analysis in R. First, an epidemic curve is constructed (Figure 7.35). Missing data with a value of 99 in the original file have been

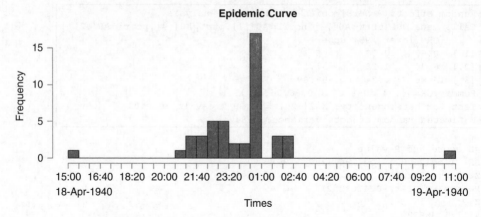

Figure 7.35   Oswego gastroenteritis data epidemic curve.

replaced with NA. Tabulations, a boxplot (Figure 7.36) stratified data analysis and logistic regression are illustrated.

```
g.d()# oswego.csv (first column is not a date column)

# Note that the date format of oswego.csv must be "dd-mmm-yyyy"
# .csv files default to eg "d-mmm-yy", "d/m/y" or "m/d/y"
# suggest change in spreadsheet using Format Cells, Custom
# to "dd-mmm-yyyy"
# Note the missing codes of 99 in oswego.csv have been replaced by NA.

datain1<-datain[datain[,5]=="1",]
dm<-as.character(datain1[,6])
tm<-as.character(datain1[,7])
s<-paste(dm,tm)
Outbreak<-strptime(s,"%d-%b-%Y %H:%M:%S")
head(Outbreak)
#[1] "1940-04-19 00:30:00" "1940-04-19 00:30:00" "1940-04-19 00:30:00"
#[4] "1940-04-18 22:30:00" "1940-04-18 22:30:00" "1940-04-19 02:00:00"
hist(Outbreak, breaks=30,freq=TRUE,xlab="Times",col="gray50", main=paste
("Epidemic Curve"))
mtext("18Apr1940",side=1,line=2,adj=0);mtext("19Apr1940",side=1,line=2,
adj=1)
# there may be a warning message but col & main appear to work
# as they appear in the documentation


oswego<-datain
#The oswego data include the following -
names(oswego)
# [1] "id"                 "age"                "sex"
# [4] "MealTime"           "ill"                "OnsetDate"
# [7] "OnsetTime"          "BakedHam"           "spinach"
#[10] "MashedPotato"       "CabbageSalad"       "jello"
#[13] "rolls"              "BrownBread"         "milk"
#[16] "coffee"             "water"              "cakes"
#[19] "VanillaIceCream"    "ChocolateIceCream"  "FruitSalad"
#
```

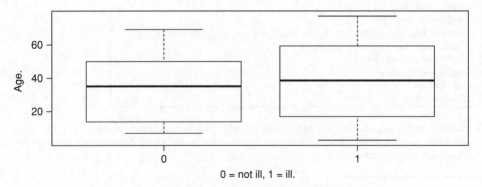

0 = not ill, 1 = ill.

Figure 7.36   Boxplot of ages, Oswego gastroenteritis data.

```
attach(oswego)
boxplot(age~ill,main="Ages.",ylab="Age.",xlab="0 = not ill, 1 = ill.")
# Figure 7.36. The people who fell ill were slightly older

t.test(age~ill)$p.value
#[1] 0.2101099
# there is no evidence of a significant difference in the ages

age1<-rep(0,length(ill))
age1[age>40]<-1 # ages grouped at 40 years
table(age1,ill)
```

```
      ill
age1   0   1
   0  21  24
   1   8  22
```

```
fisher.test(table(age1,ill))
```

```
        Fisher's Exact Test for Count Data
data:   table(age1, ill)
p-value = 0.09549
alternative hypothesis: true odds ratio is not equal to 1
95 percent confidence interval:
 0.8054664 7.5575507
sample estimates:
odds ratio
  2.378241
```

```
table(sex,ill)
```

```
     ill
sex  0   1
  F  14  30
  M  15  16
```

```
fisher.test(sex,ill)
```

```
Fisher's Exact Test for Count Data
data:  sex and ill
p-value = 0.1588
alternative hypothesis: true odds ratio is not equal to 1
95 percent confidence interval:
 0.1736485 1.4263454
sample estimates:
odds ratio
 0.5025686
```

```
# tables and fisher.tests performed on all the remaining foods.
# vanilla & chocolate ice cream the only ones showing a possible association
table(VanillaIceCream,ill)
```

```
                  ill
VanillaIceCream  0  1
              0 18  3
              1 11 43
```

```
fisher.test(table(VanillaIceCream,ill))
```

```
Fisher's Exact Test for Count Data
data:  table(VanillaIceCream, ill)
p-value = 2.597e-07
alternative hypothesis: true odds ratio is not equal to 1
95 percent confidence interval:
   5.216064 138.865034
sample estimates:
odds ratio
  22.15606
```

```
table(ChocolateIceCream,ill)
```

```
                    ill
ChocolateIceCream  0  1
                0  7 20
                1 22 25
```

```
fisher.test(table(ChocolateIceCream,ill))
```

```
Fisher's Exact Test for Count Data
data:  table(ChocolateIceCream, ill)
p-value = 0.08907
alternative hypothesis: true odds ratio is not equal to 1
95 percent confidence interval:
 0.1198724 1.2318906
sample estimates:
odds ratio
 0.4026708
```

We now employ logistic regression. Since there were 46 cases among 75 people there is only room for a small number of explanatory agents, for example, approximately one explanatory agent per 10 cases. Those identified by tabulations and Fisher exact tests included the ice creams, age and sex as being of possible interest. Therefore, it might be preferable to omit the next analysis and concentrate on the one following that involves the four agents of interest.

```
#using logistic regression
g1<-glm(ill~age1+sex+BakedHam+spinach+MashedPotato+CabbageSalad+jello+
rolls+BrownBread+milk+coffee+water+cakes+VanillaIceCream+ChocolateIceCream+
FruitSalad,family=binomial)
summary(g1)
# the sample size is really too small to permit so many explanatory
# variables with necessary power
```

```
Coefficients:
                 Estimate Std. Error z value Pr(>|z|)
(Intercept)      -2.35229    1.36233  -1.727 0.084229 .
age1              1.15357    0.82711   1.395 0.163107
sexM             -1.77901    0.77818  -2.286 0.022248 *
BakedHam          0.99936    1.72756   0.578 0.562939
spinach          -1.84788    1.62904  -1.134 0.256655
MashedPotato     -0.03679    1.03157  -0.036 0.971548
CabbageSalad      0.39925    1.02333   0.390 0.696426
jello            -0.83886    1.11996  -0.749 0.453851
rolls             0.59734    1.43311   0.417 0.676813
BrownBread        0.93923    1.08001   0.870 0.384491
milk             -2.11512    1.89891  -1.114 0.265339
coffee           -0.85398    1.16885  -0.731 0.465011
water             0.65170    1.04018   0.627 0.530967
cakes             1.21032    0.76714   1.578 0.114631
VanillaIceCream   3.92621    1.02675   3.824 0.000131 ***
ChocolateIceCream -0.16988   0.86066  -0.197 0.843523
FruitSalad        0.24298    1.35577   0.179 0.857766
    Null deviance: 97.204  on 72  degrees of freedom
Residual deviance: 58.077  on 56  degrees of freedom
AIC: 92.077
```

```
# by elimination the following remain -
g2<-glm(ill~age1+sex+VanillaIceCream+ChocolateIceCream,family=binomial)
summary(g2)
```

```
                 Estimate Std. Error z value Pr(>|z|)
(Intercept)      -1.68124    0.97778  -1.719   0.0855 .
age1              0.72231    0.67298   1.073   0.2831
sexM             -1.37175    0.67653  -2.028   0.0426 *
VanillaIceCream   3.44094    0.81735   4.210 2.56e-05 ***
ChocolateIceCream 0.01507    0.69353   0.022   0.9827
    Null deviance:  99.099  on 73  degrees of freedom
Residual deviance:  65.315  on 69  degrees of freedom
AIC: 75.315
```

```
g3<-glm(ill~sex+VanillaIceCream,family=binomial)
summary(g3)
```

```
                    Estimate Std. Error z value Pr(>|z|)
(Intercept)          -1.4254    0.6459  -2.207   0.0273 *
sexM                 -1.3253    0.6597  -2.009   0.0445 *
VanillaIceCream       3.4805    0.7797   4.464 8.04e-06 ***
      Null deviance: 100.085  on 74  degrees of freedom
Residual deviance:   67.371  on 72  degrees of freedom
AIC: 73.371
```

Clearly, vanilla ice cream was the cause of the outbreak. However, why were the males less likely to succumb? Could it be a confounder? Perhaps the men waited their turn and got a less contaminated part of the ice cream or perhaps they ate less of it. For these to be true, sex would need to be a confounder and to be associated with vanilla ice cream consumption.

```
table(sex,VanillaIceCream)
```

```
    VanillaIceCream
sex  0  1
  F 13 31
  M  8 23
```

```
fisher.test(table(sex,VanillaIceCream))
```

```
Fisher's Exact Test for Count Data
data:  table(sex, VanillaIceCream)
p-value = 0.7979
alternative hypothesis: true odds ratio is not equal to 1
95 percent confidence interval:
0.3850529 3.9429881
sample estimates:
odds ratio
1.202661
```

There is no evidence of an association. However, it is still possible that males ate less of the contaminated vanilla ice cream but, since quantities are not available, this cannot be studied. We should also check to ensure that there was no interaction, for example the ice cream effect being different in the male and female groups. It is equally clear from the following analysis that there was no evidence of interaction.

```
g4<-glm(ill~sex*VanillaIceCream,family=binomial)
summary(g4)
```

```
Coefficients:
                     Estimate Std. Error z value Pr(>|z|)
 (Intercept)          -1.2040     0.6583  -1.829 0.067405 .
sexM                 -16.3621  1398.7211  -0.012 0.990667
VanillaIceCream        3.1135     0.8487   3.668 0.000244 ***
sexM:VanillaIceCream  15.2792  1398.7213   0.011 0.991284
      Null deviance: 100.085  on 74  degrees of freedom
Residual deviance:   66.154  on 71  degrees of freedom
AIC: 74.154
```

The attack rates, shown above, displayed clearly that the vanilla ice cream was the offender. There are further examples in Myatt's Open Source Solutions–R that we mention in the Introduction. Multivariate analysis is not commonly required for dealing with hospital outbreaks.

The use of the Mantel-Haenszel stratified analysis was described in Example 1. One difficulty with mantelhaen.test occurs when there is more than one variable used in the stratification. Although age and sex do not need to be included in the analysis in this way, we illustrate the analysis using them. It is unlikely that a stratified analysis employing more than two stratification variables would be useful.

```
table(VanillaIceCream,ill,sex,age1)
```

```
, ,           sex = F, age1 = 0
                  ill
VanillaIceCream     0          1
              0     7          2
              1     3         14
, ,           sex = M, age1 = 0
                  ill
VanillaIceCream     0          1
              0     6          0
              1     5          8
, ,           sex = F, age1 = 1
                  ill
VanillaIceCream     0          1
              0     3          1
              1     1         13
#, ,          sex = M, age1 = 1
                  ill
VanillaIceCream     0          1
              0     2          0
              1     2          8
```

```
mantelhaen.test(table(VanillaIceCream,ill,sex,age1))
#Error in mantelhaen.test(table(VanillaIceCream, ill, sex, age1)) :
#  'x' must be a 3-dimensional array
```

Without using difficult data structures, the Mantel-Haenszel test requires a single stratifying variable.

```
stratum<-rep(0,length(age1))
stratum[age1==1&sex=="M"]<-1
stratum[age1==0&sex=="F"]<-2
stratum[age1==1&sex=="F"]<-3
```

```
levelA<-VanillaIceCream[stratum==0];illA<-ill[stratum==0]
# sex = M, age1 = 0
ta<-table(levelA,illA)
ta
```

```
        ill A
levelA  0   1
     0  6   0
     1  5   8
```

```
fisher.test(table(levelA,illA))
```

```
          Fisher's Exact Test for Count Data
data:  table(levelA, illA)
p-value = 0.01806
alternative hypothesis: true odds ratio is not equal to 1
95 percent confidence interval:
 1.170149        Inf
sample estimates:
odds ratio
       Inf
```

```
levelB<-VanillaIceCream[stratum==1];illB<-ill[stratum==1]
# sex = M, age1 = 1
tb<-table(levelB,illB)
tb
```

```
          illB
 levelB   0   1
      0   2   0
      1   2   8
```

```
fisher.test(table(levelB,illB))
```

```
          Fisher's Exact Test for Count Data
data:  table(levelB, illB)
p-value = 0.09091
alternative hypothesis: true odds ratio is not equal to 1
95 percent confidence interval:
 0.42098        Inf
sample estimates:
odds ratio
       Inf
```

```
levelC<-VanillaIceCream[stratum==2];illC<-ill[stratum==2]
# sex = F, age1 = 0
tc<-table(levelC,illC)
tc
```

```
          illC
 levelC   0    1
      0   7    2
      1   3   14
```

```
fisher.test(table(levelC,illC))
```

```
          Fisher's Exact Test for Count Data
data:  table(levelC, illC)
p-value = 0.008504
alternative hypothesis: true odds ratio is not equal to 1
95 percent confidence interval:
   1.662199 208.135021
sample estimates:
odds ratio
  14.06745
```

```
levelD<-VanillaIceCream[stratum==3];illD<-ill[stratum==3]
# sex = F, age1 = 1
td<-table(levelD,illD)
td
```

```
           illD
  levelD   0    1
       0   3    1
       1   1   13
```

```
fisher.test(table(levelD,illD))
```

```
        Fisher's Exact Test for Count Data
data:   table(levelD, illD)
p-value = 0.01863
alternative hypothesis: true odds ratio is not equal to 1
95 percent confidence interval:
     1.151224 2142.795321
sample estimates:
odds ratio
  25.75948
```

```
mantelhaen.test(VanillaIceCream,ill,stratum)
```

```
Mantel-Haenszel chi-squared test with continuity correction
data:   VanillaIceCream and ill and stratum
Mantel-Haenszel X-squared = 23.3354, df = 1, p-value = 1.361e-06
alternative hypothesis: true common odds ratio is not equal to 1
95 percent confidence interval:
     6.469896 180.901486
sample estimates:
common odds ratio
          34.21131
```

```
#Homogeneity and trend test (trend test illustrated but not indicated)
# numbers in some cells are small
# homogeneity and trend test are large sample tests
# inspection suggests stratified data are homogeneous
lor<-0
vlor<-0
x<-0
ta1<-ta+.5 # add .5 if any zeros
or1<-ta1[1]*ta1[4]/(ta1[2]*ta1[3])
lor[1]<-log(or1)
vlor[1]<-sum(1/ta1)
x[1]<-1
tb1<-tb+.5 # add .5 if any zeros
or2<-tb1[1]*tb1[4]/(tb1[2]*tb1[3])
lor[2]<-log(or2)
vlor[2]<-sum(1/tb1)
x[2]<-2
tc1<-tc+.5 # add .5 if any zeros
or3<-tc1[1]*tc1[4]/(tc1[2]*tc1[3])
lor[3]<-log(or3)
```

```
vlor[3]<-sum(1/tc1)
x[3]<-3
td1<-td+.5 # add .5 if any zeros
or4<-td1[1]*td1[4]/(td1[2]*td1[3])
lor[4]<-log(or4)
vlor[4]<-sum(1/td1)
x[4]<-4


# homogeneity test
alor<-sum(lor/vlor)/sum(1/vlor)
ch<-sum((1/vlor)*(lor-alor)^2)
ch
# Homogeneity test (Woolf)
#[1] 0.1378704
1-pchisq(ch,3)
#[1] .99
#

# trend test (not indicated but calculations illustrated)
w<-1/vlor
a<-sum(w*x*lor);b<-sum(w*lor);d<-sum(x*w);e<-sum(w);f<-sum(w*x^2)
Lxy<-a-b*d/e
Lxx<-f-d^2/e
ch.sq<-Lxy^2/Lxx
ch.sq
#Homogeneity trend test is illustrated although not applicable
#as stratification variable comprised of sex and agegroup
#trend not expected, trend test for illustration (Rosner)
#[1] 0.0009521514
1-pchisq(ch.sq,1)
#[1] 0.9753836
```

Finally, it is of interest to perform a stratified analysis involving sex, vanilla ice cream and illness. When the stratification is by sex, the vanilla ice cream effect is highly significant. When stratification is by the vanilla ice cream, the sex effect is not significant although the odds ratio CI does not include one. Also, the Woolf common odds ratio is calculated for vanilla ice cream with sex as the stratifying agent and a homogeneity test is performed that is not significant.

```
# vanilla ice cream effect with sex as stratifying agent
table(VanillaIceCream,ill,sex)
```

```
, , sex = F
                  ill
VanillaIceCream    0    1
              0   10    3
              1    4   27
, , sex = M
                  ill
VanillaIceCream    0    1
              0    8    0
              1    7   16
```

```
mantelhaen.test(table(VanillaIceCream,ill,sex))
```

```
          Mantel-Haenszel chi-squared test with continuity correction
data:   table(VanillaIceCream, ill, sex)
Mantel-Haenszel X-squared = 25.2769, df = 1, p-value = 4.966e-07
alternative hypothesis: true common odds ratio is not equal to 1
95 percent confidence interval:
   7.191633 197.000244
sample estimates:
common odds ratio
        37.63978
```

```
# sex effect with vanilla ice cream as stratifying agent
table(sex,ill,VanillaIceCream)
```

```
, , VanillaIceCream = 0
     ill
sex    0         1
F     10         3
M      8         0
, , VanillaIceCream = 1
     ill
sex    0         1
F      4        27
M      7        16
```

```
mantelhaen.test(table(sex,ill,VanillaIceCream))
```

```
          Mantel-Haenszel chi-squared test with continuity correction
data:   table(sex, ill, VanillaIceCream)
Mantel-Haenszel X-squared = 3.1033, df = 1, p-value = 0.07813
alternative hypothesis: true common odds ratio is not equal to 1
95 percent confidence interval:
 0.06792297 0.95936770
sample estimates:
common odds ratio
        0.2552707
```

```
# vanilla ice cream effect with sex as stratifying agent
# Woolf common odds ratio and homogeneity test
stratum<-c(rep(1,44),rep(2,31)) # Female/Male
exposure<-c(rep(1,31),rep(0,13),rep(1,23),rep(0,8)) # Vanilla ice cream
outcome<-c(rep(1,27),rep(0,4),rep(1,3),rep(0,10),rep(1,16),rep(0,7),rep(0,8))
# Ill
exp1<-exposure[stratum==1];outc1<-outcome[stratum==1]
exp2<-exposure[stratum==2];outc2<-outcome[stratum==2]
ta<-table(exp1,outc1)
tb<-table(exp2,outc2)
#Woolf stratified odds ratio plus homogeneity and trend tests
lor<-0
vlor<-0
x<-0
ta1<-ta+.5 # add .5 for zeros
or1<-ta1[1]*ta1[4]/(ta1[2]*ta1[3])
lor[1]<-log(or1)
```

```
vlor[1]<-sum(1/ta1)
x[1]<--1
tb1<-tb+.5 # add .5 for zeros
or2<-tb1[1]*tb1[4]/(tb1[2]*tb1[3])
lor[2]<-log(or2)
vlor[2]<-sum(1/tb1)
x[2]<--2
#
alor<-sum(lor/vlor)/sum(1/vlor)
valor<-1/sum(1/vlor)
OR<-exp(alor)
L95<-exp(alor-1.96*valor^.5)
U95<-exp(alor+1.96*valor^.5)
Z.score<-alor/valor^.5
P.value<-2*(1-pnorm(Z.score))
cat("Woolf OR=",round(OR,2),"\nL95=",round(L95,2),"\nU95=",round(U95,2),
"\nZ-score=",round(Z.score,2),"\nP-value=",round(P.value,5),"\n",sep="")
```

```
Woolf OR=21.4
L95=5.34
U95=85.67
Z-score=4.33
P-value=2e-05
```

```
ch<-sum((1/vlor)*(lor-alor)^2)
ch # Homogeneity test (Woolf)
#[1] 0.1722385
1-pchisq(ch,2) # P-value
#[1] 0.9174848


# sex effect with vanilla ice cream as stratifying agent
# Woolf common odds ratio and homogeneity test
stratum<-c(rep(1,21),rep(2,54)) # noice/ice
exposure<-c(rep(1,8),rep(0,13),rep(1,23),rep(0,31)) # male/female
outcome<-c(rep(0,8),rep(1,3),rep(0,10),rep(1,16),rep(0,7),rep(1,27),rep(0,4))
# Ill
exp1<-exposure[stratum==1];outc1<-outcome[stratum==1]
exp2<-exposure[stratum==2];outc2<-outcome[stratum==2]
ta<-table(exp1,outc1)
tb<-table(exp2,outc2)
#Woolf stratified odds ratio plus homogeneity and trend tests
lor<-0
vlor<-0
ta1<-ta+.5 # add .5 for zeros
or1<-ta1[1]*ta1[4]/(ta1[2]*ta1[3])
lor[1]<-log(or1)
vlor[1]<-sum(1/ta1)
tb1<-tb+.5 # add .5 for zeros
or2<-tb1[1]*tb1[4]/(tb1[2]*tb1[3])
lor[2]<-log(or2)
vlor[2]<-sum(1/tb1)
#
alor<-sum(lor/vlor)/sum(1/vlor)
valor<-1/sum(1/vlor)
OR<-exp(alor)
L95<-exp(alor-1.96*valor^.5)
```

```
U95<-exp(alor+1.96*valor^.5)
Z.score<-alor/valor^.5
P.value<-2*pnorm(Z.score)
#[1] 0.06767543
cat("Woolf OR=",round(OR,2),"\nL95=",round(L95,2),"\nU95=",round(U95,2),
"\nZ-score=",round(Z.score,2),"\nP-value=",round(P.value,5),"\n",sep="")
```

```
Woolf OR=0.32
L95=0.1
U95=1.09
Z-score=-1.83
P-value=0.06768
```

```
ch<-sum((1/vlor)*(lor-alor)^2)
ch # Homogeneity test (Woolf)
#[1] 0.1722385
1-pchisq(ch,1) # P-value
#[1] 0.67813
```

```
detach(oswego)
```

8

Hospital safety and adverse event prevention

8.1 Introduction

Although these notes are primarily about the use of statistical methods in R for the analysis of hospital infection and other adverse event surveillance data, the role of evidence-based practices and their implementation is of major importance. This supplementary chapter provides a summary of these important aspects of adverse event (AE) prevention and hospital safety (Morton[B] and colleagues, Lilford and colleagues, Vincent).

The importance of AEs in hospitals is illustrated by Ehsani and colleagues who reported that in 2003–04 in Victoria, Australia, AEs occurred in just under 7% of admissions, the patients stayed on average 10 days longer, had 7 times the mortality and cost nearly $7000 more to treat than those who did not have an AE. AEs were responsible for over 18% of total inpatient hospital budgets. It is probable that at least one third were potentially preventable.

It is an issue of concern that safety progress appears to be very slow (Landrigan and colleagues). Top-down approaches that emphasise indicators, comparisons and benchmarking dominate much QI activity. We argue that bottom-up approaches that emphasise prevention and the implementation of evidence-based systems, increasingly called bundles and checklists, together with sequential within-institution AE monitoring, are superior (Morton[C] and colleagues). While the latter approach promotes an environment that is conducive to learning from outcomes, it is important to ensure the maintenance of responsibility, accountability and discipline (Wachter and Pronovost). For example, there must be a suitable disciplinary system for dealing with staff who persistently fail to comply with well-documented evidence-based activities such as hand hygiene.

Statistical Methods for Hospital Monitoring with R, First Edition. Anthony Morton, Kerrie Mengersen, Michael Whitby and George Playford.
© 2013 John Wiley & Sons, Ltd. Published 2013 by John Wiley & Sons, Ltd.

8.2 An overview of hospital quality improvement, five pillars

It is useful to think of infection management (IM) and quality improvement (QI) in terms of the major influences that are involved. The five pillars of QI are:

```
1. The Customer,
2. The Practitioner,
3. The EVIDENCE-BASED System,
4. Change management
5. The Feedback loop.
```

8.2.1 The Customer, the first pillar

The main customer is of course the patient. However, we are all each other's customer as we request and provide services. This requires knowledge of customer needs, it demands trust that is crucially dependent on transparency, fairness and justice. Accountability and good communication are needed. The key is to treat other people as we should be treated by them.

8.2.2 The Practitioner, the second pillar

Staff need to display technical skill, judgement, knowledge and empathy, and systems are required that ensure that staff possess these characteristics. For example, regular mortality and morbidity (M&M) meetings as described by Singer are part of the fabric of good surgical units. They need to be mandatory and transparent and should be carefully documented with good feedback. Mechanisms for independent audit are necessary when possible unsatisfactory patterns exist. As described by Foot, technical skill, judgement and knowledge can be tested and improved by the use of simulators that are becoming available especially in surgery, critical care and anaesthesia.

Except in special cases (e.g. a patient with a bleeding abdominal aortic aneurysm who cannot be evacuated in time to a centre with specialists in vascular surgery), hospitals should not carry out only small numbers of complex procedures. Training and supervision of trainee staff are important. Overcrowding and staff shortages should be avoided, and support services should be adequate.

8.2.3 The System, the third and main pillar

This is the chief pillar. The hospital is a complex dynamic system and outcomes are overwhelmingly determined by system characteristics. Systems must be founded on the implementation of currently available yet continuously improving evidence, increasingly presented as bundles and checklists (also see the note on complex systems and networks in section 8.16).

8.2.3.1 Manifestations of poor systems

These include malpractice and criminal activity, substandard performance and medical error.

8.2.3.2 Malpractice and criminal activity

A good example is the late murderer, Dr Shipman. It has been suggested that statistically based surveillance could prevent such malpractice. While it is indeed important to have an effective surveillance process in place, there are several concerns with developing such a process to identify malpractice and criminal activity. If a sensitive analysis is used for early warning there would be frequent false positive signals that could require a huge costly bureaucracy to perform investigations and this could cause substantial damage to morale and practitioner-patient relationships. Alternatively, if a highly specific analysis is used to avoid false positive signals there could be long delays so genuine anomalies would not be detected in a timely manner, if at all. Furthermore, those who deliberately indulge in criminal behaviour would understand and act to defeat surveillance mechanisms, about which information is frequently available, for example, via the internet. With these data, it will usually not be possible to have both high sensitivity and high specificity as sample size cannot be controlled. In the case of Shipman it was noted that the system of death certification was unsatisfactory; therefore emphasis should be on the development of a better evidence-based system of death certification.

8.2.3.3 Substandard performance

In the case of the Bristol paediatric cardiac surgery failure there was whistle blower harassment, no evidence-based system and an inadequate safety focus. Surgical staff had inadequate training and paediatric experience. There may have been insufficient volume of work to maintain skills. Support facilities, for example preoperative workup and preparation, and postoperative care may have been suboptimal. Excellent alternative facilities would have been available; for example at that time similar patients in Perth, Western Australia, were flown to Melbourne, a substantial distance, with good results. More recently in Australia, events at the Bundaberg hospital as described by Dunbar and colleagues illustrate a not unfamiliar pattern of failure of a complex system. Dealing with substandard performance requires leadership plus management with skills to understand evidence and analyse complex systems. Management must have the resources and authority to correct system problems and prevent unsafe systems from causing patient injury. This requires understanding of systems, good leadership and management, not comparisons, benchmarking, targets, star ratings or league tables. Application of the tools for complex system analysis such as agent-based modelling and pattern (system) dynamics would improve our understanding of systems (Australian Academy of Science and CSIRO) as should the continuing development of clinical quality registries (Evans and colleagues).

8.3 Medical error

A good example is the fatal error of intrathecal administration of vincristine. 'Fail-safe' protocols have been developed. Yet the terrible error of accidental intrathecal administration of an unintended drug continues to occur. We are all prone to error, protocols can fail and, if syringes for intravenous use can be connected to spinal needles, this or a similar accident can and will recur.

8.3.1 Background of medical error (Vincent, Taylor-Adams & Vincent)

Causes include:

1. Limitations of the human nervous system.

2. Error-prone systems.

3. Low volumes of complex procedures.

4. Fatigue and sleep deprivation.

5. Distraction and complexity; having to deal with multiple problems simultaneously.

6. Communication breakdown.

7. Inadequate training and insufficient supervision.

8. Lack of physical barriers such as syringes with retractable needles.

9. Poor management, loss of trust and low staff morale resulting in violations.

10. Failure to understand self-organisation and emergent behaviour in complex systems.

8.4   Improving the system

First the system must be analysed and if necessary upgraded with emphasis on evidence-based practice. Improvement must be built into systems; it cannot be inspected in afterwards. This is why old style quality assurance often fails. Systems must be functioning in a stable, predictable way before progressive improvement is possible. Organisations, for example sporting teams or orchestras, must function predictably before they can become great. It is the same with hospitals. Finding and implementing indicators and setting targets without first attending to the relevant system does not improve quality – people just look for ways to have good indicator figures, frequently called gaming. This can damage morale and customer relationships, produce extra unproductive work with diversion from the real work of improving systems, and encourage waste. For example, when a department must meet a target, staff may be diverted from other areas and some important work may be deferred or cancelled; thus there is no quality improvement.

Conventional statistical process control (SPC) analysis of data when systems have not first been brought into control so that they can perform in a predictable way can be meaningless. A simple run chart, tabulation or chart based on a generalised additive model (GAM or spline chart) may be more useful when data display unpredictable variability and trends. Generic defences that enhance sustainability and resilience against unforeseen or unexpected AEs are important (see section 8.16 on complex systems and networks).

8.4.1   Evidence-based systems

Systems must begin to include just and transparent mechanisms to evaluate fitness to practice and to remedy deficiencies that might be revealed by this mechanism. As described in section 8.2.2, it is probable that technical skill, judgement and knowledge can be tested and improved by the use of simulators.

8.4.2   The role of bundles and checklists

It has recently become fashionable to package evidence-based systems as bundles and these now exist for a wide variety of processes. This is a welcome change as it takes emphasis away from judgemental centralised surveillance activities and places it on the systems that are responsible for outcomes. However, attention must be paid to their implementation.

Employing evidence-based bundles frequently requires behaviour change and achieving this can be difficult. Hospitals will often need a great deal of help to implement change; just telling someone to change or 'educating' them to do so seldom works. As described by Kotter, successful implementation of needed change requires continuing coordination, strong leadership, good teamwork and persistence. Using a checklist as described by Gawande in 'The Checklist Manifesto' is frequently valuable. As Evans and colleagues describe, development of epidemiologically sound and clinically relevant clinical-quality registries may aid in keeping evidence up to date. Discipline is also important: there must exist just and effective disciplinary procedures to deal with individuals who persistently flout essential evidence-based change.

An evidence-based bundle to minimise transmission of a multiple antibiotic resistant organism (MRO) would include the following:

```
1. Good hand hygiene practice,
2. Processes for screening and the detection of carriers,
3. Facilities for the isolation of carriers,
4. A clean environment, with special attention to high-touch surfaces and
   terminal cleaning.
5. Sufficient trained staff and beds to avoid overcrowding and to optimise
   patient cohorting,
6. An understanding of the role of networks in transmission,
7. Discipline in the use of antibiotics.
```

Several of these components such as the avoidance of overcrowding and provision of adequate isolation facilities and staffing are dependent on senior management decisions. When there are insufficient trained staff and beds, cohorting may become sub-optimal, hand hygiene practice may deteriorate and there may be insufficient time for thorough cleaning. As staff care for a wider range of patients and must visit patients in outlier wards, networks that potentially enhance transmission increase in size and connectedness. Staff morale is adversely affected.

Implementing bundles, for example to minimise surgical site infections (SSIs), ventilator-related pneumonia, intravenous device related bacteraemia or MRO transmission, is a complex process. It requires a deep understanding of the industrial psychology of change management, for example, as described by Kotter and Rathgerber in 'Our Iceberg is Melting', and determined ongoing coordination if it is to be sustained effectively and become a habit. IM staff in hospitals that have instituted recent advances in cleaning such as the use of bleach and black light technology would be well aware of the difficulties involved. Moreover, an evidence base needs to be established (Dancer).

There are now available excellent evidence based 'bundles' for preventing hospital-acquired infections published by the UK NHS Clean-Safe-Care program http://www.clean-safe-care.nhs.uk/index.php?pid=4, www.dh.gov.uk/en/Publicationsandstatistics/Publications/PublicationsPolicyAndGuidance/DH_078134), Health Protection Scotland (www.hps.scot.nhs.uk/haiic/ic/bundles.aspx) and The Institute of Healthcare Improvement's (www.ihi.org/) 'The Improvement Map'. Other examples include early warning score (Mitchell, Royal College of Physicians), falls prevention (Barker and colleagues) and pressure ulcer prevention systems (IHI Improvement Map[B]).

Ghaferi and colleagues have shown that hospitals with high surgical mortality may have similar complication rates to low mortality hospitals, the difference being related to the standard of postoperative care. The inexperienced junior medical officer seeing a patient with early bacteraemia in the middle of the night may underestimate severity and provide inadequate care resulting in the patient's collapse some hours later. Adherence to an evidence-based bundle, including for example, a track, trigger and response (TTR) system together with ready availability of experienced staff to whom the inexperienced person is required as part of the bundle to turn, is necessary for safe care (see Early Warning and Rapid Response in the IHI Improvement Map, the paper by Mitchell and others and most recently the Royal College of Physicians National Early Warning Score).

8.5 Error-proofing systems

This involves the re-design of systems for safety (Vincent, Batalden and Stoltz, Berwick). This can include:

```
1. Simplification,
2. Standardisation,
3. Automation,
4. Computerisation,
5. Training, including the use of simulators,
6. Behaviour change (for example hand hygiene and implementation of
   recent environmental cleaning evidence, e.g. about high-touch surfaces),
7. Physical barriers — engineering solutions that physically prevent
   errors occurring or causing harm, for example syringes with retractable
   needles,
8. Documentation of errors and near misses with use of data to further
   error-proof systems,
9. Generic defences that increase sustainability and resilience.
```

Harford describes accidents in tightly interconnected complex systems that can result in cascading failures. Orrell notes the need for redundancy, modularity, diversity and capacity for controlled shut down for resilience and sustainability in economic systems. Building some redundancy into hospital systems is required to prevent access block and other problems due to overcrowding such as premature discharge of patients.

When documenting AEs, there must be analysis, feedback and change; just documenting errors achieves little. We must learn from our data. It is important to recognise the influence of Tort Law where people are reluctant to report problems if they fear legal consequences; including suitably trained lawyers on hospital safety teams can be valuable. Trust and justice are vital for successful error reporting to occur – a judgemental or 'shoot the messenger' attitude will destroy trust and it will not be regained easily, if at all.

8.6 Discipline and accountability

A 'no blame' attitude has emerged as a counter to one that has, in the past, often been seen to be excessively judgemental. The latter may penalise staff for system problems over which they have little or no control. This is unjust; it results in lack of trust, the hiding of errors, and a failure to learn from them. Wachter and Pronovost observe that the 'no blame' culture may have gone too far. It is important to understand that discipline and accountability are essential components of a sustainable and resilient complex system. Staff (often senior) who fail to wash their hands when they know they should, leave central lines in longer than necessary for convenience or prescribe antibiotics carelessly damage systems and destroy the morale of other staff just as much as does blaming people for things that they do not control. Those who are careful to employ evidence-based procedures can feel betrayed when others fail to do so. Accountability and discipline are thus essential parts of a sustainable and resilient complex system. Perhaps we should abandon the 'no blame' versus accountability controversy and concentrate on the attributes of complex systems that result in safe self-organisation and emergent behaviour. Justice, trust and morale as well as safety are damaged when staff persist in behaviours that flaunt well-established evidence and thus disciplinary action is a necessary part of a safe complex system. Justice, trust and safety require both learning and discipline.

8.7   Limitations of imposing quality

According to Deming in 'Out of the Crisis', targets reward those who know how to use a system, not those who strive to improve it. Targets shift blame for failure to those who must meet the targets when those who set the targets have the most control over the system. Targets can discourage optimum use of data, for example their use to prove compliance with the target instead of to further improve the system. Pitches and colleagues show how they can also encourage gaming and diversion of resources from other problem areas. Targets may be incompatible with the self-organisation and emergent behaviour of safe complex systems.

Much effort has in the past and in some places still is directed at imposing quality by central authorities rather than their concentrating on helping hospital staff analyse their systems and, using currently available yet evolving best evidence, improving those systems; and seeing that they do so.

Benchmarks and league tables can encourage unhelpful comparisons of hospitals that differ in the services they provide and the populations they serve. Star ratings can reward those that appear superior when differences are dominated by predictable, often random, variation and the phenomenon of regression to the mean. Systems of reward and bonus payments can be motivated by political objectives and ideologies, and not the quality of patient care.

8.8   Performance and predictable variation

Rewards and punishments based on targets and league tables frequently reward seemingly good results that are in fact due to predictable variation and just as frequently dispense punishment such as withholding a bonus payment on outcomes that are also dominated by predictable variation, or already inadequate resources. There is the phenomenon of regression to the mean where this year's league table poor performers may be there because of predictable variation; next year they may be rated as good performers without any real change in performance. Arbitrary systems of reward and punishment damage morale, encourage tampering with sound systems and increase the probability of error.

8.9   The keys to a good system

These include (Berwick, Vincent):

```
1. Leadership,
2. Teamwork,
3. Good communication,
4. Transparency, justice and trust,
5. Mechanisms for systems analysis and implementation,
6. Understanding, modifying and changing staff behavior.
```

There must be documentation of evidence (e.g. in bundles reinforced with checklists) and evidence needs to be updated as new work appears, for example, increases in the prevalence of vancomycin-resistant *Enterococcus* (VRE) have focused attention on methods of terminal cleaning of potentially contaminated high touch patient areas. The institution of ongoing Bayesian Networks (Waterhouse and colleagues) may be a valuable adjunct to the process of updating evidence as may the development of epidemiologically sound and clinically relevant clinical-quality registries (Evans and colleagues). Managing change, as described by Kotter, is vital (e.g. improving handwashing between patient contacts and changing lifetime habits of hand hygiene).

Leadership requires involvement, competence, vigour and commitment – one cannot lead by remote control. Like good coaches, leaders do not tolerate those who lack commitment or essential skills, yet good leaders go to great lengths to provide an environment for people to develop and realise their potential. They foster innovation and organisational learning and this facilitates change. Leaders represent their team to management. Leaders understand the basics of economics; this is needed to present plans to enhance safety to management. Leaders understand the roles of learning and discipline based on trust and justice.

Teamwork promotes communication; it requires trust, fairness and justice; it fosters innovation and it encourages organisational learning and collaborative effort. Potentially destructive competition is thus discouraged. It is important to recognise the value of ownership. In most cases, collaborative bottom-up approaches to quality and safety work better than judgemental top-down ones.

The managerialist management philosophy introduced in the 1980s concentrates on individual performance and short term targets; this can cause serious problems when teamwork is vital. In hierarchies, people's responsibility to improve their systems can be lost, for example if a promising project is taken over in the pursuit of ambition and power. Moreover, those who look harder can find more problems and can appear worse than those who do not look – management may not want to know about some of the problems that are unearthed.

8.10   Analysing and implementing evidence-based systems

Multidisciplinary cross-functional teams are important in understanding and implementing evidence, understanding systems and seeking basic causes of problems. Teams can become good at gathering and understanding data and using tools for quality improvement such as brainstorming, flow charts, fishbone diagrams and Pareto charts as described in Brassard and Ritter's 'The Memory Jogger'. Teams are not committees.

Multidisciplinary teams may need to include statisticians and mathematicians who may provide the following:

1. Statistical analysis for events with a random component such as hospital infections.

2. Mathematical modelling, for example, with agent-based models (Galea and colleagues), to help identify important system and process factors such as the relationship of hand hygiene, environmental cleaning, hospital networks and the spread of hospital organisms.

3. Updating evidence, for example using Bayesian networks.

4. Operational Research can help to optimise systems.

Industrial psychologists are necessary for systems analysis, behaviour analysis and modification, for example breaking down barriers to implementation of evidence-based systems. Examples include hand hygiene between patient contacts to minimise MRSA and VRE transmission, safe care of intravenous devices and the disciplined use of antibiotics.

Economists can specify the best use of limited resources. They are also invaluable in providing a balanced approach to understanding the costs and benefits of various approaches.

Engineers can design beds to reduce pressure ulcers and physically error-proof systems, for example by making syringes with retractable needles to prevent needlestick injuries.

Lawyers are important in understanding how to deal with Tort Law and to break down the communication barriers it raises.

Information science has the crucial role of making available information and knowledge for building sustainable systems. There is a great need in some hospital systems for change from hospital information technology with its focus on hardware repair and software installation to information science with its focus on information and knowledge.

8.11   The role of patient-care staff

With the assistance of central authorities, clinical staff should define and institute systems of patient care that are evidence-based. They should then monitor processes and outcomes sequentially using surveillance and audit, and sequential statistical analysis of AEs where appropriate, to detect unforeseen problems and to ensure systems are working in a satisfactory way.

8.12   The role of central authority

The central authority has an important role in assisting hospital staff to institute optimum evidence-based systems. It must then institute process and system monitoring, for example using audits, to ensure the evidence-based systems and their within-institution monitoring are sustained and any problems that are revealed by the latter are acted upon. Central authorities must learn to be like coaches. As already described, good coaches do not tolerate players who lack commitment or essential skills. However, they go to great length to create an environment in which talented people can reach their full potential.

8.13   Change management, the fourth pillar

Hand hygiene between patient contacts is a simple yet very effective way to reduce transmission of hospital-acquired pathogens, yet it is often practiced poorly in spite of considerable publicity. Changing the hand hygiene habits of a lifetime is a complex task requiring a deep knowledge of industrial psychology, excellent leadership, communication and teamwork and a great deal of patience and determination. All change to implement evidence-based systems requires similar approaches. Change management is described by Kotter.

8.14   Feedback loops, the fifth pillar

The Shewhart/Deming (Plan, Do, Check, Act) cycle is an excellent basis. First, analyse and optimise the system using available evidence (Plan). Second, implement the system, paying particular attention to helping staff make necessary behaviour changes (Do). Next, institute surveillance and monitoring of relevant process and outcome indicators (Check step 1). This can involve:

1. Incident reporting.

2. Occurrence screening for example, employing specially trained staff to review patients' files to seek evidence of AEs.

3. Surveillance for example, employing specially trained staff to prevent and to seek evidence of AEs, especially infections, using ward and theatre contacts and pathology and radiology reports.

4. Using automated trigger tool systems to detect evidence of the occurrence of AEs (e.g. the IHI Global Trigger Tool).

5. Outbreak investigation.

6. Audit for example, using mortality and morbidity (M&M) meetings and, when needed, independent audit.

7. Surveys of patient satisfaction.

8. Development of clinical-quality registries.

Data must undergo proper analysis (Check step 2). There must be methodical study of sentinel events, for example unexpected deaths and major injuries, by independent audit if necessary (as well as discipline, transparency and justice are essential). Statistical analysis of events with a random component, for example hospital infections, is required; this will frequently involve the use of control charts. However, SPC must be used with caution when systems have not or cannot be made predictable by instituting evidence-based bundles and checklists (how can we know what monthly MRSA prevalence should be?). When there is excessive variability or a trend, spurious precision can result from the uncritical use of conventional SPC. A simple run chart, tabulation or a GAM chart will be preferable when predictable data are unavailable. There should be audit of adherence to evidence-based systems, bundles and checklists.

Finally, there should be good feedback of analysis to clinical staff, management and patients. Frequently feedback of AE data such as SSI rates results in improvement and this has been described as a Hawthorne effect (Hawthorne effects are said to be changes that result from being part of an experiment but not the change imposed by the experiment). Feedback can result in a number of changes such as seemingly minor improvements in prophylactic antibiotic therapy and hand hygiene compliance. Cumulatively, improvement following these frequently numerous but often minor interacting changes can be seen as self organisational emergent behaviour in an improving complex system.

Vincent uses Reason's analogy with Swiss cheese. In a complex system such as a hospital, adverse events (AEs) often occur as a result of a number of undesirable agents becoming aligned as in the holes in a piece of this cheese lining up and forming a tunnel. Continuing this analogy, to prevent the AE by altering one of these agents could be difficult, just as moving one of the holes in the cheese to block off the tunnel would require a considerable amount of movement, whereas relatively small simultaneous changes in the alignment of a number of agents may do so. Thus, a surgical team that is a bit lax with preoperative antibiotics, wound closure and postoperative oxygenation and temperature regulation may, after seeing feedback results, provide better supervision of the resident's antibiotic administration, more supervision of the registrar's wound closure and take more interest in the recovery room. While none of these alone may make much difference, taken together these small interacting changes may result in improved self-organisation and emergent behaviour in a complex system and thus in less SSIs. However, if the surgical team already does these things carefully, as most do, little or no change in SSI rates might be expected. This may explain one of the anomalies of public reporting where evidence of resulting improvement is controversial (Fung and colleagues, Ryan and colleagues, Landrigan and colleagues). It is the complex system that is of paramount importance, not the public reporting or lack thereof.

Public reporting is increasingly being mandated. Although the role of public reporting in improving safety has been strongly advocated (Godlee) it is in fact controversial (Fung and colleagues, Ryan and colleagues). However, it applies a useful discipline to institutions. Thus, as transparency and accountability are necessary, public reporting deserves support. However, collecting, analysing and reporting data should also involve relating them to the underlying system and using them to facilitate any needed system changes.

8.15   Implementation of the Quality Improvement Process

This process requires leadership and it is unlikely to succeed in its absence.

8.15.1   Implementation

First, see where evidence is not being applied within your institution. This may be obvious or it may require study, for example, using the IHI Improvement Map. Examine evidence-based bundles and other evidence-based systems and seek areas of poor conformance within your institution.

Then, select an area for attention, for example surveillance may have indicated unsatisfactory outcomes, an audit may have suggested that a particular aspect of patient care is not conforming to evidence-based practice or it may have been demonstrated that there has been suboptimal use of resources.

Next, if one is not already available (e.g. surveillance staff in a hospital infection management or quality improvement service) select a team and, if necessary, appoint a facilitator. Begin studying the problem area. Search the literature for details of relevant evidence-based practices (there are now available excellent evidence-based bundles for preventing hospital-acquired infections published by the UK NHS Clean-Safe-Care programme, Health Protection Scotland and The Institute of Healthcare Improvement's The Improvement Map, see section 8.4.2). Obtain further data as required using surveillance and audit, but use statistical analysis carefully; the system may be out of control so that control limits in statistical process control (SPC) charts will be meaningless (for example, when more careful data collection occurs, more adverse events may be detected without any system change).

Use a rapid improvement team approach (Alemi and colleagues). Audit results, for example using Morbidity and Mortality (M&M) Meetings, are a valuable source of data. Search for system causes, for example using SPC tools like brainstorming. Get to know the problem areas intimately; cause and effect diagrams are SPC tools that can be helpful for this purpose. Become thoroughly familiar with the processes involved; a flow chart is another SPC tool that can aid in this process analysis (Brassard and Ritter). Be careful with root-cause analysis; the aim must be to understand the system. It is preferable to employ systems analysis as described by Taylor-Adams and Vincent. Increasingly, AEs may have no root cause; they may instead represent the emergent behaviour of an unsatisfactory complex system (section 8.16). Also, beware of the Pareto principle that most problems have a few major causes. Problems can arise in complex systems due to the interaction of many agents, each of which may appear alone to be insignificant.

Now prioritise causes and actions. Keeping the comments about complex systems in mind, a Pareto analysis may enable the team to select the key changes that may be needed from the many that may be suggested. However, it is important to heed the warning given above; a problem can arise due to the interaction of a number of seemingly insignificant agents. Teams in hospitals frequently do not seem to need to use Pareto analysis and other SPC tools formally; what is wrong and what needs to be done are often clear following a careful study of the system by staff already thoroughly familiar with the relevant clinical area. Use evidence-based bundles, care maps and, where needed, prepare checklists. Then make the necessary corrections, ensure that they are implemented and document the actions taken. It may be necessary to employ an industrial psychologist to facilitate behaviour change.

Next, conduct process and outcome surveillance or audit and analyse the data – employ Taylor-Adams and Vincent's systems analysis for processes and uncommon serious adverse events. Especially in surgical units, there should be regular mandatory morbidity and mortality (M&M) meetings that are documented and there should be evidence that any shortcomings are acted upon. Use SPC charts where a random component is important, for example with hospital-acquired infections, provided it has been possible to bring the system into a predictable state, or run charts, GAM charts and simple tabulations if there is unpredictable variation.

Finally use the data to learn how to improve. Employ, for example, the Shewhart/Deming (Plan, Do, Check, Act) feedback cycle. Act to sustain improvement and to ensure ongoing application of the evidence-based system. The positive results of feedback are often dismissively called Hawthorne effects. They are probably, in fact, often the result of many small improvements that individually may seem unimportant but that by interacting result in desirable self-organisation and emergent behaviour in a complex system.

Safe hospital systems are essential and both clinical staff and central authorities have important roles to play. The role of patient care staff is, with the assistance of the central authority, to define and institute systems of patient care that are evidence-based and to monitor processes and outcomes sequentially to ensure that those systems continue to work in a satisfactory way. Then, if there is an increase in the frequency of an AE, there must be evidence that causes have been sought and, if found, that corrective action has been taken. The role of central authority should be to assist hospital staff to institute evidence-based systems and to employ process and system audit to ensure that such systems and their sequential within-institution monitoring are sustained and acted upon. The approach should be bottom-up in nature; the central authority must be prepared to assume the role of a coach. Good coaches do not tolerate players who lack commitment or essential skills but they go to great lengths to create an environment in which talented people can reach their full potential. In the hospital environment, quality and safety are thereby enhanced.

Evidence-based systems must begin to include just and transparent mechanisms to evaluate fitness to practice and to remedy deficiencies that might be revealed by this mechanism. It is probable that technical skill, judgement and knowledge can be tested and improved by the use of simulators.

8.15.2   Obtaining data

Data may be obtained by a number of methods –

```
1. M&M meetings,
2. Audit, especially independent audit,
3. Surveillance,
4. Reviews of radiology, pathology, patient records and other relevant
   databases,
5. Outbreak investigation,
6. Incident reporting
7. Occurrence screening, trigger tools
8. Patient surveys.
9. Clinical quality registries.
```

8.15.3   Special issues with QI studies

All QI studies require accurate data for decision making. However, there is frequently neither the time nor the resources available for instituting formal research methods in QI studies; neither are they necessary to answer nearly all QI questions. It is one of the aims of medical research to obtain results that can be generalised; QI studies are often most relevant to the individual institution concerned. Unlike many research projects, surveillance and audit are usually continuous or recurrent activities.

Research frequently requires the collection of considerable quantities of data to include potentially important covariates and to attain required power and this can easily overload a surveillance programme so that some data go uncollected and the quality of those that are collected deteriorates. Formal research methods are frequently neither necessary nor feasible in QI work. Tackling QI as a research activity can easily result in failure.

When deciding which of two treatments is superior, it is very important to avoid false positive results and a formal research method is required; a new treatment that is expensive and potentially toxic should not be found superior unless it is definitely so. Samples of sufficient size to provide the study with adequate power are required.

When striving to improve hospital safety it can often be more important to avoid false negative states as an undetected problem may result in potentially avoidable patient injury. To learn and improve, greater sensitivity is required so that this is achieved. In addition, surveillance data sample sizes are usually fixed and frequently small so decisions may need to be made with limited available data; specificity may thus be lowered. Unlike with community public health data, it is usually not difficult for experienced clinicians or hospital epidemiologists to determine when an occasional abnormal result in a hospital is a false positive signal.

Nevertheless, the principles from formal research for avoiding bias are equally important in QI work. The ideas described by Berwick, Batalden, Nelson and others form the basis for data collection and measurement methods in Hospital Epidemiology.

Alemi and colleagues have described rapid data collection methods. The following are important –

1. Planning for rapid data collection.

2. Collecting only data items that are needed.

3. Sampling patients using small representative samples.

4. Where relevant, relying on numerical estimates made by process owners.

Berwick has described how making changes in the processes of care is necessary for improving daily medical practice. This can often be accomplished by conducting small scale local tests using the Shewhart/Deming Cycle to learn from taking action.

Nelson and colleagues have described eight principles for measurement in QI studies:

```
1. Seek usefulness, not perfection, in measurement,
2. Use a balanced set of process, outcome and cost measures,
3. Keep measurement simple,
4. Use qualitative and quantitative data,
5. Ensure the validity, reliability and predictive value of the measures,
6. Measure small, representative samples,
7. Build measurement into daily work,
8. Develop a measurement team.
```

There is frequently a strong emphasis on outcome data. While these data do need to be analysed and reported on, it is the system that produces them that should be of primary concern. The implementation of systems based on evidence should come first. Audit of systems and processes is often of more value than outcome data. Very often AEs are uncommon even when care is suboptimal and there can be considerable delay, when reliance is placed on statistical analysis, before significance is attained. An audit that reveals a potentially unsafe system may prevent those AEs. Preventing AEs is more important than counting them (Morton[C] and colleagues).

Berwick has emphasised the importance of using measurement to learn rather than to judge. When there is an excessively judgemental approach, managements and staff direct their energies to proving that they are satisfactory, instead of using data for learning and improvement. Useful data may be suppressed and gaming and costly shifting of responsibility may occur.

Complex and often only partially effective methods of risk adjustment are frequently employed when making judgements so that comparisons can be made fair; yet in spite of this risk-adjustment, satisfactory performance can still attract blame when differences are in fact due to predictable variation or other factors that are beyond the control of the relevant staff. In addition, when measurement is used to judge, high specificity is desirable so that the risk of false positive signals is minimised. However, this can result in false negative states and this is potentially dangerous as it is frequently the undetected problem that ultimately causes most difficulty and damage. Also, unlike with community public health monitoring, occasional false positive signals can usually be tolerated in a learning environment in a hospital as their detection is in most cases straightforward.

Sequential within-institution analysis of data following the establishment of evidence-based systems is preferable for detecting adverse changes to between-institution comparisons using aggregated data. The latter usually become available at intervals of some months, by which time the cause of a run of adverse events may be difficult to discover and unnecessary patient injury may have occurred. However, the public reporting of among-institution aggregated data has value in promoting transparency and discipline, and in encouraging accountability. Risk-adjustment is simpler when used with within-institution data as between-institution variability is avoided; often it is unnecessary with within-institution data. When an evidence-based system has been instituted, AEs tend to assume a predictable pattern usually at a low rate. If an apparent run of AEs then occurs, statistical analysis, for example in control charts, complements M&M audits in early detection. In addition, the control chart should help to avoid tampering with sound systems when the AEs are in fact occurring at a predictable rate.

It is important to decide what data to collect and to analyse. Increasingly collection of indicator data is mandated. However, it is more important to understand precisely what is happening within the relevant system than it is to automatically collect data. To achieve this objective, relevance is paramount. We should heed Montgomery's dictum: 'to know the system'. SSIs are a useful example. Short length of stay (LOS) means that many SSIs occur after discharge yet no practicable system exists for detecting superficial post-discharge SSIs reliably (Whitby and colleagues), many of which are in any case minor. Therefore post-discharge SSI data can be misleading both because of difficulty with ascertainment and variation in LOS. However, complex (deep or organ-space) SSIs can be identified readily as readmission is necessary and, although they represent only a subset of all SSIs, their monitoring can provide reliable information (Anderson and colleagues). In addition, they are clinically and economically of greatest importance. When studying bacteraemias, some blood cultures identify organisms that are of doubtful significance. It is better to concentrate on definite pathogens such as *Staphylococcus aureus* and definite pathogens associated with devices such as intravenous lines and urinary catheters. Although only a subset of all bacteraemias (definite, probable or possible), counts of definite bacteraemias, sometimes classified as criterion one bacteraemias, and changes in their occurrence rates can be relied upon to provide information that is of practical relevance. As Evans and colleagues describe, development of epidemiologically sound and clinically relevant clinical-quality registries may aid in deciding what needs to be measured.

8.16   The hospital as a network

Hospitals can be thought of as networks of complex dynamic systems. This has profound consequences for understanding hospital safety. Some outcomes, for example excessive LOS and severity of medication errors, can some times appear to have fractal (power law) distributions. Simple practical statistical analysis of these data is complicated (see Length of Stay in Chapter 7). Also in practical terms, being a complex system means that, while many AEs are preceded by potentially identifiable system problems, some can be unpredictable and of major importance. For example, these could range from the relatively minor need to close a ward temporarily due to a norovirus outbreak or one of a number of other minor AEs, through to more major problems. VRE is becoming much more prevalent. *Clostridium difficile* is potentially a major problem and the New Delhi metallo-beta-lactamase-1 (NDM-1) gene and enzyme may be a future major problem. There is widespread occurrence of the ESBL enzyme that confers antibiotic resistance due, in part, to the use of antibiotics in farming. The Hendra/Nipah viruses can unpredictably produce severe illness. A virulent virus may spring, seemingly from nowhere. There may be natural disasters like earthquakes, floods, industrial or transportation accidents or terrorist events. The next major AE may be due to something we do not know anything about at present.

When and where will the next of these strike? No-one knows. What will it be? This cannot be known. What is the probability of it occurring? This cannot be computed. How can it be defended against? We may be able to take specific steps to minimise the potential damage due, for example, to VRE but in general there is no way to prepare in specific terms for a presently unknown future event. We can only take general steps to make systems as sustainable and resilient as possible so that damage is minimised, for example, as we describe in Chapter 7, there are well-defined processes for the investigation and control of epidemics.

Hospitals are complex systems. Such systems exhibit self-organisation and emergent behaviour. We advise caution in the use of root-cause analysis to study AEs as they may represent the emergent behaviour of a defective complex system.

It is a characteristic of complex systems that, as they become more efficient, they simultaneously become more unstable and more vulnerable to failure. For years, efficiency and productivity have been the guiding principles of the economic management of hospitals. Yet we know that such emphasis results in increasing AEs such as those that arise when there is access block or when premature discharge becomes necessary. When patients are in outlying wards, staff must traverse extended networks and when they are moved between wards, continuity of care can suffer. It would be a useful exercise to find out how much of the work of a super-efficient hospital involves dealing with adverse events that result from that super-efficiency. As Eshani and colleagues have reported, AEs can account for up to 18% of some hospital inpatient budgets.

How can we defend against AEs that retrospective analysis has revealed are preceded by a characteristic trail of pre-existing anomalous performance? Pattern or system dynamics (Australian Academy of Science and CSIRO) is a generic process for understanding the processes that lead up to thresholds beyond which systems change. Its employment in research on hospital safety may aid in the prevention of potentially preventable AEs. Transmission of multiple antibiotic resistant organisms (MROs) in hospitals is of immense importance. Understanding the hospital as a network and using the characteristics of the network to minimise contact between carriers and susceptible patients and staff is vital to reducing MRO prevalence.

Complex systems display emergent behaviour and self-organisation. It is important to understand these processes. A complex system can be much more than a collection of its component parts. These behaviours can be modelled using complex simulations in a process known as agent-based modelling (Australian Academy of Science and CSIRO). Better understanding of the characteristics of hospital systems could aid in improving safety.

Since some AEs are unexpected and unpredictable, what are the defences against unknown future disasters? These must be generic and aimed at making systems more sustainable and resilient. Resilient systems can absorb disturbance without changing to a new and possibly dangerous state. Network science has some answers. As described by Orrell, they are modularity, diversity, redundancy and capacity for controlled shutdown. This means the following.

```
1. Modularity and diversity. Avoiding 'putting all our eggs in one basket',
2. Conducting research to understand and improve systems, especially the
   network of staff-patient contacts,
3. Avoiding things we know about such as poor hand hygiene, inadequate
   terminal cleaning of potentially contaminated and high-touch areas,
   leaving central lines in place for convenience and access block due to
   overcrowding,
4. Having as much backup facility as possible and being able to shut areas
   down when necessary.
```

As described by Taleb, some redundancy is of key importance. In advocating redundancy, we recognise that network science has learnt its value from nature. Therefore, a major need is to find the balance between efficiency and redundancy that is optimal for a hospital.

References

Adap, P., Rouse, A., Mohammed, M. and Marshall, T. (2002) 'Performance league tables: the NHS deserves better.' *British Medical Journal* 324:95–98.

Altman, D., Machin, D., Bryant, T. and Gardner, M. (2000) *Statistics with Confidence*, London: BMJ Books, 2nd ed. (A).

Altman, D. and Bland, M. (2011) 'How to obtain a P value from a confidence interval.' *British Medical Journal* 343:d2304. (B)

Alemi, F., Moore, S., Headrick, L., Neuhauser, D., Hekelman, F., and Kizys, N. (1998) 'Rapid Improvement Teams.' *Journal on Quality Improvement* 24:119.

American College of Cardiology Foundation/American Heart Association Task Force on Performance Measures (Writing Committee to Develop a Position Statement on Composite Measures) ACCF/AHA 2010 'Position Statement on Composite Measures for Healthcare Performance Assessment.' *Journal of the American College of Cardiology* 55:1755–1766.

Anderson, D., Chen, L., Sexton, D. and Kaye, K. (2008) 'Complex surgical site infections and the devilish details of risk adjustment: important implications for public reporting.' *Infection Control and Hospital Epidemiology* 29:941–946.

Armitage, P., Berry, G. and Matthews, J. (2002) *Statistical Methods in Medical Research*, Oxford: Blackwell Science, 4th ed.

Assareh, H. and Mengersen, K. (2012) 'Change point estimation in monitoring survival time' PLoS ONE 7:e33630.

Australian Academy of Science and CSIRO. www.science.org.au/nova/092/092key.htm, www.science.org.au/nova/094/094key.htm and www.csiro.au/science/CABM.html.

Barker, A., Kamar, J., Morton, A. and Berlowitz, D. (2009) 'From evidence to practice: review of an acute hospital inpatient falls program.' *Quality and Safety in Health Care* 18:467–472.

Batalden, P. B., Stoltz, P. K. (1993) 'A framework for the continual improvement of health care: building and applying professional and improvement knowledge to test changes in daily work.' *Joint Commission Journal on Quality Improvement* 19: 424–452.

Bartko, J. (1966) 'Approximating the negative binomial.' *Technometrics* 8:345–350.

Beiles, B. and Morton, A. (2004) 'Cumulative sum control charts for assessing performance in arterial surgery.' *Australian and New Zealand Journal of Surgery* 74:146–151.

Benneyan, J. (2001) 'Number between g-type statistical quality control charts for monitoring adverse events.' *Health Care Management Science* 4:305–318.

Berwick, D. (1998) 'Developing and testing changes in delivery of care.' *Annals of Internal Medicine* 128:651.

Bissell, A. (1970) 'Analysis of data based on incident counts.' *The Statistician* 19:215–247. (A)

Bissell, A. (1973) 'Monitoring event rates using varying element sample sizes.' *The Statistician* 22:43–58. (B)

Bland, J. and Altman, D. (1986) 'Statistical methods for assessing agreement between two methods of clinical measurement.' *Lancet* 50:1088–1101.

Brassard, M. and Ritter, D. (2010) *The Memory Jogger^{TM} 2*, 2nd ed. GOAL/QPC.

Breslow, N. and Day, N. (1980) *Statistical Methods in Cancer Research*, Volume 1, Lyon: IARC.

Campbell, M. and Swinscow, T. (2009) *Statistics at Square One*, London BMJ Books/Wiley-Blackwell 11th ed.

Champ, C. and Rigdon, S. (1997) 'An analysis of the run sum control chart.' *Journal of Quality Technology* 29:407.

Christiansen, C. and Morris, C. (1997) 'Improving the statistical approach to health care provider profiling.' *Annals of Internal Medicine* 127(8S) Supplement:764–768.

Clayton, D. and Hills, M. (1998) *Statistical Methods in Epidemiology*, Oxford: Oxford Science Publications.

Clements, A., Tong, E., Morton, A. and Whitby, M. (2007) 'Risk stratification of surgical site infections in Australia: evaluation of the US National Nosocomial Infection Surveillance risk-index.' *Journal of Hospital Infection* 66:148–155.

Cohen, G., Yang, S-Y (1994) 'Mid-P confidence intervals for the Poisson expectation.' *Statistics in Medicine* 13:2189–2203.

Collignon, P., Wilkinson, I., Gilbert, G., Grayson, L. and Whitby, M. (2006) 'Health care associated Staphylococcus aureus bloodstream infections: a clinical quality indicator for all hospitals.' *Medical Journal of Australia* 184:404–406.

Cook, D., Coory, M. and Webster, R. (2011) 'Exponentially weighted moving average charts to compare observed and expected values for monitoring risk-adjusted hospital indicators.' *BMJ Quality and Safety* 20:469–474. (A)

Cook, D., Duke, G., Hart, G., Pitcher, D. and Mullany, D. (2008) 'Review of the application of risk-adjusted charts to analyse mortality outcomes in critical care.' *Critical Care and Resuscitation* 10:239–251. (B)

Cook, D., Steiner, S., Cook, R., Farewell, V. and Morton, A. (2003) 'Monitoring the evolutionary process of quality: risk-adjusted charting to track outcomes in intensive care.' *Critical Care Medicine* 31:1676–1682. (C)

Cook, D. (2000) 'Performance of APACHE III models in an Australian ICU.' *Chest* 118:1732–1738. (D)

Cook, R. and Rasmussen, J. (2005) 'Going solid: a model of system dynamics and consequences for patient safety.' *Quality and Safety in Health Care* 14:130–134.

Crawley, M. (2003) *Statistical Computing*, Chichester, John Wiley and Sons.

Crawley, M. (2005) *Statistics An Introduction using R, Chichester*, John Wiley and Sons.

Crawley, M. (2007) *The R Book*, Chichester, John Wiley and Sons.

Dalgaard, P. (2008) *Introductory Statistics with R*, New York, Springer, 2nd ed.

Dancer, S. (2011) 'Hospital cleaning in the 21st century.' *European Journal of Clinical Microbiology and Infectious Diseases* 30:1473–1481.

De Maria, R., Mazzoni, M., Parolini, M., Gregori, D., Bortone, F., Arena, V. and Parodi, O. (2005) 'Predictive value of EuroSCORE on long term outcome in cardiac surgery patients: a single institution study.' *Heart* 91:779–784.

Deming, W. (1982) *Out of the Crisis*, Cambridge University Press.

derSimonian, R. www.niaid.nih.gov/about/organization/dcr/BRB/staff/Pages/rebecca.aspx. (A)

derSimonian, R. and Kacker, R. (2007) 'Random-effects model for meta-analysis of clinical trials: An update.' *Contemporary Clinical Trials* 28:105–114. (B)

Dunbar, J., Reddy, P. and May, S. (2011) *Deadly Healthcare*, Bowen Hills: Australian Academic Press.

Ehsani, J., Jackson, T. and Duckett, S. (2006) 'The incidence and cost of adverse events in Victorian hospitals 2003–04.' *Medical Journal of Australia* 184:551–555.

Evans, S., Scott, I., Johnson, N., Cameron, P. and McNeil, J. (2011) 'Development of clinical-quality registries in Australia: the way forward.' *Medical Journal of Australia* 194:360–363.

Everitt, B. (2003) *Modern Medical Statistics*, London, Arnold, Chapter 4.

Everitt, B. and Hothorn, T. (2010) *A Handbook of Statistical Analyses Using R*, Boca Raton, CRC Press, 2nd Ed.

Faris, P., Ghali, W. and Brant, R. (2003) 'Bias in estimates of confidence intervals for health outcome report cards.' *Journal of Clinical Epidemiology* 56:553–558.

Farsky, P., Graner, H., Duccini, P., Zandonadi, E., Anger, J., Sanches, A., Abboud, C. (2011) 'Risk factors for sternal wound infections and application of the STS score in coronary artery bypass graft surgery.' *Brazilian Journal of Cardiovascular Surgery* 26(4):624–629.

Fleiss, J. (1981) *Statistical Methods for Rates and Proportions*, New York: John Wiley and Sons 2nd ed.

Foot, C. (2007) Australian Anaesthesia; www.anzca.edu.au/resources/college-publications/pdfs/books-and-publications/Australasian%20Anaesthesia/australasian-anaesthesia-2007/Foot.pdf

Fung, C., Lim, Y., Mattke, S., Damberg, C. and Shekelle, P. (2008) 'Systematic review: the evidence that publishing patient care performance data improves quality of care.' *Annals of Internal Medicine* 148:111–123.

Galea, S., Riddle, M. and Kaplan, G. (2010) 'Causal thinking and complex system approaches in epidemiology.' *International Journal of Epidemiology* 39:97–106.

Gan, F. and Tan, T. (2010) 'Risk-adjusted number-between failures charting procedures for monitoring a patient care process for acute myocardial infarctions.' *Health Care Management Science* 13:222–233.

Gawande, A. (2010) *The Checklist Manifesto*, London: Profile Books.

Gebhardt, F. (1969) 'Some numerical comparisons of several approximations to the binomial distribution.' *Journal of the American Statistical Association* 64:1638–1646.

Gelman, A. and Hill, J. (2007) *Data Analysis Using Regression and Multilevel/Hierarchical Models*, Cambridge University Press.

Ghaferi, A., Birkmeyer, J. and Dimick, J. (2009) 'Variation in hospital mortality associated with inpatient surgery.' *New England Journal of Medicine* 361:1368–1375.

Giesecke, J. (2002) *Modern infectious disease epidemiology*, London, Arnold, 2nd ed.

Goodman, S. (1999) 'Toward evidence-based medical statistics 2: the Bayes Factor.' *Annals of Internal Medicine* 130:1005–1013.

Graham, P., Mengersen, K. and Morton, A. (2003) 'Confidence limits for the ratio of two rates based on likelihood scores: non-iterative method.' *Statistics in Medicine* 22:2085.

Grant, J. (1991) 'The fetal heart rate is normal, isn't it? Observer agreement of categorical assessments.' *The Lancet* 337:215–218.

Graves, N., Halton, K., Paterson, D., Whitby, M. (2009) 'Economic rationale for infection control in Australian hospitals.' *Healthcare Infection* 14:81–88.

Graves, N., Harbarth, S., Beyersmann, J., Barnett, A., Halton, K. and Cooper, B. (2010) 'Estimating the cost of health care-associated infections: Mind your p's and q's.' *Clinical Infectious Diseases* 50:1017–1021.

Gross, M. (1976) 'Oswego County revisited.' *Public Health Reports* 91:160–170.

Grunkemeier, G., Jin, R. and Wu, Y. (2009) 'Cumulative sum curves and their prediction limits.' *Annals of Thoracic Surgery* 87:361–364.

Harford, T. (2011) *Adapt*, London: Little Brown.

Hart, M., Lee, K., Hart, R. and Robertson, J. (2003) 'Application of attribute control charts to risk-adjusted data for monitoring and improving health care performance.' *Quality Management in Health Care* 12:5–19. (A)

Hart, M., Robertson, J., Hart, R. and Lee, K. (2004) 'Application of variables control charts to risk-adjusted time-ordered healthcare data.' *Quality Management in Health Care* 13:99–119. (B)

Hart, M., Robertson, J., Hart, R. and Schmaltz, S. (2006) 'Z and S charts for health care comparisons.' *Quality Management in Health Care* 15:2–14. (C)

Horan, T., Gaynes, R., Martone, W., Jarvis, W., Emori, T. (1992) 'CDC definitions of nosocomial surgical site infections, 1992: a modification of CDC definitions of surgical wound infections.' *Infection Control and Hospital Epidemiology* 13:606–608.

Institute for Healthcare Improvement 'IHI Global Trigger Tool Guide'. www.IHI.org. (A)

Institute for Healthcare Improvement 'IHI Improvement Map'. www.IHI.org. (B)

Johnson, N. (2007) *Simply Complexity*, Oxford: Oneworld.

Jones, H., Ohlssen, D. and Spiegelhalter, D. (2008) 'Use of false discovery rate when comparing multiple health care providers.' *Journal of Clinical Epidemiology* 61:232–240.

Jones, M. and Steiner, S. 'Assessing the effect of estimation error on risk-adjusted CUSUM chart performance.' *International Journal of Quality in Health Care* 24:176–181.

Kirkwood, B. and Sterne, J. (2003) *Essential Medical Statistics*, 2nd ed. Oxford: Blackwell Science.

Koetsier, A., de Keizer, N., de Jonge, E., Cook, D. and Peek, N. (2012) 'Performance of risk-adjusted control charts to monitor in-hospital mortality of intensive care unit patients: A simulation study.' *Critical Care Medicine* 40:1799–1807.

Kotter, J. (1996) *Leading Change*, Boston: Harvard Business Review Press.

Kotter, J. and Rathgerber, H. (2006) *Our Iceberg is Melting*, London: Macmillan.

Kulkami, P., Tripathi, R. and Michalek, J. (1998) 'Maximum (Max) and mid-P confidence intervals and p values for the standardized mortality and incidence ratios.' *American Journal of Epidemiology* 147:83–86.

Kunadian, B., Dunning, J., Roberts, A., Morley, R., Twomey, D., Hall, J., Sutton, A., Wright, R., Muir, D., de Belder, M. (2008) 'Cumulative funnel plots for the early detection of interoperator variation: retrospective database analysis of observed versus predicted results of percutaneous coronary intervention.' *British Medical Journal* 336:931–934.

Landrigan, C., Parry, G., Bones, C., Hackbarth, A., Goldmann, D., Sharek, P. (2010) 'Temporal trends in rates of patient harm resulting from medical care.' *New England Journal of Medicine* 363:2124–2134.

Leandro, G., Rolando, N., Gallus, G., Rolles, K. and Burroughs, A. (2005) 'Monitoring surgical and medical outcomes: the Bernoulli cumulative sum chart. A novel application to assess clinical interventions.' *Postgraduate Medical Journal* 81:647–652.

Lilford, R., Mohammed, M., Spiegelhalter, D. and Thomson, R. (2004) 'Use and misuse of outcome data in managing performance of acute medical care: avoiding institutional stigma.' *Lancet* 363:1147–1154.

Loke, C. and Gan, F. (2012) 'Joint monitoring scheme for clinical failures and predisposed risks.' *Quality Technology and Quantitative Management* 9:3–21.

Lovegrove, J., Valencia, O., Treasure, T., Sherlaw-Johnson, C., and Gallivan, S. (1997) 'Monitoring the results of cardiac surgery by variable life-adjusted display.' *The Lancet* 350: 1128.

Lucas, J. and Crosier, R. (1982) 'Fast initial response for CUSUM quality control schemes.' *Technometrics* 24:199–205.

Maindonald, J. and Braun, J. (2010) *Data Analysis and Graphics Using R*, Cambridge University Press.

McGrath, G. and Morton, A. (1986) 'A study of postoperative respiratory complications' Unpublished Social and Preventative Medicine Project, University of Queensland.

McLaws, M-L and Berry, G. (2005) 'Nonuniform risk of bloodstream infection with increasing central venous catheter-days.' *Infection Control and Hospital Epidemiology* 26:715–719.

Miettinen, O. (1985) *Theoretical Epidemiology*, Chichester: Wiley Medical.

Mitchell, I., Kulh, M. and McKay, H. (2011) 'Use of the modified early warning score in emergency medical units.' *Medical Journal of Australia* 195:448.

Mohammed, M. and Laney, D. (2006) 'Overdispersion in health care performance data: Laney's approach.' *Quality and Safety in Health Care* 15:383–384. (A)

Mohammed, M., Rathbone, A., Myers, P., Patel, D., Onions, H. and Stevens, A. (2004) 'An investigation into general practitioners associated with high patient mortality flagged through the Shipman inquiry: retrospective analysis of routine data.' *BMJ* 328:1474–1477. (B)

Montgomery, D. (2005) *Introduction to Statistical Quality Control*, 5th edition, New York: John Wiley and Sons.

Morton, A., Clements, A., Doidge, S., Stackelroth, J., Whitby, M. (2008) 'Surveillance of hospital-acquired infections in Queensland, Australia: Lessons from the first 5 years of data collection.' *Infection Control and Hospital Epidemiology* 29:695–701. (A)

Morton, A., Clements, A. and Whitby, M. (2009) 'Hospital adverse events and control charts: the need for a new paradigm.' *Journal of Hospital Infection* 73:225–231. (B)

Morton, A., Cook, D., Mengersen, K., Waterhouse, M. (2010) 'Limiting risk of hospital adverse events: avoiding train wrecks is more important than counting and reporting them.' *Journal of Hospital Infection* 76:283–286. (C)

Morton, A., Mengersen, K., Rajmokan, M., Jones, M., Playford, G. and Whitby, M. (2011) 'Funnel plots and risk-adjusted count data adverse events. A limitation of indirect standardization.' *Journal of Hospital Infection* 78:260–263. (D)

Morton, A., Mengersen, K., Waterhouse, M., Steiner, S. (2010) 'Analysis of aggregated hospital infection data for accountability.' *Journal of Hospital Infection* 76:287–291. (E)

Morton, A., Mengersen, K., Waterhouse, M., Steiner, S., Looke, D. (2010) 'Sequential analysis of uncommon adverse outcomes.' *Journal of Hospital Infection* 76:114–118. (F)

Morton, A., Smith, S., Mullany, D., Clarke, A., Wall, D. and Pohlner, P. (2011) 'An application of outcomes monitoring for coronary artery bypass surgery 2005–2008 at TPCH.' *Heart Lung and Circulation* 20:312–317. (G)

Morton, A., Waterhouse, M., Playford, G., Mengersen, K. (2011) 'Using centers for disease control national nosocomial infections surveillance surgical site infection risk-adjustment for a group of related orthopaedic procedures.' *Healthcare Infection* 16:89–94. (H)

Morton, A., Whitby, M., McLaws, M-L., Dobson, A., McElwain, S., Looke, D., Stackelroth, J. and Sartor, A. (2001) 'The application of statistical process control charts to the detection and monitoring of hospital acquired infections.' *Journal of Quality in Clinical Practice* 21:112–117. (I)

Myatt, M. (2005) 'Open Source Solutions–R' (http://www.brixtonhealth.com/.)

Nam, J. (1995) 'Confidence limits for the ratio of two binomial proportions based on likelihood scores: non-iterative method.' *Biometrics Journal* 37:375.

Nelson, E., Splaine, M., Batalden, P., and Plume, S. (1998) 'Building measurement and data collection into medical practice.' *Annals of Internal Medicine* 128:460.

Nelson, L. (1999) 'Notes on the Shewhart control chart.' *Journal of Quality Technology* 31:124–126.

Newcombe, R. (1998) 'Interval estimation for the difference between independent proportions.' *Statistics in Medicine* 17:873.

Nolan, T. and Berwick, D. (2006) 'All-or-none measurement raises the bar on performance.' *JAMA* 295:168–170.

Orrell, D. (2010) *Economyths*, London: Icon Press.

Ostrowsky, B. and Jarvis, W. (2003) 'Efficient management of outbreak investigations' in Wenzel, R. *Prevention and Control of Nosocomial Infections*, Philadelphia, Lippincott Williams and Wilkins, 4th ed.

Papadopoulos, M., Hadjitheodossiou, M., Chrysostomou, C., Hardwidge, C., and Bell, A. (2001) 'Is the national health service at the edge of chaos?' *Journal of the Royal Society of Medicine* 94:613–616.

Pearse, R., Holt, P. and Grocott, M. (2011) 'Managing perioperative risk in patients undergoing non-cardiac surgery.' *British Medical Journal* 343:d5759.

Pelecanos, A., Ryan, P. and Gatton, M. (2010) 'Outbreak detection algorithms for seasonal disease data: a case study using Ross river virus disease.' *BMC Medical Informatics and Decision Making* 10:74.

Pettitt, A. (1979) 'A non-parametric approach to the change-point problem.' *Journal of the Royal Statistical Society*. Series C (Applied Statistics)28:126–135.

Pilcher, D., Hoffman, T., Thomas, C., Ernest, D. and Hart, G. (2010) 'Risk-adjusted continuous outcome monitoring with an EWMA chart: could it have detected excess mortality among intensive care patients at Bundaberg Base Hospital?' *Critical Care and Resuscitation* 12:36–41.

Pitches, D., Burls, A. and Fry-Smith, A. (2003) 'How to make a silk purse from a sow's ear – A comprehensive review of strategies to optimise data for corrupt managers and incompetent clinicians.' *British Medical Journal* 327:1436.

Plsek, P. and Greenhalgh, T. (2001) 'The challenge of complexity in health care.' *British Medical Journal* 323:625–628.

Rajmokan M., Morton A., Marquess J., Playford G., and Jones M. 'Development of a risk-adjustment model for antimicrobial utilization data in 21 public hospitals in Queensland, Australia (2006–11).' *Journal of Antimicrobial Chemotherapy* (to appear).

Reingold, A. (1998) 'Outbreak investigations-a perspective.' *Emerging Infectious Diseases* 4:21–27.

Reynolds, M. and Stoumbos, Z. (1999) 'A CUSUM chart for monitoring a proportion when inspecting continuously.' *Journal of Quality Technology* 32:87–108.

Rosner, B. (2006) *Fundamentals of Biostatistics*, Belmont, Thomson, 6th ed., page 779.

Rossi, G., Del Sarto, S. and Marchi, M. 'A Simple Risk-Adjusted CUSUM chart for monitoring binary health data.' Proceedings of the 46th Scientific Meeting of the Italian Statistical Society (USB stick), Rome 2012, Cleup, ISBN 978 886129 882 8.

Rothman, K. and Boice, J. (1979) 'Epidemiologic analysis with a programmable calculator', Washington DC, NIH Publication, pp. 79–1649.

Royal College of Physicians 2012. www.rcplondon.ac.uk.

Runger, G. and Willemain, T. (1995) 'Model-based and model-free control of autocorrelated processes.' *Journal of Quality Technology* 27:283–292.

Ryan, T. (2011) *Statistical Methods for Quality Improvement*, Hoboken: John Wiley and Sons, 3rd ed. 2011.

Ryan, A., Nallamothu, B. and Dimick, J. (2012) 'Medicare's public reporting initiative on hospital quality had modest or no impact on mortality from three key conditions.' *Health Affairs* 31:585–592.

Scheaffer, R. and Levenworth, R. (1976) 'The negative binomial model for counts in units of varying size.' *Journal of Quality Technology* 8:158–163.

Siegel, S. and Castellan, N. (1988) *Nonparametric Statistics for the Behavioral Sciences*, 2nd ed. Singapore, McGraw-Hill.

Silcocks, P. (1994) 'Estimating confidence limits on a standardized mortality ratio when the expected number is not error free.' *Journal of Epidemiology and Community Health* 48:313–317.

Simpson, J., Evans, N., Gibberd, R., Heuchan, A. and Henderson-Smart, D. (2003) 'Analyzing differences in clinical outcomes between hospitals.' *Quality and Safety in Health Care* 12:257–262.

Singer, A. (2000) 'Mandatory regular meetings of hospital staff would complement medical audit and revalidation.' *British Medical Journal* 320:1072.

Smith, I., Garlick, B., Gardner, M., Brighouse, R., Foster, K. and Rivers, J. (in press) 'Use of graphical statistical process control tools to monitor and improve outcomes in cardiac surgery.' *Heart, Lung and Circulation.*

Spiegelhalter, D. (1985) 'Statistical methodology for evaluating gastrointestinal symptoms.' *Clinics in Gastroenterology* 14:489–515. (A)

Spiegelhalter, D. (2002) 'Funnel plots for institutional comparison.' *Quality and Safety in Health Care* 11:390–391. (B)

Spiegelhalter, D. (2005) 'Funnel plots for comparing institutional performance.' *Statistics in Medicine* 24:1185–1202. (C)

Spiegelhalter, D. (2005) 'Handling over-dispersion of performance indicators.' *Quality and Safety in Health Care* 14:347–351. (D)

Spiegelhalter, D., Grigg, O., Kinsman, R. and Treasure, T. (2003) 'Risk-adjusted sequential probability ratio tests: applications to Bristol, Shipman and adult cardiac surgery.' *International Journal for Quality in Health Care* 15:7–13. (E)

Spiegelhalter, D., Abrams, K., Myles, J. (2004) *Bayesian Approaches to Clinical Trials and Health-Care Evaluation*, Chichester: John Wiley and Sons. (F)

Steiner, S., Cook, R., Farewell, V. and Treasure, T. (2001) 'Monitoring surgical performance using risk adjusted cumulative sum charts.' *Biostatistics* 2:441.

Taleb, N. (2010) *The Black Swan*, New York: Random House, 2nd ed.

Taylor-Adams, S. and Vincent, C. 'Systems Analysis of Clinical Incidents, the London Protocol' Clinical Safety Research Unit, Imperial College London. http://www.patientensicherheit.ch/de/projekte/londonprotocol_e.pdf.

Temime, L., Opatowski, L., Pannet, Y., Brun-Buisson, C, Boelle, P., and Guillemot, D. (2009) 'Peripatetic health-care workers as potential superspreaders.' Proceedings of National Academy of Sciences 106:18420–18428.

Thornton, J. and Lilford, R. (1995) 'Decision analysis for medical aanagers.' *British Medical Journal* 310:791.

Tong, E., Clements, A., Haynes, M., Jones, M., Morton, A. and Whitby, M. (2009) 'Improved hospital-level risk adjustment for surveillance of healthcare-associated bloodstream infections: a retrospective cohort study.' *BMC Infectious Diseases* 9:145.

Toumpoulis, I., Anagnostopoulos, C., DeRose, Jr J. and Swistel, D. (2005) 'The impact of deep sternal wound infection on long-term survival after coronary artery bypass grafting.' *Chest* 127:464–471.

Ueno, T. and Masuda, N. (2008) 'Controlling nosocomial infection based on structure of hospital networks.' *Journal of Theoretical Biology* 254:655–666.

US Centers for Disease Control. www.cdc.gov/hai/.

van der Tweel, I. (2005) 'Repeated looks at accumulating data: to correct or not to correct.' *European Journal of Epidemiology* 20:205–211.

Venables, W. and Ripley, B. (2002) *Modern Applied Statistics with S*, New York, Springer, 4th ed.

Verzani, J. (2005) *Using R for Introductory Statistics*, Boca Raton, CRC Press.

Vincent, C. (2010) *Patient Safety*, Chichester: Wiley, 2nd ed.

Vollset, S. (1993) 'Confidence intervals for a binomial proportion.' *Statistics in Medicine* 12:809–824.

Wachter, R. and Pronovost, P. (2009) 'Balancing no blame and accountability in patient safety.' *The New England Journal of Medicine* 361:1401–1406.

Wadsworth, H., Stephens, K. and Godfrey, B. (2002) *Modern Methods for Quality Control and Improvement*, New York, Wiley, 2nd ed.

Waterhouse, M., Smith, I., Assareh, H. and Mengersen, K. (2010) 'Implementation of multivariate control charts in a clinical setting.' *International Journal for Quality in Health Care* 22:408–414. (A)

Waterhouse, M., Morton, A., Mengersen, K., Cook, D., Playford, G. (2011) 'Investigating the role of overcrowding in MRSA transmission using a Bayesian network. Results for a single public hospital.' *Journal of Hospital Infection* 78:92–96. (B)

Webster, R. (2008) 'Development of statistical methods for the surveillance and monitoring of adverse events which adjust for differing patient and surgical risks.' PhD thesis, Queensland University of Technology. http://eprints.qut.edu.au/view/types/qut=5Fthesis/2008.html#group_W.

Whitby, M., McLaws, M-L., Collopy, B., Looke, D., Doidge, S., Henderson, B., Selvey, L., Gardner, G., Stackelroth, J. and Sartor, A. (2002) 'Post-discharge surveillance: can patients reliably diagnose surgical wound infections?' *Journal of Hospital Infection* 52:155–160.

Winkel, P. and Zhang, N. (2007) *Statistical Development of Quality in Medicine*, Chichester: John Wiley & Sons.

Woodworth, G. (2004) *Biostatistics A Bayesian Introduction*, New York: John Wiley and Sons.

Zou, G. and Donner, A. (2008) 'Construction of confidence limits about effect measures: A general approach.' *Statistics in Medicine* 27:1693–1702.

Index

Statistical Methods for Hospital Monitoring with R, First Edition. Anthony Morton, Kerrie Mengersen, Michael Whitby and George Playford.
© 2013 John Wiley & Sons, Ltd. Published 2013 by John Wiley & Sons, Ltd.

Statistics in Practice

Human and Biological Sciences

Welton, Sutton, Cooper and Ades – Evidence Synthesis for Decision Making in Healthcare
Whitehead – Design and Analysis of Sequential Clinical Trials, Revised Second Edition
Whitehead – Meta-Analysis of Controlled Clinical Trials
Willan and Briggs – Statistical Analysis of Cost Effectiveness Data
Winkel and Zhang – Statistical Development of Quality in Medicine

Earth and Environmental Sciences

Buck, Cavanagh and Litton – Bayesian Approach to Interpreting Archaeological Data
Chandler and Scott – Statistical Methods for Trend Detection and Analysis in the Environmental Statistics
Glasbey and Horgan – Image Analysis in the Biological Sciences
Haas – Improving Natural Resource Management: Ecological and Political Models
Haas – Introduction to Probability and Statistics for Ecosystem Managers
Helsel – Nondetects and Data Analysis: Statistics for Censored Environmental Data
Illian, Penttinen, Stoyan, H and Stoyan D – Statistical Analysis and Modelling of Spatial Point Patterns
Mateu and Müller (Eds) – Spatio-temporal design: Advances in efficient data acquisition
McBride – Using Statistical Methods for Water Quality Management Webster and Oliver – Geostatistics for Environmental Scientists, Second Edition
Wymer (Ed) – Statistical Framework for Recreational Water Quality Criteria and Monitoring

Industry, Commerce and Finance

Aitken – Statistics and the Evaluation of Evidence for Forensic Scientists, Second Edition
Balding – Weight-of-evidence for Forensic DNA Profiles
Brandimarte – Numerical Methods in Finance and Economics: A MATLAB-Based Introduction, Second Edition
Brandimarte and Zotteri – Introduction to Distribution Logistics
Chan – Simulation Techniques in Financial Risk Management
Coleman, Greenfield, Stewardson and Montgomery (Eds) – Statistical Practice in Business and Industry
Frisen (Ed) – Financial Surveillance
Fung and Hu – Statistical DNA Forensics
Gusti Ngurah Agung – Time Series Data Analysis Using EViews
Kenett (Eds) – Operational Risk Management: A Practical Approach to Intelligent Data Analysis
Kenett (Eds) – Modern Analysis of Customer Surveys: With Applications using R
Kruger and Xie – Statistical Monitoring of Complex Multivariate Processes: With Applications in Industrial Process Control
Jank and Shmueli (Ed.) – Statistical Methods in e-Commerce Research Lehtonen and Pahkinen – Practical Methods for Design and Analysis of Complex Surveys, Second Edition
Ohser and Mücklich – Statistical Analysis of Microstructures in Materials Science

Pasiouras (Ed.) – Efficiency and Productivity Growth: Modelling in the Financial Services Industry

Pourret, Naim & Marcot (Eds) – Bayesian Networks: A Practical Guide to Applications

Taroni, Aitken, Garbolino and Biedermann – Bayesian Networks and Probabilistic Inference in Forensic Science

Taroni, Bozza, Biedermann, Garbolino and Aitken – Data Analysis in Forensic Science